D1551556

CELLULAR ENERGY METABOLISM
AND ITS REGULATION

CELLULAR ENERGY METABOLISM
AND ITS REGULATION

DANIEL E. ATKINSON

Biochemistry Division
Department of Chemistry
University of California
Los Angeles, California

ACADEMIC PRESS   New York   San Francisco   London   1977

A Subsidiary of Harcourt Brace Jovanovich, Publishers

ACADEMIC PRESS, INC.
111 Fifth Avenue, New York, New York 10003

United Kingdom Edition published by
ACADEMIC PRESS, INC. (LONDON) LTD.
24/28 Oval Road, London NW1

Library of Congress Cataloging in Publication Data

Atkinson, Daniel E
    Cellular energy metabolism and its regulation.

    Bibliography: p.
    Includes index.
    1.   Cell metabolism.   2.   Energy metabolism.
3.   Cellular control mechanisms.   I.   Title.
QH634.5.A84   574.8'761   77-9522
ISBN 0–12–066150–0

To Elsie

Contents

Preface

The potential readers I primarily had in mind when I wrote this book were graduate students in biochemistry, physiology, microbiology, and related fields, although I hope it will be useful also to senior undergraduate students and to more advanced workers who have a direct or peripheral interest in energy metabolism. Thus, I assume a general familiarity with the material covered in a standard biochemistry textbook as well as some knowledge of such related areas as genetics. When elementary points are considered it is for the sake of illustration or in an attempt to suggest a point of view that may be novel for some readers. An extensive bibliography is not provided. Information that may be found in a good textbook is not usually referenced. Citations are illustrative rather than exhaustive; this is not a review of the literature. If the proportion of papers from my own laboratory seems large, it should be realized that they report experiments that were planned to test or illustrate the concepts with which this book deals.

Reviewers sometimes praise a book by saying that the author has carefully distinguished between well-established concepts and speculation. More often, they complain that this distinction has not been made. Similarly, some authors note in their prefaces that they have taken care to label speculation, as distinct from accepted generalizations. I think that such comments are inappropriate in the context of science, and I make no such claim for this book. Presumably the implication of "well-established" or "accepted" is that the concept thus described is favored by a majority of scientists in relevant fields. Majority opinion has not historically been an infallible guide to validity in science, and there is no reason to believe that is more likely to be so today. I do, naturally, indicate which possibilities seem to me to be more likely than others, but this will be one man's opinion at one particular time. I do not attempt to indicate the majority position on any issue, both because I am not clairvoyant and because this information would be of little, if any, value.

Many of the concepts discussed in this book were first presented in research papers that were submitted to scientific journals for publication. In nearly every case at least one reviewer objected strenuously to the ideas and voted against publication of the manuscript. That aspect of the history of the concepts says nothing as to their value or lack of value, but only that they differ in some respects from what was taught in graduate courses in biochemistry ten or twenty years earlier. If about half of the present crop of scientific referees is receptive to publication of papers containing some novelty, we are probably doing as well as at any time in the past. But it may be well to warn timid and consensus-seeking readers that they may wish to stop here; some of the ideas proposed in this book have not received the imprimatur of universal acceptance. They must stand or fall on their own merits, as all scientific ideas should, with no Establishment authority to prop them up.

At any time some new and speculative concepts are sounder than many aspects of the conventional scientific wisdom. Until recently, nearly all introductory chemistry texts listed the inability of the "noble" gases to form compounds among the best-established generalizations. Current editions of those same texts describe several compounds of xenon. The shape of the South Atlantic, as shown in a fifth-grade geography book, suggested the concept of continental drift to me and doubtless to thousands of other elementary-school children not yet encrusted with scientific caution. It is not surprising that my teacher derided the idea, but it is more depressing to realize that almost any professional American geologist would have reacted similarly, even though the idea and much evidence for it had been published years earlier. An overwhelming confluence of evidence of the most diverse types was needed before the great majority of geologists would admit the idea to be a respectable hypothesis, much less one that they could accept. Darwin was vehemently opposed not only by bishops but by many of the most eminent scientists of his day. At about the same time, Liebig was staunchly upholding firmly established chemical principles while ridiculing the fanciful and unscientific notion that microorganisms might be involved in fermentation.

Unfortunately, examples of the resistance of scientific authorities to new ideas would, if covered in any detail, fill a sizable chapter, and the history of biochemistry has more than its share. Several are discussed by Krebs in a delightful essay [Krebs, H. A. (1966). *In* "Current Aspects of Biochemical Energetics" (N. O. Kaplan and E. P. Kennedy, eds.), p. 83. Academic Press, New York] that should be read by every graduate student in any field of science.

In fields far from our own areas of competence we must to a considerable extent rely on the weight of informed opinion. But an important mark of the professional is independence of judgment in his own field. This is a characteristic that graduate students should be consciously working toward. On finishing graduate school, or within a few years, a scientist or other scholar should be able and willing to sustain a well thought-out viewpoint even if it is opposed by all the leaders in his field. But of course support of a scientific point of view should be intellectual, flexible, and subject to change, rather than emotional and rigid.

A book such as this should supply generalizations to aid a reader in mentally ordering the observations in the field with which the book deals and in planning further experiments. But no particular pattern of conceptual ordering should inhibit thinking about possible modifications or alternatives. Indeed, a major benefit of a conceptual treatment of a scientific subdiscipline should be the induction in the minds of imaginative younger readers of new questions that had not occurred to the author or his contemporaries.

I am indebted to the graduate and undergraduate research students, technicians, postdoctoral fellows, and visiting scholars with whom I have been associated during the past dozen years. Without their experimental work and their intellectual contributions the concepts presented here could not have been developed. I am also grateful for many discussions with colleagues both at UCLA and other institutions, which have identified points of difficulty and forced me to focus on them. I thank Martha O'Connor for excellent and patient help in the preparation of the manuscript.

Finally, like everyone who has been involved with academic science in this country, I must thank the Congress and people of the United States for their generous and unprecedented support of scientific research during the past three decades, while hoping that problems and needs in other areas will not cause future Congresses to lose sight of the long-range wisdom of adequate public support of basic research.

Work in my laboratory relevant to the material discussed in this book was supported by research grants from the National Institute of Arthritis, Metabolism and Digestive Diseases, National Institutes of Health, and from the National Science Foundation.

Daniel E. Atkinson

1

Introduction: Evolutionary Design

Biochemistry may be described as the study of living systems, using the methods of chemistry and physics. Life is a complex of interrelated chemical reactions. Even the structural features on which taxonomic classifications are mainly based are the products of chemical reactions. In any case, structure, since it survives nearly intact when a cell or organism dies, is clearly not life, although a high degree of structure is probably required for life. Disruption of the interrelated chemical activities of an organism is death; by the same token, these chemical activities, collectively, are life.

If life is chemical activity, it may seem to follow that a straightforward chemical approach is all that will be necessary to explain biological phenomena. We might predict that classical biology and biologists will become increasingly irrelevant while chemists and physicists, with their quantitative and tough-minded approach, take over the study of living systems. This claim, or something similar, is quite often heard. It is a prediction conceived in ignorance and often delivered with arrogance. Since organisms are chemical systems, the *methods* of chemistry are essential to their study, and there is hardly any important area of biological interest to which chemical methodology cannot make important contributions. But certain of the *concepts* of the physical sciences have long hindered conceptual advance in biology, and may well have been the most serious obstacle to the development of a rational scientific approach to biological problems.

In the nonliving world, function and purpose are irrelevant concepts. If a landslide dams a river, we may say that the landslide caused a lake to form, but it would be meaningless to say that production of the lake was the *function* of the landslide. In elementary courses in the physical and earth sciences, students are, quite rightly, warned to avoid statements that imply function and "why" questions that imply purpose. These warnings are merely simple, common-sense observations as to the nature of the inanimate world. But, by a historical quirk, they have become widely accepted as fundamental tenets of science. Thus students are usually indoctrinated with the dogma that science does not deal with function, that there are no "why" questions in science, and the like. In fact this dogma applies only to some areas of scientific interest, and is totally inapplicable and incorrect in other areas. Function and purpose are clearly evident everywhere around us in all aspects of the living world, but some scientists refuse to see them. Textbooks sometimes (less often now than formerly) resort to absurd circumlocutions to avoid seeming teleological. Some that did not have been taken to task in articles that view with alarm the infiltration of biological texts by teleological wording and hence, it is claimed, by unscientific concepts. One is reminded of the professors of the Middle Ages who solemnly taught anatomy from ancient texts despite the evidence before their own, and their students' eyes.

Consistency is basic to any logical process, and development of a consistent world view is a major aim of science. But the imposition of a concept— afunctionality—that is valid in one field onto another where it is clearly inapplicable is an excellent example of the foolish consistency that Emerson described as the hobgoblin of little minds.

The basis for the difference between the living and the nonliving worlds is that organisms have been designed by the evolutionary processes of mutation and selection. These processes can occur only in systems that reproduce with a high, but not perfect, degree of fidelity. They are in the present world confined to living organisms and quasiliving systems such as viruses; thus they constitute a difference in kind between the living and nonliving worlds. This is not, of course, to imply that an unbridgeable gap exists between these worlds. It must once have been bridged—that is, reproduction with its concomitant processes of mutation and selection must itself have evolved. But the early transitional forms have long since been lost, and at present we may well take evolutionary design as the touchstone of living systems.

Although evolutionary design and its products—living organisms—differ in kind from naturally occurring inanimate objects, they differ only in degree from the products of human design, with which they share the fundamental attributes of function and purpose. Evolutionary design is in fact very similar to engineering design. Both involve the trial of variants and selection of those that work. An engineer calls on his cumulative experience and on the various principles and equations that represent the accumulated experience of past engineers and scientists in selecting from among many possible designs those that he considers worthy of trial; thus the fraction of his trials that are successful is far higher than in evolution, where mutations occur at random and the overwhelming majority are deleterious and are thus quickly abandoned. Nevertheless the two processes are fundamentally very similar. No modern technological device has been designed solely on the basis of

fundamental physical principles; they have all evolved through experience—
that is, through trial and error. The sequence from the models in the Wright
brothers' primitive wind tunnels to the latest supersonic planes is marked
by a long line of advances based on experience with airfoils and models in
wind tunnels and with actual planes in flight. The increasing use of slide
rules, and more recently computers, in aeronautical design has been based
far more solidly on information obtained from these earlier tests than on
physical fundamentals like the kinetic theory of gases. Thus one function
of computers is to simulate trials and select those design changes that are
worthy of actual trial in a model or prototype. The screening will be more
or less valid (that is, will give answers corresponding more or less closely
to those that would have been obtained by actual trial) according to how
adequate are the codified generalizations obtained from past experience. In
principle, computer simulation is imaginary testing done as a preliminary
to the real thing, and it corresponds to the intuitive testing and rejection of
alternative possibilities that is the essence of the design of even the simplest
devices. Evolution differs from engineering design in lacking intuition and
computers. The compensating factor, of course, is the enormous number of
trials that are possible, and in fact inevitable, in the course of evolution. As
an inexorable consequence of differential reproduction, those changes that
are advantageous to the organism are favored and become fixed in the population, while those that are deleterious are abandoned. Thus the results of
the more successful trials become the norm against which further variation
is tested.

   The close analogy between evolutionary design and human design is in-
structively illustrated by the many cases in which progress in understanding
biological function has been aided by comparison with a technological device
that serves a somewhat analogous function. In some cases the analogies were
direct and were utilized consciously; in others they were unconscious, but
probably no less important for merely being derived from general knowledge
of current technology. In few, if any, cases has much progress been made
toward understanding any extensive biological function until after the development of a technological system, however crude, that could supply at least
a distant analogy. Large and small examples abound. Structures that we now
know are valves were seen in mammalian hearts and veins much earlier, but
their function, and thus the fact that the blood circulates, was not recognized
until after the development by mining engineers of pumps with analogous
checkvalves (2). The study of metabolic regulation has profited importantly
from the principles of simple electronic control systems, and such analogies
were mentioned in the two papers in which regulation at the molecular level
was first demonstrated (118, 127). Information processing by the central
nervous system can be considered in ways that would not have been possible

before the development of computers, and these approaches may prove useful in understanding brain function. It is unlikely that the splitting of arteries supplying part of the skeletal muscles of tunas into strange networks of small vessels that are intimately mixed with a similar network of small vessels subdivided from the veins draining the same muscles would have been recognized as a device to allow the muscle to be stabilized at a temperature similar to that of mammals, although the blood must cool in the gills to the temperature of the ambient water, unless heat exchangers identical in principle had been in use technologically. The idea of a linear genetic message was certainly derived directly from linear writing of verbal messages, as is amusingly evident from such terms as "translation," "transcription," and "genetic dictionary," and the frequent references, especially in the early literature, to "code words" or to "letters in the genetic alphabet."

Even the most important biological generalization—that of evolution as a consequence of variation and selection—was conceived as a result of conscious analogy with purposeful human activities. Many current elementary textbooks give the impression that Darwin was guided by the fossil record, but that record, because of its incompleteness, was in fact a serious embarrassment to him. His reading of Malthus' essay on population and his observations of differences between the finches on different islands in the Galapagos contributed to his ideas. But his central contribution was not the idea of changes in species; that was accepted by many, though by no means all, biologists of his time and earlier. The importance of Darwin's contribution was that he supplied a plausible *mechanism* by which such changes might, and indeed must, occur. He consciously and explicitly based his concept of natural selection on the artificial selection that had led to such wide variations among breeds of domestic dogs, agricultural livestock, and fowl.

Since the designs developed by evolution are so similar in principle to those that would be reached by a conscious designer, and since biological progress in the past has been strongly dependent on analogies, explicit or implicit, with engineering practice, it seems reasonable to suggest as a general approach to biological problems that the investigator should ask himself what are the essential functions involved and how might a designer provide for them. This approach, which could have no relevance or meaning in the study of the inanimate world, seems highly promising in biology.

Heritable changes of many types have contributed to the evolution of contemporary organisms. These changes include, among others: deletions of blocks of DNA or transpositions of such blocks to other positions in the chromosome; incorporation of genetic information from other organisms as a consequence of ingestion; parasitism, or other processes by which DNA from two organisms comes to be present in the same cell; and, especially in plants, hybridization with stabilization of nuclei containing all or most of the chromosomes of two or more parental species. Some of these processes may have been of very great importance. For example, much evidence suggests that mitochondria and chloroplasts may have been derived from free-living organisms; if so, incorporation of these organisms into eukaryotic cells was one of the most significant developments in evolutionary history. Nevertheless, all processes of the type listed above are secondary. They involve redistribution of information rather than the development of new information. On the basis of present evidence it seems likely that the development of new information occurs mainly by the selection of mutations in the strict sense—single-base changes in DNA leading to alterations of single amino acid residues in proteins. If this is true, any protein of a contemporary organism, with its incredibly complicated functional properties, is the product of evolutionary design operating through selection from among an unimaginably large number of individual changes in amino acid composition that have occurred during the history of the protein.

But point mutations and selection alone cannot lead to the large-scale development of new information. In general, these processes lead only to modification of the properties of a protein. They could in principle cause conversion of a functional protein to one of different function, but this would be substitution of information rather than development of additional information (or function). Even such substitution would be highly unlikely unless the old function had ceased to matter, since changes that diminished the old function would be disadvantageous and thus not likely to survive. Clearly an additional type of genetic change is needed. On the basis of genetic and cytological evidence, it has been known for many years that genes or larger blocks of genetic material are occasionally duplicated. This process is believed to be the additional factor needed for the evolution of new functions. When a gene has been duplicated, so that each haploid genome contains two copies, selective pressure is almost totally relaxed. Since either copy of the gene can supply an adequate level of the protein that it specifies, changes in either will have no serious adverse consequences. When one has changed in such a way as to significantly affect the functionality of the corresponding protein, the full force of functional selection will be reimposed on the other. The altered gene, however, is free to change further in a random manner; thus properties such as substrate specificity may be altered. Whenever the properties of the altered protein become slightly advantageous to the organism (for example, the protein may feebly catalyze a reaction chemically similar to that catalyzed by the "parent" enzyme, but involving a different substrate), the usual processes of mutation and selection may be expected to produce an enzyme as exquisitely adapted for catalysis and regulation of the new reaction as is the parent enzyme for the old reaction.

   As techniques for determining amino acid sequences of proteins are simplified and come to be more widely applied, and as more three-dimensional
structures are determined, one of the exciting prospects is that we should
soon know to what extent an array of enzymes catalyzing chemically related
reactions—dehydrogenases, for example—show vestiges in their structures
and amino acid sequences of common origin of this type. One of the most
general such findings to date is the fascinating discovery by Rossmann and
colleagues (*102*) of a complex nucleotide-binding site consisting of an array
of β-sheets. This structure seems to be present wherever nucleotides are
bound, and mathematical analysis supports the intuitive belief that such a
complex feature must have been conserved rather than reinvented. In other
words, at least a portion of each enzyme that binds nucleotides must be coded
for by a segment of DNA that shares a common ancestry with the corresponding segment for each other such enzyme.
   An inexperienced designer often finds it necessary to overcome a tendency
toward overdesign of components. He may lavish much loving care on the
design of a truly superior variable-reluctance, temperature-compensated,
self-orienting widget, but this perfection of one part may detract from the
utility of the device in which it is to be used—perhaps by excessive weight,
size, or power requirement, or perhaps merely by increasing the cost of production with no corresponding improvement in overall performance. Such
overdesign is impossible in evolution, since the component part is never
tested in isolation, but only as a functioning element in the overall system,
which is the organism. Mutation is expressed at the level of the individual
protein, but selection is at the level of the whole organism. Thus the design
of any component of a living system will reflect functional utility for the
organism rather than improvement of the component as such. For example,
high affinity for substrate, which allows the catalyzed reaction to proceed
at an effective rate even though the substrate concentration is low, is evidently
a desirable feature for enzymes in general, and high affinity is in fact characteristic of enzymes. But it does not follow that increase of affinity without limit
would be advantageous. Like any other phenotypic characteristic of an
organism, the affinity of an enzyme for its substrate is the result of compromise in design, and we may infer that further increase in affinity would
be as harmful to the organism as a decrease. The relative importance of the
factors involved in the compromise will differ with different enzymes. In
some cases the decisive factors may relate to the functioning of the enzyme
itself. An increase in affinity might necessarily involve a concomitant decrease in catalytic activity or in ease of dissociation of the product that more
than balanced otherwise advantageous consequences of increased substrate
affinity. Probably more often, in the complexly integrated metabolism of
contemporary organisms, increased affinity as such would have unfavorable
effects on the overall functioning of the organism. As we will discuss in later

chapters, enzymes interact in metabolism in various ways, of which the two most obvious are a producer-consumer relation, where the product of one enzyme is substrate for another, and competition, where two or more enzymes compete for the same substrate. It is evident that in either of these situations a change in affinity of one enzyme for substrate might well be disruptive.

In the enormous literature on evolution, one may find almost every possible statement as to the relation between purpose and Darwinian evolution. Thus we may read that Darwin drove the last nails into the coffin of teleology or that he firmly established the importance of teleology in biology. One author will say that Darwin put purpose back into biology, whereas others insist that there is no purpose in evolution. As with many other apparently contradictory views, the differences here are primarily in the meanings attached to the words employed. Probably all of these statements are correct in the sense in which their authors meant them, but this could obviously not be so if "teleology" and "purpose" had the same significance in each case. The point at issue is the place at which purpose enters. We should be able to agree that there is no *preexisting* purpose in evolution. This is the valid sense in which one may deny the validity of teleology in biology or the existence of function in evolution. This is perhaps the most significant difference between engineering and evolutionary design—the engineer typically has a definite function in mind at the time he begins to design a device. In evolution, on the other hand, *the function evolves with the design features that will serve it*. Flight, for example, has evolved independently at least three times—in insects, in mammals, and in the reptilian ancestors of birds. But of course it would be preposterous to assume that there was a preexisting need to fly, and that evolution set about to plan how to do it. Whatever random changes allowed an organism to extend a leap slightly by gliding might increase his chances of escape from a predator, or perhaps his chance of capturing prey. Further modification and perfection of gliding ability would follow, as long as the organism's ability to survive and reproduce was enhanced by the changes. Steerability would almost certainly be advantageous, and this might lead, by imperceptible changes, to true flight. Each step on the evolutionary sequence must have been characterized by a greater degree of functionality than those that preceded it. Thus function and functionality evolved together. This must always be the case.

Function can be considered on different levels. Flight itself is functional in many ways. It aids the flying organism in obtaining food by following prey organisms into the air (bats and insect-eating birds), by the speed and effectiveness of striking from the air (hawks), or simply by the much wider range over which food may be sought; it may aid an organism in escaping from predators; it permits the vulnerable egg and nestling stages to be passed in nests built in locations that are inaccessible to many predators, and so on.

On another level, each of the characteristics of the organism that contribute to the capacity for flight is functional. Many of the features of the skeleton (or exoskeleton) and musculature of a flying organism are specific adaptations for efficient flight, and this is true also of many other large and small phenotypic characteristics.

Similar comments apply equally to any other evolved functional ability. Our remote ancestors benefitted from the possession of primitive eyespots that allowed them to orientate themselves with respect to incident light, to move toward or away from illumination, or to synchronize their activities with the diurnal light-dark cycle. Improvement in the sensitivity and other operational characteristics of the eyespots developed because of their immediate advantages to the organisms in which they evolved, not because of the ultimate advantage to us, their distant descendants. The long, slow development of sensitive color-discriminating image-forming eyes of high resolution occurred because of the slight advantages conferred by each change. The functions of eyes evolved along with their structure. These functions necessarily coevolved with those of the central nervous system and the musculature; a highly developed eye would be of very little use to a mushroom.

The concept of function is inseparable from that of organic evolution. *All products of evolution are functional (or have been functional), and only products of evolution are functional.* (We must, of course, consider functional devices made by man or other organisms to be secondary products of evolution.) Thus in the abstract we may say that functionality is *the* product of evolution, and a product uniquely of evolution, since it simply cannot exist—it would have no meaning—aside from evolution. Evolution is the purposeless process by which purpose and function arise. Functionality is the basis of each evolutionary decision, but at each stage it is function itself that is being evolved. In no sense except the theological could any meaning whatever be ascribed to the concept of a biological function that does not yet exist or a need not yet fulfilled. Needs, as well as functions, can arise only through the mutations and selective processes that satisfy them.

Resistance to the concept of teleology in biology arises in some cases from foolish consistency, and in other cases from semantic differences in the meanings given to the word. In the sense that implies some type of guidance by which evolution was caused to solve preexisting problems, fulfill preexisting functional needs, and ultimately achieve the production of man, teleology evidently has no place in a rational view of biology. But in the more restricted sense of simple functionality, a teleological orientation is essential to any rational view of biological systems. In an attempt to avoid these semantic difficulties, Pittendrigh (*92*) proposed that the latter type of teleological concepts—those denoting mere functionality—be termed "teleonomic." There is something to be said for this distinction, but in this book "evolutionary teleology" will be used with the restricted meaning of simple functionality. In this evolutionary sense, teleological concepts are basic to the consideration of all features of biological systems, from the shapes of bones or shells to the details of biosynthetic processes. Krebs (67) was the first to point out forcefully the necessity for a teleological point of view in the study of metabolism.

A dichotomy between functional and evolutionary biology has been discussed in many articles and seminars. (More recently, the contrasting adjectives have often been molecular and evolutionary.) Sometimes the motivation has been to extol the supposed superior intellect or the more scientific orientation of the functional or molecular biologist, who has even been said to bring a different logical approach to the study of nature (93); more often it has been to man the dikes of classical biology against the rising tide of functional or molecular biology. Even very eminent biologists who have made important contributions to the study of evolution have written articles of the second type. This is to be regretted. It must be evident that any attempt to deal separately with function and evolution is a particularly unfortunate example of the establishment of a distinction where there is no difference. As the preceding discussion has attempted to demonstrate, function and evolution lie equally at the heart of biology and are virtually synonymous. Evolution occurs through selection of function. There can be no evolution without function, and no function without evolution. A paleontologist or taxonomist whose only concern is with the details of structure for their own sake, without regard to function, is as limited in his view as is a biochemist who is interested only in the physical or kinetic properties of enzymes, without regard to the significance of those properties in the complex evolved interrelations of the living cell. Both have arbitrarily walled themselves off from the biologically significant aspects of the systems that they study. Both may obtain results that contribute to advances in biology, but neither is dealing with his chosen material on its own terms—those of evolved biological function.

The aim of science is the advance of understanding, not the accumulation of facts. The descriptive phase of any science, during which facts are gathered almost at random, is necessary to later development, since generalizations can only be arrived at on the basis of facts. But in later stages experiments are designed on the basis of hypotheses, and facts are useful chiefly as they disprove or support these hypotheses. There is always need for relatively undirected mining for facts, but facts should be sought not so much for their own sake as to supply the basis for new hypotheses. Generally speaking, facts are important in science because of their relation to generalizations.

It goes without saying, on the other hand, that a scientific hypothesis is valuable only if it is consistent with the relevant facts (at least with those that are really true). It is desirable for a hypothesis to be subject to direct experimental test, but this is by no means necessary. Indeed, the more extensive and important the generalization, the less likely is the possibility of a definite test. The concept that organisms evolve as a consequence of mutation and differential reproduction is by far the most fundamental generalization of biology. It is consistent with thousands of observations and thousands of experiments, but it is evidently not subject to any single definitive test. This in no way limits the validity or usefulness of the concept. But the new hypotheses that we deal with in everyday science are not of the magnitude of the concept of evolution. They are small vantage points cantilevered out from facts, and it is very comforting if they suggest experiments capable of generating new facts to prop them up. This desirability of experimental testability has led to a damaging and misleading cliche. The only value of a hypothesis, it is sometimes said, is to suggest new experiments. This dictum misses the point of what science is about, and demeans the whole scientific endeavor to a make-work operation. It amounts to saying, in effect: "Here are all these people trained to be scientists; we must keep them occupied doing experiments; a hypothesis would help to do that, so let's see if we can produce one." The scientific search for understanding is much more intellectually meaningful than that.

Some areas of science outgrow the descriptive phase faster than others. In large part, the differences reflect the relative complexities of the areas: the greater the complexity, the longer an essentially undirected search for facts will be useful. Biology is the most complex of the natural sciences, and some types of descriptive biology continue to be important. It is still useful to catalogue a new species or a new enzyme. Such activities are not useful for their own sakes, however, but because of the possibility that knowledge of the new species or new enzyme may contribute to better understanding of ecology and evolution in the one case, or metabolism in the other. Unfortunately, some biologists and biochemists cling nostalgically to the idea that such cataloging, along with descriptions of life cycles or kinetic properties, is the main aim of science. The preference for description rather than correlation and synthesis is closely related to the anti-functional attitude that was referred to earlier in this chapter; together they tend to discourage innovation and to coerce young investigators into safe and unimaginative projects that have a high probability of yielding an impressive quantity of publishable results just like those being published by dozens of their contemporaries. In our greatly expanded scientific community, no single individual has the power to delay for years the acceptance of a valid generalization, as did such *Geheimräte* of the past as Hoppe-Seyler (the participation of cytochromes in respiration) or Willstätter (the protein nature of enzymes). But the collective conservatism of members of editorial boards, study sections, and grant committees can have the same deadening effect.

To some readers, especially biologists, this chapter will seem to belabor the obvious. But many graduate students enter biochemistry or molecular biology after taking an undergraduate degree in chemistry or physics with little exposure to biology and, consciously or unconsciously, retain an anti-functional orientation. It seems necessary to emphasize at the outset that everything that follows is based on the concept that evolution is a process of functional design, and that the characteristics of an organism, whether morphological or molecular, have been selected because of functional advantage to the organism's ancestors. If that concept is not accepted, this book will seem totally irrelevant. When it is accepted, it follows that enzyme molecules are important only in terms of the reactions that they catalyze, that reactions are important only in terms of the sequences in which they participate, and the sequences only in terms of their interrelations with other sequences in the overall economy of the organism. Study of an enzyme, a reaction, or a sequence can be biologically relevant only if its position in the hierarchy of function is kept in mind. This book deals with some aspects of metabolism from that point of view.

2

Conservation of Solvent Capacity
and of Energy*

The origin of life and the early stages in the evolution of biological macro-molecules, of the genetic code, and of metabolic sequences, have been discussed by many authors. These topics are of the greatest scientific interest, but they are outside the range of this book.

CONSERVATION OF SOLVENT CAPACITY

Our consideration will begin at a time when organisms had developed highly precise self-replication with occasional mutations, and possessed at least rudimentary metabolic systems. As evolution proceeded and metabolic patterns became increasingly complex, the number of enzymes and inter-mediates in the cell solution increased. This development must have posed a threat to further evolution. The solvent capacity of water is finite and the amount of material in solution cannot increase without limit. Clearly the evolution of further complexity in metabolism was possible only if very stringent limitations on the concentrations of individual compounds were developed. The existence of the contemporary living cell containing several thousand enzymes and several thousand metabolic intermediates indicates that such limitations have evolved and are in operation. If one thousand metabolites were each present at an average concentration of 0.1 M, which would be considered a relatively low concentration in many contexts, and if the average molecular weight were 100, there would be 10^4 g of metabolites per liter, with a density of 10 g/cm^3. Quite aside from the solvent capacity of

* Some of the concepts in this chapter have been discussed in a previous paper (7).

water, and even assuming that no water or protein were present, such a total concentration is clearly impossible; the densities of most metabolic compounds are close to 1 g/cm³. A similar situation exists in the case of enzymes. Several enzymes catalyzing reactions in major pathways occur at concentrations near 10^{-5} M, but the levels of most enzymes must be considerably lower. One thousand enzymes at an average concentration of 10^{-5} M with an average molecular weight of 10^5 would sum to 1 kg/liter, or a density of 1 g/cm³. This would correspond approximately to the density of dry protein, and could be attained only if all water and other cell constituents were excluded. The existence of functioning viable cells containing enough water to hold thousands of metabolic compounds and nearly as many enzymes in solution is evidence that concentrations are very effectively limited.

Enzyme Concentrations

Present knowledge of the location and state of enzymes *in vivo* is unsatisfactory. It seems likely, however, that many or most enzymes are not in solution, but are attached to intracellular membranes. If so, solubility considerations are not directly relevant, but the total amount of protein must still be held well below 1 g/cm³ in order that space may be available for water, other macromolecules such as nucleic acids, dissolved metabolites, and insoluble structural and storage compounds such as lipids and polysaccharides. Typical cells may contain about 50 mg/cm³ of protein, which thus, disregarding associated water, occupies about 5% of the available space. The deleterious consequences of exceeding that level must put serious constraints on the options that are open in evolution of further metabolic complexity. Long ago, at a time so remote that common ancestors of all present-day organisms were alive, organisms must have reached a point where an increase in the level of protein would have been injurious. Since that time, the evolution of further complexity (new sequences and new reactions, hence, new enzymes) has been possible only at the expense of either deletion or decrease in amount of preexisting enzymes. Decrease in amount of an enzyme, if its function is retained, requires an increase in catalytic effectiveness; thus there must have been rather strong selective pressure for improvement of enzymes in this regard. Deletion of an enzyme is possible only if its function can be dispensed with. When an organism obtains its carbon and energy by consuming other organisms, some of the basic pathways of intermediary metabolism become superfluous. In eating enough plant or animal matter to meet its energy demands, an organism will almost certainly obtain an adequate supply of such building blocks as amino acids. It is striking that many heterotrophic organisms, especially highly developed ones such as vertebrates, have lost all of the amino acid synthetic pathways that consist of long sequences of reactions and thus require many enzymes. They retain the ability to produce only the amino acids that can be reached from glycolytic or citrate cycle intermediates in one or very few steps. These losses may have been passive, in the sense that if a complex function is not needed mutations that impair it will not be eliminated by selection and may accumulate until the function is totally lost. It is at least possible, however, and seems to me probable, that there has been active selection for removal of nonessential enzymes. If the protein concentration of typical cells is at the level where any increase has a deleterious effect on the cell's overall metabolic economy, a new function cannot become established in the face of selection against an increase in protein level unless it is quite advantageous even in early stages of its development. Deletion of unnecessary protein would relax the counterselection and thus facilitate evolution toward greater complexity. This beneficial result will follow only if the enzyme is actually deleted, not merely changed. One or a few mutations leading to single amino acid substitution might cause the production of an altered protein with no catalytic activity and thus delete the metabolic sequence, but this would, of course, not clear the way for the addition of new enzymes (unless the altered protein failed to assume a tight globular conformation and was thus subject to rapid hydrolysis by intracellular proteolytic enzymes). Deletion of the approximately 50 enzymes that participate in the synthesis of the 10 or 11 amino acids that mammals do not synthesize could allow for the addition of many new metabolic reactions without a net increase in protein level. Amino acids are used at relatively very high rates and the enzymes in their synthetic pathways must therefore be present at high levels. In contrast, most of the reactions involved in the later development of metabolic complexity proceed at relatively very low rates, and the enzymes catalyzing them are thus required at corresponding low levels. Deletion of one enzyme of an amino acid synthetic pathway may thus allow the addition of many new enzymes. Evolution of vertebrates was not characterized, as sometimes used to be said, by loss of biosynthetic functions; rather, it was characterized by gain in biochemical function and complexity. If along the way it has often been possible to replace one enzyme from the bulk-chemical sector of the cell's economy by 10 or 100 enzymes that perform new fine-chemical interconversions, the result is clearly an increase in functional flexibility and complexity.

Some metabolic sequences are needed under certain conditions, but are dispensable at other times. In many such cases, repression-derepression and induction mechanisms have evolved to adjust production of the enzymes of the sequence to momentary need for the product of the sequence. Like the total loss of ability to make an enzyme, these regulatory mechanisms have the double advantage of limiting total protein level (since not all of these enzymes will be induced under any single set of conditions) and of preventing the expenditure of energy and building blocks in the production of unnecessary proteins, although in these cases the organism retains the ability to make the enzyme when its activity would be advantageous.

Little is known of the factors that determine the levels of enzymes that are not under obvious repression-induction control, but it is evident that the production of each, and hence the total protein concentration, is tightly controlled. This book deals primarily with the concentrations of metabolites of low molecular weight, however, and the problem of control of protein levels will not be dealt with further except in terms of the effects of enzyme levels on the concentrations of metabolic intermediates.

Metabolite Concentrations

The concentrations of metabolites must be controlled for at least two reasons: (a) as noted above, if several thousand compounds are to coexist in the same solution, their average concentration must be very low; and (b) the higher the concentration of an individual metabolite, the greater the possibility of undesirable side reactions. Many metabolic intermediates are rather reactive compounds. The tight control of metabolism that is essential to a viable cell would be impossible if nonenzymatic, and hence unregulated, reactions occurred to any significant degree. The low concentrations of metabolites, especially of the more reactive ones, aid in guarding against side reactions. Even a reaction with a moderately large rate constant (the velocity when both reactants are at unit activity) may be insignificant under metabolic conditions. If two compounds are each at a concentration of 10^{-5} M, for example, the reaction between them, assuming that it is first order in each, will go at 10^{-10} times the rate under standard conditions. The amount of reaction that would occur in one second if both reactants were at unit activity will require about 317 years in the dilute system. The protection against dangerous side reactions that the cell gains from simple dilution is obvious. Protection against uncontrolled excessive occurrence of the same reactions that participate in metabolism is a less obvious need, but may be equally important; regulation is essential to a viable cell. It is also evident that a dynamic chemical system operating at typical biological rates can be constructed with all intermediates at concentrations in the nanomolar to millimolar range only by the use of very effective catalysts; it is noteworthy that many enzymes catalyze reactions at rates of 10^{10} to 10^{16} times those of corresponding nonenzymatic conversions.

One might ask why it was necessary to evolve the rapid reaction rates that characterize living systems. What would be the disadvantages of metabolizing one-billionth as fast as we now do, and presumably living a billion times as long? Two answers are obvious. The absolute rates of metabolic reactions may not be important in themselves, but the relative rates (compared to non-enzymatic reactions of the same metabolites at the same concentrations) must, as noted above, be very high to permit the channeling and control of metabolic reaction sequences that are essential to life. In addition, selection must often, especially in the early stages of evolution, have been a simple matter of growth rate. It is easy to show that if two cells are similar except that cell A grows 1% faster than cell B, the descendents of A will outnumber those of B by a factor of 2 after 100 generations of B, by a factor of 4 after 200 generations, and so on. Descendents of the more slowly growing cell would be overgrown more rapidly, of course, if the difference in growth rate were greater. Without further discussion of the point, it is evident that the development of very high catalytic activity has been of enormous evolutionary significance.

Activation of Intermediates

The necessity to hold concentrations of all intermediates at low levels poses both kinetic and thermodynamic difficulties. We have noted above that the kinetic problems have been taken care of by the evolution of enzymes capable of catalyzing reactions at rapid rates even at typical metabolite concentrations. The thermodynamic problems require a different solution—the avoidance of intermediates that are unduly stable with regard to later compounds in the sequence; more strictly speaking, the avoidance of reactions with highly unfavorable equilibrium constants, for which the value of $\Delta G'$ is large and positive.* For any such reaction to proceed, however effective the catalyst, the concentrations of the reactants must be much greater than those of the products. In order to maintain a suitable concentration of product in such cases, the reactant concentrations would necessarily be relatively very high, with all of the consequent disadvantages.

The many activating groups that are found in metabolism have as a primary function the avoidance of thermodynamically unfavorable reactions. A few examples will be considered in this chapter. This function overlaps with that of providing stoichiometric coupling between reaction sequences, which is the subject of the next chapter. Thus ATP is the most important and ubiquitous coupling agent, being either consumed or regenerated in every metabolic sequence. It is also valid to consider ADP as the activating group for phosphate (an alternative and probably more meaningful statement is that AMP is a carrier for the phosphate-pyrophosphate system).

---

* In this book, $\Delta G'$ specifies the free energy change for a reaction when all reaction components are at their conventional standard states, except that the standard pH is taken as 7, rather than 0 as is usual in physical chemistry.

Finally, in most cases where ATP is consumed its immediate function is the avoidance of a high concentration of some other metabolite. In considering ATP as the basic coupling agent, as activated phosphate, and as a means of holding down metabolic concentrations, we are merely looking at three aspects of the same phenomenon. The latter two will be discussed below; the first is the subject of Chapter 3.

Activation of Phosphate

Transfer of phosphate from phosphoenolpyruvate to glucose to form glucose 6-phosphate would go nearly to completion; that is, the equilibrium constant is large and $\Delta G'$ is large and negative. This transfer could proceed in any of three general ways: (a) by direct donation (by attack of glucose oxygen at the phosphorus atom, displacing enolpyruvate); (b) by way of orthophosphate; that is, phosphoenolpyruvate could be hydrolyzed and the orthophosphate formed could react with glucose; and (c) by way of activated phosphate; that is, phosphate could be accepted by a carrier or activating group and in turn transferred to glucose. In each case the equation for the overall process would be that shown in 2-1. The values of $\Delta G'$ (about

$$\text{phosphoenolpyruvate} + \text{glucose} \rightleftharpoons \text{glucose 6-P} + \text{pyruvate} \qquad (2\text{-}1)$$

-10 kcal/mole) and K_{eq} (about 10^7) would be identical in all three cases. Yet the route that is actually observed in general metabolism—transfer by way of an activated form of phosphate—is greatly to be preferred. The general advantages of coupling agents over direct transfer will be discussed in the next chapter. Here we will compare possibilities (b) and (c). If (b) were used, we would have reactions 2-2 and 2-3. From the value of K for reaction

$$\text{phosphoenolpyruvate} + H_2O \rightleftharpoons \text{pyruvate} + P_i \qquad \begin{array}{l} \Delta G' = -13\,\text{kcal/mole};\ (2\text{-}2) \\ K = 2 \times 10^9 \end{array}$$

$$P_i + \text{glucose} \rightleftharpoons \text{glucose 6-P} + H_2O \qquad \begin{array}{l} \Delta G' = 3\,\text{kcal/mole};\ (2\text{-}3) \\ K = 7 \times 10^{-3} \end{array}$$

2-3, it follows that at equilibrium $(P_i) = (G6P)/(7 \times 10^{-3})(\text{glucose})$. In order to maintain a ratio of glucose 6-P to free glucose of 10, which is certainly a reasonable requirement, the concentration of P_i would need to be about 1400 M. There is of course not nearly room enough in one liter of space for 1400 moles of phosphate. On the other hand, if a phosphate concentration of 500 mM could be tolerated—a highly optimistic assumption— the ratio of glucose 6-P to glucose could not exceed 1/300. Note that these are thermodynamic limitations and that they could not be circumvented by any improvement of the enzyme catalyzing the phosphorylation. Clearly the route by way of free orthophosphate is not feasible; a useful ratio of glucose 6-P to glucose could not be established or maintained in this manner.

Using the activating carrier route, we have reactions 2-4 and 2-5. For each

$$\text{PEP} + \text{ADP} \rightleftharpoons \text{pyruvate} + \text{ATP} \qquad \Delta G' = -5 \text{ kcal/mole}: K = 3.6 \times 10^3 \quad (2\text{-}4)$$

$$\text{ATP} + \text{glucose} \rightleftharpoons \text{ADP} + \text{glucose 6-P} \qquad \Delta G' = -5 \text{ kcal/mole}: K = 3.6 \times 10^3 \quad (2\text{-}5)$$

step, K_{eq} is about 3600, and it is evidently quite feasible to maintain the glucose 6-P/glucose ratio at almost any desired value. For example, an ATP/ADP ratio of 5 is quite typical *in vivo*. This ratio could in principle be sustained even at PEP/pyruvate ratios smaller than 0.002. Conversely, when the ATP/ADP ratio is 5 the equilibrium ratio of glucose 6-P to glucose is about 18,000. Thus it would be impossible to phosphorylate glucose effectively by route (b), but simply by route (c). No thermodynamic legerdemain is involved. The overall equilibrium constant, which may be thought of as the ratio of glucose 6-P/glucose to phosphoenolpyruvate/pyruvate, is the same in each case (being about 10^7, it is for all practical purposes infinitely large). The difference between the two routes is that in one case nearly all of the phosphate would accumulate as free orthophosphate, while in the other it is transferred smoothly to glucose without the accumulation of high concentrations of any intermediates.

Activation of Organic Intermediates

The avoidance of high concentrations of intermediates is a characteristic of metabolic pathways of all types, and is probably the reason that a wide variety of metabolic activating agents have been evolved. Activation in the organic synthetic laboratory may play both a kinetic role (in accelerating the rate of the reaction) and a thermodynamic role (in increasing the yield of product at equilibrium). Thus the synthesis of an ester (reaction 2-6) may be made to go more rapidly if the acid is activated (reactions 2-7 and 2-8); at the same time the portion of the alcohol that may be esterified is greatly increased. It is evident that the overall reaction shown in equation 2-9,

$$\text{RCOOH} + \text{HOR}' = \text{RCOOR}' + \text{HOH} \qquad (2\text{-}6)$$

$$\text{RCOOH} + \text{PCl}_5 = \text{RCOCl} + \text{POCl}_3 + \text{HCl} \qquad (2\text{-}7)$$

$$\underline{\text{RCOCl} + \text{HOR}' = \text{RCOOR}' + \text{HCl}} \qquad (2\text{-}8)$$

$$\text{RCOOH} + \text{HOR}' + \text{PCl}_5 = \text{RCOOR}' + \text{POCl}_3 + 2 \text{ HCl} \qquad (2\text{-}9)$$

actually carried out as indicated by equations 2-7 and 2-8, could also be broken down to partial reactions in other ways, one of which is shown in equations 2-10 and 2-11. Here equation 2-10 is identical to equation 2-6 and equation 2-11 shows the hydrolysis of PCl_5. Such a representation may be

$$\text{RCOOH} + \text{HOR}' = \text{RCOOR}' + \text{HOH} \qquad (2\text{-}10)$$

$$\underline{\text{PCl}_5 + \text{HOH} = \text{POCl}_3 + \text{HCl}} \qquad (2\text{-}11)$$

$$\text{RCOOH} + \text{HOR}' + \text{PCl}_5 = \text{RCOOR}' + \text{POCl}_3 + 2 \text{ HCl} \qquad (2\text{-}12)$$

useful for the thermodynamic purposes; for example, if the $\Delta G'$ values and equilibrium constants for equations 2-10 and 2-11 are known, they may be used to calculate $\Delta G'$ and K_{eq} for reaction 2-12, which is the same as reaction 2-9. Since reaction 2-10, which is identical to 2-6, has an unfavorable K_{eq}, whereas reaction 2-12, which is identical to 2-9, is highly favorable, one might be led to say that the esterification (reaction 2-10) has been driven by the free energy of hydrolysis of PCl_5 (reaction 2-11). Just such a statement is made in many biochemistry texts in connection with the role of ATP in similar cases. Unless carefully qualified and explained, this statement is seriously misleading. The esterification actually proceeds as shown in equations 2-7 and 2-8, and no hydrolysis of PCl_5 is involved. Such hydrolysis, if it did occur (reaction 2-11), could not conceivably cause reaction 2-10 to go to a new equilibrium ratio. Indeed, hydrolysis of PCl_5 would obviously be an undesirable side reaction that would wastefully remove PCl_5, and the reaction is therefore always run in the absence of water. Reaction 2-7 is favorable because of the stability of $POCl_3$ relative to PCl_5; similarly, reaction 2-8 is favorable because the acyl chloride is unstable (the chloride ion is a good leaving group). The overall free energy change accompanying the actual esterification (reactions 2-7 and 2-8) must be identical with that calculated to accompany any other path by which the same conversion might be represented, whether or not the path is feasible. Reactions 2-10 and 2-11 make up one such path. The free energy change of reaction 2-11 is an indication of the same relative stabilities of $POCl_3$ and PCl_5 that cause reaction 2-7 to be favorable. Thus reactions 2-11 and 2-7 have something in common, but there is no sense in which it is correct to say that reaction 2-11 "drives" reaction 2-10. Neither of these reactions in fact occurs.

Reaction 2-9 could also be broken down as shown in reactions 2-13, 2-14, and 2-15. Reactions 2-13 and 2-14 are analogous to the incorrect treatment of the kinase-catalyzed transfer of a phosphoryl group that was illustrated

$$PCl_5 + HOH = POCl_3 + 2\,HCl \qquad (2\text{-}13)$$

$$RCOOH + HCl = RCOCl + HOH \qquad (2\text{-}14)$$

$$\underline{RCOCl + HOR' = RCOOR' + HCl} \qquad (2\text{-}15)$$

$$RCOOH + HOR' + PCl_5 = RCOOR' + POCl_3 + 2\,HCl \qquad (2\text{-}16)$$

in equations 2-2 and 2-3. Again the problem is mainly one of concentrations; the concentration of HCl that would be required for nearly quantitative conversion of RCOOH to RCOCl is unattainable.

Almost any metabolic sequence could be used to illustrate the generalization that the primary function of activation in metabolism is the avoidance of high concentrations. In most metabolic acylations, coenzyme A esters at very low concentrations are used instead of free acids, which would require high concentration. Biotin-CO_2 at a low concentration, rather than CO_2 at a high concentration, is used in many carboxylations. Many cells are able to make nucleotides from free purine and pyrimidine bases if they encounter them. Ribose 5-P is not added directly, however, but is first activated to 1-pyrophospho-5-phosphoribose (PRPP) at the expense of ATP. An impossibly high concentration of ribose 5-P would be required for the direct reaction (equation 2-17), but the use of PRPP, and indirectly of ATP, avoids the need for high concentrations of any intermediates (equations 2-18 and 2-19). Maintenance of low concentrations is one of the most important consequences of the participation of ATP in metabolic sequences.

$$R5P + base = nucleotide + HOH \qquad (2\text{-}17)$$

$$R5P + ATP = PRPP + AMP \qquad (2\text{-}18)$$

$$\underline{PRPP + base = nucleotide + PP_i} \qquad (2\text{-}19)$$

$$R5P + base + ATP = nucleotide + AMP + PP_i \qquad (2\text{-}20)$$

A slightly more complex example of the importance of the activation of intermediates may be seen in the conversion of pyruvate and oxaloacetate (OAA) to citrate (equation 2-21). This conversion could be represented as proceeding by various paths, including the two nonphysiological sequences specified in reactions 2-22 through 2-25 and 2-26 through 2-30 and the true metabolic sequence of reactions 2-31 through 2-36.*

$$pyruvate + OAA + NAD^+ + HOH = citrate + NADH + CO_2 + H^+ \qquad (2\text{-}21)$$

$$pyruvate = acetaldehyde + CO_2 \qquad (2\text{-}22)$$

$$acetaldehyde + NAD^+ + HOH = acetic\ acid + NADH + H^+ \qquad (2\text{-}23)$$

$$\underline{acetic\ acid + OAA = citrate} \qquad (2\text{-}24)$$

$$pyruvate + OAA + NAD^+ + HOH = citrate + CO_2 + NADH + H^+ \qquad (2\text{-}25)$$

$$pyruvate = acetaldehyde + CO_2 \qquad (2\text{-}26)$$

$$acetaldehyde + NAD^+ + HOH = acetic\ acid + NADH + H^+ \qquad (2\text{-}27)$$

$$acetic\ acid + HSCoA = acetyl\text{-}SCoA + HOH \qquad (2\text{-}28)$$

$$\underline{acetyl\text{-}SCoA + OAA + HOH = citrate + HSCoA} \qquad (2\text{-}29)$$

$$pyruvate + OAA + NAD^+ + HOH = citrate + CO_2 + NADH + H^+ \qquad (2\text{-}30)$$

$$pyruvate + TPP = HETPP + CO_2 \qquad (2\text{-}31)$$

$$HETPP + lip_{ox} = acetyl\text{-}lip_{red} + TPP \qquad (2\text{-}32)$$

$$acetyl\text{-}lip_{red} + HSCoA = acetyl\text{-}SCoA + lip_{red} \qquad (2\text{-}33)$$

$$lip_{red} + NAD^+ = lip_{ox} + NADH + H^+ \qquad (2\text{-}34)$$

$$\underline{acetyl\text{-}SCoA + OAA + HOH = citrate + H\ 'CoA} \qquad (2\text{-}35)$$

$$pyruvate + NAD^+ + OAA + HOH = citrate + CO_2 + NADH + H^+ \qquad (2\text{-}36)$$

* Abbreviations used in equations 2-31 to 2-36 are TPP, thiamin pyrophosphate; HETPP, hydroxyethyl thiamin pyrophosphate ("active acetaldehyde"); lip_{ox} and lip_{red}, oxidized and reduced lipoic acid.

The sequences corresponding to equations 2-22 through 2-35 are presented in road map style in Figure 2-1. In this figure the vertical coordinate is a generalized representation of free energy, not drawn to scale. A reaction arrow tending downward indicates a reaction with a negative value of $\Delta G'$, and hence a favorable equilibrium constant; arrows directed upward represent reactions with positive values of $\Delta G'$, and unfavorable equilibrium constants. As in the case of the illustration involving activation by the use of PCl_5, all of the overall reactions (2-25, 2-30, and 2-36) are identical. Therefore the values of K_{eq} and $\Delta G'$ are the same for all three paths, and at equilibrium at any given pH, the ratio (citrate)(CO$_2$)(NADH)/(pyruvate)(OAA)(NAD$^+$) would necessarily be the same in each case. The difference between the paths is, as in the previous illustration, that the relative stability of acetate is such that in paths involving this compound nearly all of the carbon introduced as C-2 and C-3 of pyruvate would accumulate as acetate at equilibrium and very little citrate could be formed. In other words, the equilibrium for the conversion of pyruvate to acetate and CO_2 and that for the reaction of acetate and OAA to form citrate would also apply. The equilibrium concentration of acetate would be very large compared to those of pyruvate and citrate. Since acetate does not appear in the overall equilibrium expression, the *ratio* of citrate to pyruvate at equilibrium is independent of acetate concentration. But the actual concentrations of both must, of course, vary with the level of acetate when a path including acetate is taken.

In the actual path (equations 2-31 through 2-35 and upper path of Figure 2-1), the metabolic function of lipoate and of coenzyme A is the avoidance of stable intermediates that would accumulate to high concentrations—spe-

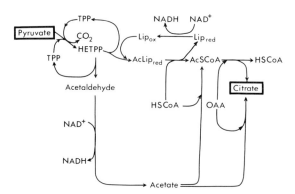

Figure 2-1.   Schematic diagram of the free energy relationships of the three routes from pyruvate to citrate discussed in the text (equations 2-22 to 2-24, 2-26 to 2-29, and 2-31 to 2-35). The vertical coordinate schematically indicates relative free energies, but is not drawn to scale. Adapted from Atkinson (7).

cifically, the avoidance of acetate. Thus their role, like that of most metabolic activating groups, is purely thermodynamic. All of the reactions of the lower paths of Figure 2-1 (equations 2-22 through 2-24 and 2-26 through 2-29) are kinetically feasible, and are catalyzed by known enzymes. Acetate can be formed by the hydrolysis of acetyl-SCoA or the cleavage of citrate, and enzymes catalyzing these reactions must be kinetically capable of catalyzing their reversal, but the free energy relations are such that net reversal would never be possible in a living cell.

Thiamin pyrophosphate may be considered to be an arm of pyruvate decarboxylase, participating in the catalysis of the reaction. Decarboxylation of an α-keto acid is an unlikely reaction because of the energetic instability of the intermediate aldehyde carbanion. The reaction can proceed only if this intermediate is stabilized by attachment of a strongly electron-withdrawing group to the carbonyl carbon. This function is served by cyanide in the analogous benzoin condensation; in metabolic decarboxylation of α-keto acids, thiamin pyrophosphate is the stabilizing group. Thiamin pyrophosphate participates in providing a reaction path with a much lower barrier than would otherwise be available. It is thus, in effect, a part of the enzyme and plays a largely kinetic role, in contrast to the thermodynamic roles of typical metabolic activating groups.

The only known metabolic function of lipoate is the avoidance of free acetate or succinate in the oxidative decarboxylations of pyruvate and α-ketoglutarate. The acetyl group is generated as the thiol ester acetyl lipoate, which in the presence of water is thermodynamically very unstable relative to acetate and lipoate. For simplicity in the essentially qualitative comparison that we wish to make, we will assume that $\Delta G'$ for hydrolysis of acetyl lipoate is -7 kcal/mole, corresponding to a K_{eq} of 10^5 M. The actual value may be somewhat higher. As in the case of ATP, the free energy of hydrolysis is of use to us only as an indication of the ease with which lipoate may be replaced by another group; no reaction is "driven by the free energy of hydrolysis of acetyl lipoate," but this compound is thermodynamically very reactive in other reactions for the same reasons that make its hydrolysis thermodynamically favorable.

After reduced lipoate is displaced by coenzyme A, the electrons that were gained from the 2-carbon fragment in its oxidation from the aldehyde to the acyl level are transferred to NAD^+, and the oxidized lipoate thus regenerated is ready to participate in generation of another acetyl group. In metabolic terms, the acetyl group may be said to have been transferred from lipoate to coenzyme A. For the sake, again, of simplicity, we will assume the $\Delta G'$ and K_{eq} values for hydrolysis of acetyl-SCoA to be identical with those of acetyl lipoate. Again it would not be valid to say that the free energy of hydrolysis of acetyl-SCoA "drives" condensation with oxaloacetate. However, if K_{eq} for the hydrolysis of acetyl-SCoA is 10^5 M, and the physiological concentration of free HSCoA is 10^{-5} M, we may consider an acetyl group to be thermodynamically as available from acetyl-SCoA at 10^{-10} M as from 1 M acetic acid, since the equilibrium ratio of the two compounds is 10^{10} (see below). Thus even if its physiological concentration is 10^{-5} M, acetyl-SCoA is 100,000 times as effective an acetyl donor as 1 M acetic acid. This comparison illustrates rather dramatically the importance of lipoate, coenzyme A, and similar activating agents in the avoidance of the necessity for high concentrations of reagents in order to obtain needed levels of products.

On the basis of an assumed value of 10^5 M for the equilibrium constant for the hydrolysis of acetyl-SCoA (reverse direction of reaction 2-28) we may illustrate the problems associated with the pathway shown in equations 2-26 to 2-29. The relation between the concentrations of acetyl-SCoA and free HSCoA (equation 2-38) at equilibrium follows from the equilibrium expression (equation 2-37). If we assume that 10^{-5} M is a reasonable physi-

$$K_{eq} = \frac{(AcOH)(HSCoA)}{(AcSCoA)} = 10^5 \ M \tag{2-37}$$

$$\frac{(AcSCoA)}{(AcOH)} = \frac{(HSCoA)}{10^5} \tag{2-38}$$

ological value for (HSCoA), the equilibrium ratio (AcSCoA)/(AcOH) would be 10^{-10}. If an acetyl-SCoA concentration of 1 μM were to be maintained by means of reaction 2-28, an acetate concentration of 10,000 M would be be necessary. This is over 500 times the concentration of pure acetic acid. Or, if the maximal tolerable concentration of acetate were 1 mM, the concentration of acetyl-SCoA could not exceed 10^{-13} M, and there would be less than one chance in a thousand of finding a single molecule of this intermediate in a bacterial cell at any given time. These calculations illustrate again that although the ratio of the concentrations of the products of a sequence to the concentrations of reactants is independent of the pathway, the very important question of whether nearly all of the material accumulates as intermediates is totally dependent on the pathway taken. Living systems are able to maintain all intermediates at low concentrations, and therefore have the capacity for proliferation of pathways, only because they have evolved the use of a group of activating agents as a means of avoiding stable intermediates that would necessarily accumulate to high concentrations.

The energy profile for a nonbiological reaction sequence will consist of an arrangement of peaks and valleys like that illustrated in greatly simplified form in Figure 2-2a. The higher an energy barrier, the smaller the velocity constant for the corresponding reaction; the lower the valley corresponding to a stable intermediate, the higher the steady-state concentration of that

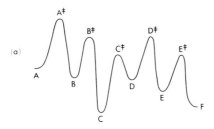

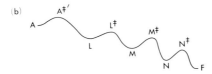

Figure 2-2. Schematic energy profiles for conversion of compound A to compound F: (a) by a sequence of nonenzymatic reactions; (b) by a sequence of enzyme-catalyzed reactions, with avoidance of overly stable intermediates. Adapted from Atkinson (7).

intermediate will be. The height of a peak is meaningful mainly in terms of its relation to the valley immediately preceding it, and the velocity constant of the corresponding reaction will depend on this valley-to-peak height. When a sequence of reactions (equation 2-39) is proceeding at a steady state the net velocities of all reactions are necessarily equal. For homogeneous systems, ignoring back reactions, we may then relate the steady-state concentrations of intermediates and the reaction rate constants as in equation 2-40. From this equation it follows that steady-state concentrations of in-

$$A \xrightarrow{k_A} B \xrightarrow{k_B} C \xrightarrow{k_C} D \xrightarrow{k_D} P \qquad (2\text{-}39)$$

$$\text{Velocity} = k_A(A) = k_B(B) = k_C(C) = k_D(D) \qquad (2\text{-}40)$$

termediates in a sequence of first-order homogeneous reactions are inversely proportional to the velocity constants of the following reactions (equation 2-41).* It is also seen that each concentration is directly proportional to the

$$(A) = \text{vel}/k_A; \quad (B) = \text{vel}/k_B; \quad (C) = \text{vel}/k_C; \quad (D) = \text{vel}/k_D \qquad (2\text{-}41)$$

---

* The terms in equation 2-40 give the velocities of the forward reactions. These will be equal to the net rates, making equation 2-41 valid, only if ΔG for each reaction is large and negative under steady-state conditions—that is, if each reaction is so far from equilibrium that the rate of the back reaction can be ignored. Equation 2-41 thus has no general applicability to the real world, but it is useful in contrasting nonbiological reaction sequences with sequences of enzyme-catalyzed reactions.

velocity; thus if a new and higher steady-state flux were established, the concentrations of all intermediates would necessarily rise in proportion. If, for example, the reaction sequence illustrated in Figure 2-2a were accelerated by an increase in the concentration of the starting material A, in a simplified treatment we may consider that each valley would fill to a somewhat higher level with the intermediate, thus decreasing the height of the corresponding activation barrier, and increasing the rate of each reaction until a new steady state was ultimately reached.

The characteristic property of an enzyme, as a catalyst, is its ability to provide a reaction path in which the highest-energy intermediate (the transition state) is at a very much lower energy level than that for the corresponding nonenzymic reaction—so much lower that the reaction is typically accelerated by a factor of 10^{12} or greater. When the reactions of a sequence are considered together, it is almost equally striking, and probably fully as important in the design of a living cell, that enzymes direct metabolic sequences along routes that avoid any unduly stable intermediates, such as acetate in the conversion of pyruvate to citrate, or intermediate C in the schematic illustration of Figure 2-2a. Thus the energy profile for a typical metabolic sequence, shown schematically in Figure 2-2b, contains neither high peaks, which would impede the progress of the sequence, nor low valleys, in which high concentrations of an intermediate would accumulate.

The general considerations of Figure 2-2 are applied to the specific case of the conversion of pyruvate to acetyl-SCoA in Figure 2-3. This figure is schematic and not drawn to scale, but it illustrates the major point under consideration: the use of activating groups such as lipoate and coenzyme A allows organisms to avoid high concentrations of any intermediate.

Some important activated intermediates are listed in Table 2-1. All of these resemble AcSCoA in the important feature that the activated group is attached to the remainder of the molecule by a bond that is characterized by a large negative value of the standard free energy of hydrolysis. They all play similar roles in avoiding the need for high concentrations of metabolic intermediates.

Although the point is somewhat peripheral to our present considerations, it is interesting to note that each of the activating molecules either is attached covalently to an enzyme molecule or bears a nucleotide group at the end of the molecule remote from that at which the activated group is bound. These nucleotide groups presumably serve as recognition signals for the appropriate enzymes, and their interactions with specific groups on the enzymes probably provide an important part of the binding energy for formation of the enzyme-intermediate complex.

In some senses, NADH, NADPH, and $FADH_2$ could be considered to be activated forms of electron pairs; they are at any rate carriers of electrons.

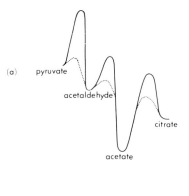

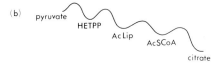

Figure 2-3. Schematic energy profiles for the conversion of pyruvate to citrate: (a) by way of acetaldehyde and acetate. Broken lines indicate that enzymic catalysis of these reactions could reduce the activation energy peaks and thus accelerate the reactions, but could not affect the accumulation of acetate; (b) by way of acetyl lipoate and acetyl coenzyme A. Rates are high because of the relatively low activation barriers, and no intermediates accumulate because the enzyme-directed path avoids thermodynamically stable intermediates. Adapted from Atkinson (7).

It is notable that these electron carriers resemble the activating or carrier molecules of Table 2-1 in their possession of AMP enzyme recognition groups.

CONSERVATION OF ENERGY

Lipmann (74) was the first to point out clearly the importance in metabolism of activated intermediates, in which groups are held by weak bonds and are thus thermodynamically highly available. (It is thus appropriate that he received his Nobel Prize, years later, for the discovery of one of the most important such intermediates, acetyl-SCoA). As discussed in the preceding section, the standard free energy changes for many reactions of such intermediates, including hydrolysis, are large and negative. Thus, in the presence of water, the activated intermediates may be thought of as being at higher energy levels than their hydrolysis products, as schematically indicated in Figure 2-1. They have thus come to be spoken of as "high-energy" intermediates. Their production in the course of metabolism is sometimes termed

TABLE 2-1

Some Activated Metabolic Intermediates

Compound or group activated	Activated form	Type of unstable compound	Carrier or enzyme recognition group
Orthophosphate	ATP	Pyrophosphate	AMP
Carboxylic acid	Acyl-SCoA	Thiol ester	AMP
Carboxylic acid	Acyl lipoate	Thiol ester	Covalent[b]
Carboxylic acid	Acyl-ACP[a]	Thiol ester	Covalent[b]
Carboxylic acid	Acyl-AMP	Mixed anhydride	AMP
Aminocarboxylic acid	Aminoacyl-tRNA	Ester	tRNA
CO_2	Biotin-CO_2	N-substituted carbamate	Covalent[b]
Ribose 5-P	PRibPP[a]	Acetal phosphate	—
Hexoses, hexosamines, uronic acids, and other hexose derivatives	NDP-sugar[a]	Acetal phosphate	UMP, AMP, or GMP
Phosphatidic acids	CDP-diacylglycerides	Pyrophosphate	CMP
Choline	CDP-choline	Pyrophosphate	CMP
Ethanolamine	CDP-ethanolamine	Pyrophosphate	CMP

[a] Abbreviations: ACP, pantotheine-bearing acyl carrier protein; PRibPP, 1-pyrophospho-ribose 5-phosphate; NDP-sugar, nucleoside diphosphate compound of hexose or hexose derivative.

[b] Covalently bonded to enzyme.

conservation of energy, in the sense that part of the free energy decrease that would accompany the conversion of pyruvate to acetate, for example, does not occur when the product is instead acetyl-SCoA. If used with restraint, the concept of energy conservation is useful. The metabolic path from pyruvate to acetyl-SCoA, the upper path in Figure 2-1, somewhat resembles that of a hiker who tries to conserve altitude by following elevation contours instead of going down into a valley from which he would later have to climb out. Thus, since the vertical coordinate is a schematic free energy scale, the path may by analogy be said to conserve free energy.

To avoid misunderstandings that might arise from this analogy, it is important to remember that free energy is not a physical entity in the same sense as heat or mass. Free energy is a function of concentrations, and the molar free energy change of a reaction is not fixed, but depends on concentrations. As a reaction proceeds toward equilibrium, the amount of heat evolved per micromole of product formed remains constant, but the negative change in free energy per micromole decreases steadily and becomes zero at equilibrium. As discussed in Chapter 3, when we speak of a chemical system as storing energy, we mean that it contains compounds whose concentration ratio is different from what it would be at equilibrium of some feasible reaction. Conservation of energy thus, in a chemical context, can only mean conservation of nonequilibrium concentration ratios. The physiological concentrations of such compounds as acetyl-SCoA and acetyl lipoate, although low, are very far above the concentrations that would be in equilibrium with water and the hydrolysis products at their physiological concentrations. It is in this sense that they store or conserve energy.

The term conservation of energy is most commonly used in connection with the phosphorylation of ADP associated with glycolysis or respiration. Part of the free energy change of these processes is said to be conserved in ATP (or, sometimes, in ATP bond energy). The concept of storing energy in a bond and releasing it on rupture of the bond has no meaning in chemistry or common sense; energy is always required, rather than released, in breaking a bond. Otherwise there would be no bond. But when ADP is phosphorylated the ATP/ADP concentration ratio is moved farther from its hydrolysis equilibrium value, so the statement that part of the free energy of respiration is conserved in the maintenance of a nonequilibrium ATP/ADP ratio would be acceptable.

The central point of our discussion of conservation of energy is that since chemical energy is always a function of concentration ratios, anything that can reasonably be termed conservation of chemical energy must deal with conservation or maintenance of concentration ratios. This must be true, of course, also for the activated derivatives listed in Table 2-1. Concentrations and free energies are closely related, thus much of the discussion of conservation of solvent capacity in the preceding sections could be paraphrased in terms of free energy. As we noted in connection with equation 2-37, if the intracellular level of HSCoA is 10^{-5}, any concentration of AcSCoA may be considered to be equivalent thermodynamically to acetate at 10^{10} times that concentration. This is equivalent to saying that the AcSCoA system stores (or conserves) chemical energy by virtue of the fact that the concentration ratio AcSCoA/HSCoA is far from its equilibrium value. Similar statements could be made about each of the other activated compounds listed in Table 2-1. This alternative way of looking at activation is a major topic of the next chapter.

SUMMARY

Both the space requirements of matter and the solvent capacity of water limit the amounts of enzymes and metabolic intermediates that can exist in a cell (or in any volume element of a cell). Mechanisms for maintenance of low concentrations of both enzymes and intermediates are thus essential. Low concentrations of intermediates are essential also for another reason—

they limit nonenzymatic reactions to insignificant rates and thus make integrated and regulated enzyme-controlled metabolic systems possible.

If concentrations are to be kept low, intermediates of relatively low free energies of formation, which would necessarily accumulate to high concentrations, must be avoided. This is accomplished by utilization of activated derivatives of such compounds. Formation of these activated intermediates is the metabolic role of most of the compounds that are conventionally termed cofactors.

Avoidance of transition states of high free energy (by participation of enzymes that specify reaction pathways in which all transition states are at relatively low energy levels) and avoidance of high concentrations of intermediates (by participation of activating cofactors) are two of the major chemical features of metabolic sequences. Both are essential for an ordered metabolism and hence for life.

3

Functional Stoichiometric Coupling
and Metabolic Prices*

All living cells have three fundamental requirements: energy (ATP), reducing power (NADPH), and starting materials for biosynthesis. The most fundamental metabolic distinction between organisms—that between autotrophs and heterotrophs—relates to the ways in which these needs are satisfied (Table 3-1). Autotrophs obtain all three from the inorganic environment without recourse to compounds produced by other organisms. Thus all of their carbon compounds must be synthesized from the only important available inorganic compound of carbon, carbon dioxide. Different kinds of chemoautotrophs can obtain reducing power by oxidation of a wide variety of inorganic materials such as hydrogen and reduced compounds of sulfur and nitrogen (each species is usually quite specific as to the electron donors that it can utilize). The same reduced compounds supply electrons for regeneration of ATP by electron transfer phosphorylation. Photoautotrophs obtain ATP by electron transfer phosphorylation during the cycling of a photochemically excited electron back to ground-state chlorophyll, and are also able to use these excited electrons for the reduction of $NADP^+$, while obtaining electrons from water to replace them in the chlorophyll system. They have thus achieved independence of all sources of energy except the sun and of all sources of electrons except water. For this reason, photoautotrophic fixation of carbon dioxide is the predominant base of the food chain both on land and in the sea.

Ordinary heterotrophs depend on preformed organic compounds for all three primary needs. Although some carbon dioxide is fixed in heterotrophic metabolism, notably in the synthesis of amino acids, the heterotrophic cell

* Some of the concepts in this chapter have been discussed in earlier papers (9, 10).

TABLE 3-1

Metabolic Classification of Organisms

hexo	Source of ATP	Source of NADPH	Source of carbon
Chemoautotroph	Oxidation of inorganic compounds	Oxidation of inorganic compounds	CO_2
Photoautotroph	Sunlight	H_2O	CO_2
Photoheterotroph	Sunlight	Oxidation of organic compounds	Organic compounds
Heterotroph	Oxidation of organic compounds	Oxidation of organic compounds	Organic compounds

functions at the expense of compounds formed by other cells, and is not capable of net fixation of carbon dioxide. Some bacteria are able to regenerate ATP photochemically, but cannot supply electrons to $NADP^+$ as a result of photochemical reactions. These photoheterotrophs are thus as dependent as other heterotrophs on preformed organic compounds. They should, however, be able to incorporate nearly all of the organic matter that they obtain into cellular components. They differ in this respect from typical heterotrophs, which must oxidize much of the organic material that they take up to provide the ATP required for incorporation of the remainder. From their photochemical apparatus, photoheterotrophs thus gain greater efficiency in use of organic food, but not independence of such food.

Although all are dependent on preformed organic compounds, heterotrophs differ markedly in the number of compounds required. Some bacteria and fungi can make all of the compounds of the cell when supplied with any suitable single carbon source, but many other species, including many microorganisms, have lost some or many biosynthetic capabilities. Mammals require about half of their amino acids preformed, and are also unable to make several metabolic cofactors (hence the nutritional requirement for vitamins). Some bacteria and some parasites have even more extensive nutritional requirements than this.

FUNCTIONAL COUPLING

The popular large metabolic maps, designed for wall display, correspond roughly to schematic diagrams of electronic devices. At the cost of considerable complexity, they include all of the major and many of the quantitatively minor pathways. They are unable, however, to convey a clear idea of the functional relationships that are the heart of metabolism. As with electronic devices, the overall operational aspects of metabolism may be clarified by block diagrams that omit details and focus on functional relationships. Such a functional block diagram for a typical heterotrophic aerobic cell is shown in Figure 3-1, in which the metabolism of such a cell is symbolized by only three functional blocks:

(a) *Catabolism, or degradative metabolism:* Foods are oxidized to carbon dioxide. Most of the electrons liberated in this oxidation are transferred to oxygen, with concomitant production of ATP (electron transport phosphorylation). Other electrons are used in the regeneration of NADPH, the reducing agent for biosynthesis. The major pathways in this block are the glycolytic sequence and the citrate cycle. These same sequences, with the pentose phosphate pathway, also supply the starting materials for all of the cell's biosynthetic processes.

(b) *Biosynthesis, or anabolism:* This block includes much greater chemical complexity than the first. The starting materials produced by glycolysis and the citrate cycle are converted into hundreds of cell components, with NADPH serving as a reducing agent when necessary, and with ATP as the universal coupling agent or energy transducing compound.

(c) *Synthesis of macromolecules and growth:* Among the products of the second block are the building blocks for synthesis of the complex macromolecules on which biological functionality depends: proteins, nucleic acids, components of membranes, and so on. Most macromolecular syntheses use

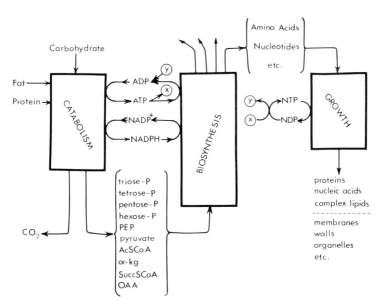

Figure 3-1. Schematic block diagram of metabolism of a heterotrophic aerobic cell. From Atkinson (*12*).

ATP indirectly, through the mediation of GTP, UTP, or CTP. This special-
ization of function among the nucleoside triphosphates will be discussed
in Chapter 6. It is probably important for efficient regulation of metabolism
and for appropriate allocation of ATP among different metabolic needs,
but our present considerations are not affected by whether ATP is used
directly or indirectly.

Each block in Figure 3-1 represents a variety of complex reactions and
interrelations, but perhaps the most noteworthy aspect of the figure is the
small number of connections between the blocks, that is, the small number of
compounds that are produced or regenerated in one block and used in another. Only about ten compounds, supplied by glycolysis, the pentose phosphate pathway, and the citrate cycle, are used in the many and varied biosynthetic processes, or at least in the synthesis of the quantitatively major
components of the cell. (In this count, isomeric metabolites interconvertible
by simple reactions are counted as a single compound.) They are four sugar
phosphates: triose phosphate (dihydroxyacetone phosphate and 3-phospho-
glyceraldehyde), tetrose phosphate, pentose phosphate, and hexose phosphate; three α-keto acids: pyruvate, oxaloacetate, and α-ketoglutarate;
two activated carboxylic acids: acetyl-SCoA and succinyl-SCoA; and
phosphoenolpyruvate.

The starting materials just listed are consumed in biosynthetic sequences
and must be continuously replaced by catabolic processes. The functions of
NADPH and ATP are very different. When they contribute to biosynthesis,
these coupling agents are converted to $NADP^+$ and ADP or AMP. Thus
they must be merely regenerated—reduced or rephosphorylated—at the
expense of substrate oxidation in the catabolic block of reactions. As the
figure indicates, ATP and NADPH are the only fundamental coupling agents
in metabolism—the only compounds that have primary roles in coupling
between the major functional blocks. The functions of other coupling agents
are essential but less broad in scope. NADH and $FADH_2$, for example,
participate within the catabolic block in the transfer of electrons from substrate to oxygen in electron transfer phosphorylation, but are not significantly involved in coupling between major functional blocks.

The block diagram of Figure 3-1 obviously does not represent the total
metabolism of organisms other than aerobic heterotrophs. The photochemical production of ATP in photoheterotrophs would require the addition of
a photochemical block, with ATP production in the catabolic block being
deleted. For a photoautotroph, two blocks are needed in addition to those
shown in Figure 3-1. One, the photochemical block, regenerates ATP and
reduces $NADP^+$ to NADPH, while consuming water and producing a
stoichiometric amount of oxygen. The second, that representing the "dark

reactions" of photosynthesis, uses ATP and NADPH produced by the first block in the reduction of carbon dioxide to various products, which might be represented by fructose 6-P or glucose. These photosynthetic products provide the input to the catabolic block, which in this case serves only one function—the production of the starting materials for synthesis. Of course such diagrams involve some oversimplification. Most photoheterotrophs and autotrophs are capable of ordinary heterotrophic metabolism; thus the catabolic block will, when necessary, lead to the regeneration of both NADPH and ATP. The assumption that photosynthesis supplies only hexose is also probably an oversimplification. It is probable that triose phosphate and perhaps some other intermediates, as well as some amino acids, might appropriately be considered to be primary products of photosynthesis. But these points do not significantly affect the general pattern of functional relationships that are illustrated by Figure 3-1 and the similar diagrams that may be drawn for other types of organisms.

TYPES OF METABOLIC STOICHIOMETRIES

Each metabolic sequence uses or regenerates ATP, and the functional relationships between sequences depend in large part on the stoichiometries of ATP consumption and production. We must therefore consider the nature of metabolic stoichiometric relationships, which are of three essentially different types. Of these, the first two are familiar and do not differ in any way from the stoichiometric relationships dealt with in other areas of chemistry. The third is unique to living cells and other functionally designed systems.

1. *Reaction stoichiometry.* This could also be termed simple conservation stoichiometry. Any valid equation, whether for a single reaction or an extended metabolic sequence, must have the same number of atoms of each type on each side of the arrow. This obvious kind of stoichiometry is learned in high school chemistry classes, and it is included here only for completeness and for comparison with the two types of coupling stoichiometries. As applied to respiration, stoichiometric considerations of this type tell us only that if glucose is converted quantitatively to carbon dioxide, 6 moles of carbon dioxide will be produced from each mole of glucose used.

2. *Obligate coupling stoichiometry.* In some kinds of interactions between metabolic sequences, the stoichiometric relationships are fixed by the chemical nature of the processes. The most important examples of this type involve oxidation and reduction, with one sequence providing electrons and the other consuming them. The simple balanced equation for respiration of

glucose (equation 3-1) tends to obscure the fact that we deal here with two

$$C_6H_{12}O_6 + 6\,O_2 \rightarrow 6\,CO_2 + 6\,H_2O \qquad\qquad (3\text{-}1)$$

quite different sequences, which are subblocks within the catabolic block of Figure 3-1, and which are coupled by biological electron carriers (equations 3-2 and 3-3). The stoichiometry of such coupling is evidently fixed by

$$C_6H_{12}O_6 + 10\,NAD^+ + 2\,FAD + 6\,H_2O$$
$$\rightarrow 6\,CO_2 + 10\,NADH + 10\,H^+ + 2\,FADH_2 \quad (3\text{-}2)$$
$$10\,NADH + 10\,H^+ + 2\,FADH_2 + 6\,O_2 \rightarrow 10\,NAD^+ + 2\,FAD + 12\,H_2O \quad (3\text{-}3)$$

elementary chemical considerations, and oxidation-reduction balancing is in principal the same whether we deal with one simple reaction or with inter-relationships between two extended sequences. If we know the amount of oxidation occurring in one sequence and the amount of reduction occurring in the other we can easily calculate the stoichiometric ratio between the rates of the two sequences. This ratio is determined by chemical considerations, and cannot be altered by evolution.

   3. *Evolved coupling stoichiometries.* The adenine nucleotides participate in every metabolic sequence (in some cases the participation is indirect). This participation, however, is fundamentally different from that of the pyridine nucleotides or flavins. The stoichiometry of the adenylates is not fixed by any chemical necessity; it is entirely under evolutionary control. The oxidation of a mole of glucose is coupled, for example, to the phosphorylation of 36 or 38* moles of ADP. The overall process is represented by equation 3-4. The coefficients in this equation illustrate the three types of stoichiometry discussed here. The 6 moles of carbon dioxide produced per mole of glucose,

$$C_6H_{12}O_6 + 6\,O_2 + 38\,ADP + 38\,P_i \rightarrow 6\,CO_2 + 6\,H_2O + 38\,ATP \qquad (3\text{-}4)$$

and the 6 moles of oxygen required for the process, are chemically fixed; the production of 38 moles of ATP is a biological adaptation. It depends on no chemical necessity, and *cannot be predicted from any chemical consideration whatever.* The importance of this last statement can hardly be overempha-sized. It illustrates the difference between the world of chemistry, physics, geology, and the other nonbiological sciences on the one hand and the world of functional design, which includes all living organisms and the functional

---

   * As discussed later in this chapter, the uncertainty results from the question of whether the 2 moles of cytoplasmic NADH produced in glycolysis for each mole of glucose metabolized give rise to 2 or 3 moles of ATP each when they are oxidized. Since a definite answer is not available, we will for the sake of simplicity assign a value of 3 ATP equivalents to every mole-cule of NADH, whether in the cytoplasm or in a mitochondrion. If the true value for cyto-plasmic ATP turns out to be 2, the corrections required will be very minor.

products of their activities, on the other. Products of functional design differ in the most fundamental ways from other objects, and in the broadest sense it does not matter whether the design is directly determined by evolutionary processes, as in the case of a protein; is indirectly determined by means of evolutionary designed behavioral programs genetically built into an organism, as in the case of a termite mound; or is the product of conscious design by an organism genetically programmed to be capable of such activity.

For our present purposes, we need only emphasize that whenever we deal with the products of design, whether the design be conscious or evolutionary, we can hope to *explain* and *understand* the designed object by the approaches of chemistry and physics, but that no knowledge of chemistry and physics, however complete, could even in principle permit *prediction* of the properties of that object. The assertions of some astronomers to the contrary notwithstanding, a planet containing water, carbon dioxide, and phosphates on its surface does not contain thereby the seeds of manlike organisms, any more than the properties of a jet plane could be predicted from careful study of a number of ores. Any process of design makes use of the properties of the materials that are used, but the functional relationships added by design become a fundamental part of the product, and one that is to a considerable degree independent of the properties of the starting materials and totally unpredictable from them.

Stoichiometric relatio. hips of types 1 and 2 require no further discussion here. Type 3 stoichiometry, on the other hand, is of fundamental interest to us. This type of stoichiometry, being functional, is a product of design in the sense discussed in the preceding paragraph. Such functional stoichiometry is unique to metabolism and to man-designed systems. The remainder of this book is devoted mainly to discussion of type 3 stoichiometry and some of its consequences.

The evolution of any phenotypic character must involve compromise. Such gross morphological features as the size of an animal or the length of its limbs result from a balance between the advantageous and disadvantageous consequences of increased size or longer legs, arms, or wings. Evolved coupling stoichiometries are phenotypic characters and, like other characters, must reflect such a balance between positive and negative consequences. Some of the factors involved in this compromise are obvious. Since the free energy of hydrolysis of ATP under physiological conditions is large and negative, a change in the ATP stoichiometry of a sequence would change the apparent equilibrium constant for the overall sequence. This change must have been balanced against the changed profit or cost (in terms of ATP produced or consumed) of the sequence. Thus for glycolysis an increase in the ATP yield would have the desirable effect of increasing the amount of ATP obtained from a given amount of glucose, but also the undesirable result that the equilibrium constant would be reduced. As a consequence, the minimal levels of glucose or oxygen that could be effectively utilized would increase. An organism that obtained more than 38 moles of ATP per mole of glucose would thus use glucose more efficiently when it was present in good supply, but might be unable to compete for it as effectively when the supply was limited. Since competition may be expected to be especially stringent when the food supply is limited, such organisms would be at a severe disadvantage. It would therefore be expected that the ATP yield of a primary energy-transforming sequence like respiration would have become fixed at a low enough level to establish a very high overall equilibrium constant, and thus to allow for use of substrates at very low levels. This clearly has happened in the case of respiration. If the free energy of hydrolysis of ATP under physiological conditions is taken as -11.5 kcal/mole (125), the free energy change corresponding to equation 3-4 (with other reactants and products at unit concentrations, and at pH 7) should be about 240 kcal. (The value of ΔG^0 for the oxidation of a mole of glucose to carbon dioxide is about -677 kcal.) The equilibrium constant for the whole process, including the production of 38 moles of ATP, is then about 10^{170}. Clearly the compromise in evolutionary design has favored a large equilibrium constant over a high yield of ATP.

Other factors, in addition to the advantage of utilizing substrates at very low concentrations, make large overall equilibrium constants desirable. The most obvious is the need for metabolic control points. For effective kinetic control, a reaction should be far from equilibrium at physiological concentrations of the reactants and products. Since the ratio of these physiological concentrations is seldom very large or very small, it is thus desirable that the equilibrium constant for each reaction catalyzed by a regulatory enzyme be large. When a sequence, like respiration, contains several reactions catalyzed by regulatory enzymes, the product of these several large equilibrium constants will necessarily contribute to the overall equilibrium constant of the sequence. Very large values for such overall constants are thus logically necessary. But even when all apparent advantages of large values are considered, it is still impossible to rationalize entirely satisfactorily such inconceivably large constants as 10^{170}. At any rate, the fundamental pattern of aerobic metabolism must have become fixed, by some interplay of chance and selective advantage, at least a billion years ago when conditions were quite unlike those today. Once established, the ATP yield would be very unlikely to change, because any change would require simultaneous alterations in several components of a system that is functioning very effectively as it is.

Other factors besides the equilibrium constant for the overall sequence affect the ability of an organism to compete for very low levels of substrate.

The most obvious of these additional factors are the affinities for substrate of the transport systems that bring the substrate into the organism and of the enzyme that catalyzes the first metabolic reaction of the substrate. It is no accident that the first step in the utilization of carbohydrates is phosphorylation. Conversion of a sugar to a phosphate ester may hinder its leakage out through the cell membrane, as has often been proposed, but it also allows for considerable increase in concentration. Since the equilibria of the reactions catalyzed by hexose kinases and by phosphofructokinase lie far toward the sugar phosphates, the concentration of these derivatives can be maintained at much higher levels than those of the free sugars from which they are derived. When the phosphoryl group is supplied directly from phosphoenolpyruvate, as in some sugar uptake mechanisms (*101*), the overall equilibrium constant is even larger. Hence enzymes catalyzing later steps need not deal with extremely low concentrations of intermediates. It should be noted that the two phosphate groups of fructose diphosphate, which are derived from ATP, have no apparent role in later steps in glycolysis. The net yield of ATP in glycolysis comes from the 3-phosphoglyceraldehyde dehydrogenase and 1,3-diphosphoglycerate kinase reactions, which incorporate inorganic phosphate and transfer it to ADP. (The ADP-derived phosphates of fructose diphosphate are ultimately recovered as ATP at the pyruvate kinase step; thus intermediates are tagged with phosphoryl groups with no net gain or loss of ATP being involved.) There is no reason to believe that the phosphate groups of fructose diphosphate are necessary for the aldol cleavage of fructose, for the subsequent oxidation of triose with incorporation of phosphate to form acyl phosphate, or for the transfer of this phosphate to ADP. That is, enzymes corresponding to aldolase, 3-phosphoglyceraldehyde dehydrogenase, and 1,3-diphosphoglyceric acid kinase, but not requiring phosphorylated substrates, should be as effective in obtaining a net yield of 2 moles of ATP per mole of hexose glycolyzed as are the enzymes actually observed. Thus we may abandon earlier ideas that these phosphate groups somehow activate the sugar for further reaction or provide handles for the convenience of later enzymes. (It has been suggested that the phosphate groups at the two ends of the fructose molecule might be compared to the handles sometimes attached to the ends of an ear of sweetcorn to protect the fingers of fastidious diners from contact with the kernels. Unfortunately, this appealing analogy seems not to be relevant.) The phosphate groups of fructose diphosphate have, I think, already fulfilled their function—the increase of concentration of substrate. All that remains for them is to be fed back into the ATP pool without loss. Even this use of ATP is a form of energy coupling. The free energy decrease in a late step in glycolysis (the conversion of phosphoenolpyruvate to pyruvate) is used to increase the concentrations of early intermediates of the sequence. This increase in concentration may even, as in the case of phosphoenolpyruvate-linked transport, involve movement across a membrane.

The degree of involvement of ATP in metabolism has come to be recognized over the past 30 or 40 years, and is now taken for granted. We therefore tend not to realize how remarkable it is that this one compound should be involved in virtually every extended metabolic sequence in the cell. Clearly the role of the adenine nucleotide pool (ATP, ADP, and AMP) is entirely unique; no other metabolites even approach the metabolic ubiquity of the adenylates. Their participation would often not seem to be advantageous if only an isolated sequence were considered. This is especially true for catabolic sequences. Glycolysis, for example, would proceed as well (and with a larger negative free energy change) if the adenylate-coupled steps were eliminated. The role of the adenylates, however, is not specific to any single pathway, but rather is completely general—the coupling and correlation of all of the metabolic activities of the cell, as illustrated in Figure 3-1. It is this coupling that underlies biological homeostasis and the functionality that is the most fundamental characteristic of life. Glycolysis would proceed as well, it is true, but to little metabolic purpose, if it were not coupled to the regeneration of ATP.

Coupling Coefficients

Since stoichiometric coupling by ATP underlies all metabolic functionality, the evolved stoichiometric relationships are of fundamental concern in any realistic discussion of metabolism. We will discuss these relationships in terms of the ATP *coupling coefficients* of reactions or of sequences, defined as the number of moles of ATP or ATP equivalents produced per mole of substrate converted in the reaction or sequence. Thus the coupling coefficient for the respiration of glucose is 38; the coupling coefficient for the pyruvate kinase reaction in the physiological direction is 1; and the coupling coefficient for the hexokinase reaction, which consumes ATP, is -1. The evolved stoichiometric relationship between any two reactions or sequences is directly evident from their coupling coefficients. In addition, the coupling coefficients may be taken as the basis for further consideration of metabolic stoichiometry in terms of metabolic prices, costs, and yields.

The metabolizing cell resembles in many ways a complex economic system. The use of ATP in metabolism has often been compared with the use of money. Some of the advantages that the cell gains by the use of ATP resemble the advantages of a money economy over a barter economy. Thus if an organism with a barter-type metabolism had 6 primary phosphate-donating reactions and 200 phosphate-consuming reactions, 1200 enzymes would be required for complete flexibility—to provide that phosphate from any one of the phosphate-donor reactions could be transferred to any one of the phosphate acceptors. In ATP-based metabolism, this number is reduced to only 206 enzymes—6 for the ATP-producing reactions and 200 for those using ATP. This saving in the number of enzymes that must be synthesized should in itself confer very great selective advantage as compared to a barter type of metabolism. But a cell or organism also gains other and probably much more important benefits from the use of ATP. These relate to regulation and the maintenance of biological homeostasis. One need only consider the problems of regulating the 1200 enzymes mentioned above, catalyzing 1200 reactions with no common reactant, to realize how enormously the problem of regulation is simplified by the use of ATP. When all sequences are stoichiometrically coupled by ATP, they may all be regulated through ATP interactions. The types of metabolic correlation and control mechanisms that have evolved, based on the ATP/ADP/AMP system, will be discussed in Chapters 4 and 6.

Metabolic Prices

In a money economy, goods and services have prices. If the analogy with a money economy is to provide us with any useful insight into the operation of metabolic systems, we must consider how prices are to be assigned to metabolites and costs assigned to metabolic conversions. It is evident at the outset that the unit of exchange—that is, of the pricing system—must be based on ATP. The cell gains ATP by carrying out certain metabolic sequences, and spends it on others. Just as different goods and services can be evaluated or symbolized in a money economy in terms of price, metabolic intermediates and metabolic conversions can be evaluated in terms of ATP requirement or yield. The statement that ATP is either earned or spent in nearly every activity of a cell is, of course, equivalent to the more chemical statement that ATP is the ubiquitous stoichiometric coupling agent in living cells. Because of this ubiquity, a value in ATP units can be assigned to the conversion effected by any metabolic sequence, and hence a price can be assigned to each of the metabolites participating in these sequences.

The ATP Equivalent

The metabolic unit of exchange, which will be termed the *ATP equivalent*, is the conversion of ATP to ADP or of ADP to ATP. Thus when ATP is used in a reaction catalyzed by a kinase, the amount of metabolic energy expended is one ATP equivalent. In a number of reactions, mostly in biosynthetic sequences but including the activation of fatty acids for degradation, ATP is converted to AMP. Two phosphorylations are required for regeneration of ATP from AMP; thus the cost of the regeneration is two ATP equivalents. As we will discuss later, the expenditures of two ATP equivalents in these reactions can be seen to be desirable when they are considered in their metabolic contexts.

Prices of Coupling Agents

All other metabolic conversions can be chemically related to the conversion of ATP to ADP, and thus they can all be evaluated or priced in terms of ATP equivalents. Because of their intimate relation to ATP regeneration, it is reasonable to begin with the internal coupling agents of catabolism, NADH and $FADH_2$. The value of NADH is evidently the familiar P/O ratio. Three molecules of ATP are produced for each molecule of NADH oxidized by the electron transfer phosphorylation system; hence, the value of NADH is 3 ATP equivalents. Similarly, the oxidation of one molecule of $FADH_2$ leads to the regeneration of two molecules of ATP; the price of $FADH_2$ is thus 2.*

The price to be assigned to NADPH is less immediately obvious. One of the most striking examples of biological specificity is the sharp functional distinction between NAD and NADP. The two compounds differ only by a phosphate group on carbon 2 of the ribose attached to adenine, which thus modifies the AMP enzyme recognition group of the molecule. Nearly all dehydrogenases are specific for one or the other of these cofactors, and these specificities conform to a pattern that is one of the great generalizations of metabolic chemistry—NAD participates in degradative metabolism and NADP in biosynthetic sequences. This generalization has been stated above, in different words, in the statement that NADP is a primary coupling agent, linking degradative sequences to reductive biosynthesis, whereas NAD plays a more local role within the degradative portion of metabolism.

The functional distinction between NAD and NADP supplies an excellent illustration of the resemblance of living systems to consciously designed mechanisms. The phosphate group on the adenosine of NADP has no significant effect on the reactivity of the nicotinamide ring or on the reduction potential of the compound. In any ordinary chemical context, NAD and NADP would be entirely equivalent as oxidation-reduction agents. The

---

* It is obvious that these prices represent changes in value accompanying oxidation or reduction, rather than the cost of actually synthesizing the molecule. It would cost many ATP equivalents to synthesize a molecule of NAD *de novo*. But we deal here only with the price of NADH relative to that of NAD^+. Such prices, which are appropriate for metabolic coupling agents, may be termed conversion prices to distinguish them from costs of synthesis.

extra phosphate of NADP seems to function strictly as a recognition code, and dehydrogenases have evolved conformations that allow them either to require a phosphate at that position or to reject a molecule containing it.

Since the reduction potentials of NAD and NADP are essentially identical, functional specificity in their use would by itself confer no advantage. The advantage of this specificity depends on similar specificity in regeneration, by which NADP in the living cell is maintained at a more reduced level than NAD. This difference has been repeatedly confirmed with respect to the cytoplasm, where most biosyntheses occur, although estimates of the magnitude of the difference vary widely. It appears that various types of cells, as well as various intracellular compartments, probably differ in this regard. The difference may be especially small in mitochondria (70). Nevertheless, there seems no doubt of the validity of the generalization, at least for cytoplasm. The difference in degree of reduction of the two pyridine nucleotide coenzymes clearly facilitates their metabolic functions. Although the $\mathscr{E}^0$ values for the two systems are virtually identical, it is evident that the more reduced system will be the stronger reducing agent, and conversely. The thermodynamic reducing power as a function of the standard electrode potential and the concentrations of the oxidized and reduced forms is given by the Nernst equation (equation 3-5), where R is the gas constant and $\mathscr{F}$ the faraday. In the cell, NADPH is a stronger reducing agent than NADH, and

$$\mathscr{E} = \mathscr{E}^0 + \frac{RT}{n\mathscr{F}} \ln \frac{[\text{ox}]}{[\text{red}]} \tag{3-5}$$

thus better suited for biosynthetic reductions, by virtue of the relative degrees of reduction of the two couples. Conversely, NAD^+ is a stronger oxidizing agent than $NADP^+$.

Several metabolic conversions are made thermodynamically favorable by being coupled to the transfer of a pair of electrons from NADPH to NAD^+, rather than by the use of ATP. As one example, the carbohydrate of mammalian semen is predominantly fructose. Since the equilibrium ratio of fructose to glucose is not far from unity, a quantitative conversion of glucose to fructose can occur only as a consequence of coupling to some reaction with a large negative free energy change. The reactions used are shown by equations 3-6 and 3-7. The overall equation (3-8) shows that the driving force for essen-

$$\text{glucose} + \text{NADPH} + \text{H}^+ \rightarrow \text{sorbitol} + \text{NADP}^+ \tag{3-6}$$

$$\underline{\text{sorbitol} + \text{NAD}^+ \rightarrow \text{fructose} + \text{NADH} + \text{H}^+} \tag{3-7}$$

$$\text{glucose} + \text{NADPH} + \text{NAD}^+ \rightarrow \text{fructose} + \text{NADP}^+ + \text{NADPH} \tag{3-8}$$

tially quantitative conversion of glucose to fructose is provided by the reduction of NAD^+ at the expense of NADPH. This electron transfer serves the metabolic function that is usually satisfied by ATP. Thus the organism may be considered to have expended 1 ATP equivalent by oxidizing NADPH and producing NADH. NADPH is therefore metabolically equivalent to NADH + ATP; since the potential yield of the NADH → NAD$^+$ conversion is 3 ATP equivalents, the price of NADPH must be 4 ATP equivalents greater than that of NADP$^+$. Thus a value of 4 is assigned to the NADPH → NADP$^+$ conversion.

The second argument for this price assignment is based on the regeneration, rather than the expenditure, of NADPH. NADP$^+$ is reduced in several metabolic reactions, and our information as to the relative importances of these reactions *in vivo* is at present extremely unsatisfactory. (Naturally, we know even less about the regulatory processes by which the NADPH/ NADP$^+$ ratio is controlled.) Among the known reactions in which NADP$^+$ is reduced, the one of special importance to us here is the ATP-driven transphosphorylation reaction discovered by Danielson and Ernster (*43*), which is shown in equation 3-9. The reduction of one mole of NADP$^+$ by this re-

$$\text{NADH} + \text{NADP}^+ + \text{ATP} + \text{H}_2\text{O} \rightarrow \text{NAD}^+ + \text{NADPH} + \text{ADP} + \text{P}_i \qquad (3\text{-}9)$$

action requires the oxidation of 1 mole of NADH (3 ATP equivalents) and the expenditure of 1 mole of ATP; hence the price of NADPH is 4 ATP equivalents greater than that of NADP$^+$, and a value of 4 is assigned to the NADPH → NADP$^+$ conversion. Although we do not know at present what fraction of NADPH regeneration occurs by way of this reaction (and the fraction doubtless varies with metabolic conditions), the existence of the reaction furnishes strong support for our belief that NADPH is metabolically 1 ATP equivalent more valuable than NADH. It seems likely that mitochondria produce NADPH at the expense of NADH and one equivalent of potential ATP; that is, some chemical or conformational high-energy state may be used either in the regeneration of ATP or the transfer of electrons from NADH to NADP$^+$. This possibility obviously does not alter the price to be assigned to NADPH.

As Krebs (*70*) has pointed out, his inference of a relatively low NADPH/ NADP$^+$ ratio inside mitochondria casts some doubt on the relevance of the Danielson-Ernster reaction in the maintenance of a high NADPH/NADP$^+$ ratio in the cytoplasm. It seems somewhat unlikely that an organelle with a low ratio would be responsible for the high ratio seen elsewhere. This objection, however, is not necessarily fatal to the hypothesis that mitochondria might be an important source of NADPH for biosynthesis; a great deal more must be known concerning intramitochondrial compartmentation, location of enzymes, and vectorial processes across membranes, before the importance of the Danielson-Ernster reaction can be evaluated.

TABLE 3-2

Metabolic Prices of Coupling Agents[a]

Coupling agents	ATP equivalents
Primary	
$ATP \rightarrow ADP$	1
$ATP \rightarrow AMP$	2
$NADPH \rightarrow NADP^+$	4
Secondary	
$NADH \rightarrow NAD^+$	3
$FADH_2 \rightarrow FAD$	2

[a] Prices are expressed in ATP equivalents corresponding to the coupling reaction shown.

It is clear that the transhydrogenase reaction (equation 3-9a), often ob-

$$NADPH + NAD^+ \rightleftharpoons NADP^+ + NADH \qquad (3\text{-}9a)$$

served in cell-free preparations, either must not exist in intact cells (at least in the cytoplasm) or must be inactive under nearly all conditions. This reaction would bring the reduction levels of NAD and NADP to the same value. The teleological argument that this would amount to short-circuiting an energy supply would alone be an excellent basis for doubting the existence of this enzymatic activity; the actual observation of a large difference between the reduction levels *in vivo* appears to settle the matter. Quite likely the transhydrogenase activity observed in disrupted systems is an artifact resulting from fragmentation of some integrated enzyme system, probably that responsible for the Danielson-Ernster reaction.

The conversion prices for coupling agents that have been discussed are shown in Table 3-2.

Prices of Metabolic Intermediates

In contrast to conversion prices, the actual price of a compound is defined as the number of moles of ATP or ATP equivalents obtained on oxidizing the compound to carbon dioxide (in anaerobes, the number obtained on complete fermentation of a compound) or as the number of ATP equivalents required in the synthesis of the compound. These two prices will nearly always be different, just as buying and selling prices are different for goods in an actual economic system. These differences between the degradation prices and the cost of synthesis do not indicate any inefficiencies or imperfections in the system; rather, they are the basis for the fundamental and essential property of metabolic unidirectionality that will be discussed in a later section.

Prices of the intermediates in glycolysis and the citrate cycle are shown in Figure 3-2. They are based on the number of ATP equivalents that could be produced at the expense of the oxidation of the compound in question. Since one turn of the citrate cycle oxidizes acetyl-SCoA totally to CO_2 and, in conjunction with the electron transport phosphorylation system, produces 12 moles of ATP per mole of acetate oxidized, the price of acetyl-SCoA can be set at 12 ATP equivalents. All of the other prices shown are derived from that for acetyl-SCoA. For example, the conversion of pyruvate to acetyl-SCoA and CO_2 involves the regeneration of NADH, with a value of 3; thus the value of pyruvate must be set at 15. Pyruvate can be carboxylated to oxaloacetate with the consumption of one ATP; thus the value of oxaloacetate is 16. Condensation of oxaloacetate with acetyl-SCoA involves no ATP or other coupling agent; thus the value of citrate is the sum of the values of the substrates, or 28. The other prices in the figure are obtained similarly.

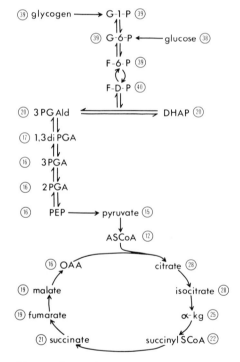

Figure 3-2.   Prices of intermediates of glycolysis and the citrate cycle, expressed in ATP equivalents. Each price is the number of moles of ATP that will be produced when 1 mole of the substrate is oxidized to CO_2. Modified from Atkinson (10).

There is some uncertainty as to the ATP yield that accompanies the oxidation of NADH produced in the cytoplasm of eukaroytic cells (for example, that resulting from the reaction catalyzed by 3-phosphoglyceraldehyde dehydrogenase). If mitochondrial membranes *in vivo* are impermeable to NADH, a shuttle system involving smaller molecules must be used to transport the electrons into the mitochondria. In some of the shuttle systems that have been proposed, a small molecule is reduced in the cytoplasm at the expense of NADH, enters the mitochondrion, and reduces a flavin. For any cell in which such a system actually functions, the value of cytoplasmic NADH is obviously the same as that of mitochondrial reduced flavin, or 2 ATP equivalents. As a consequence, the value of triose phosphate would be one ATP equivalent lower, and those of hexoses and hexose phosphates 2 ATP equivalents lower, than the values we have assigned. Since these slightly lower values would make no significant difference in any of the discussions in this book, we will for convenience consider NADH, wherever formed, to have a value of 3 ATP equivalents relative to NAD^+.

Storage and Transfer of Chemical Energy

Before going on to further discussion of the coupling coefficients of sequences or the prices of metabolites, both expressed in ATP equivalents, it seems desirable to consider the chemical basis for coupling of this type.* Biochemistry texts, monographs, and reviews have used a variety of approaches and terms in connection with energy metabolism, not all of which appear to have chemical or physical meaning.

A system may be considered to contain chemical potential energy if there is some chemical transformation available to the system, and it is not at equilibrium with respect to that transformation. In order to be a useful supplier of chemical energy, the system must be kinetically inert until its energy is needed. Thus the primary requirements for a chemical fuel are that it be thermodynamically unstable but kinetically stable under storage conditions, and that there be a feasible means of overcoming or circumventing the kinetic barrier when the fuel is to be used. A gasoline-air mixture, for example, is thermodynamically highly unstable. A great deal of heat is obtained when gasoline and oxygen react to form carbon dioxide and water, and some of the heat can be converted into mechanical energy. Under storage conditions at all ordinary temperatures, however, gasoline is so kinetically stable, even in contact with air, that it is transported and stored in nearly complete safety. The energy-releasing reaction is initiated, when desired, simply by

---

* A brief introduction to some relevant aspects of chemical thermodynamics is presented in Appendix A.

the heat of an electric arc between spark plug terminals. The situation is closely similar for the primary biological fuels. Carbohydrate, fat, and protein are thermodynamically unstable in contact with air, but are kinetically very stable. They are utilized as needed through enzymic catalysis of the appropriate reactions.

An energy-coupling agent such as ATP has many characteristics and requirements in common with fuels, and indeed may appropriately be considered a fuel for those reactions or sequences that utilize it. In order to serve as a source of energy—that is, to cause the reaction to proceed farther than it would in the absence of the coupling agent—the coupling agent must, like other fuels, be thermodynamically unstable. This merely means that it must be far from equilibrium with regard to some feasibly useful conversion. In the case of ATP, the feasible conversion is hydrolysis, and the reaction $ATP + H_2O \rightleftharpoons ADP + P_i$ is far from equilibrium. The system meets the second requirement of a useful energy storage system, in that it is kinetically inert. Solutions of ATP in water are quite stable kinetically. Finally, the energy can be used when needed as a consequence of enzymatic catalysis. In muscle contraction and in some active transport systems operating across membranes, direct ATP hydrolysis, linked tightly to contraction or to substrate movement, probably occurs. However, the reactions in which ATP is used need not involve direct hydrolysis as such. In fact, in the very nature of the types of energy coupling that occur in most metabolic contexts, direct hydrolysis not only would serve no purpose, but would be a simple waste of metabolic energy. But, as will be discussed below, any conversion, even if several reactions are involved, in which ATP is converted to ADP has received a thermodynamic push equivalent to the free energy of hydrolysis of ATP.

For a chemical reaction at constant temperature and pressure, the change in free energy is given by a standard equation of elementary thermodynamics (3-10). Q is the reaction parameter $(C)(D)/(A)(B)$, where the letters in paren-

$$\text{For} \quad A + B \rightleftharpoons C + D \qquad \Delta G = -RT \ln K + RT \ln Q \qquad (3\text{-}10)$$

theses denote the chemical activities (essentially concentrations if the solution is dilute and if ionic and other interactions are small). K, the equilibrium constant, is merely the value of Q at equilibrium. R is the gas constant, T is the absolute temperature, and ΔG is the change in free energy associated with the conversion of 1 mole each of A and B to C and D, with no change in concentration (strictly, activity) of any component. That is, the activities in the term for Q are assumed to be unchanged during the reaction.

When the terms on the right-hand side of equation 3-10 are combined, the resulting equation (3-11) emphasizes the property of ΔG that is nearly always the one of interest with regard to metabolic processes: it is a simple measure of how far a system is from equilibrium, and on which side. Converting to

$$\Delta G = RT \ln Q/K \qquad (3\text{-}11)$$

base-10 logarithms and inserting the values of R and T (0.002 kcal mole^{-1} degree^{-1} and about $300°$ at room temperature) we obtain equation 3-12, which is perhaps a satisfactory, although minimal, basis for understanding most applications of thermodynamics to simple metabolic processes. It is

$$\Delta G = 1.4 \log (Q/K) \text{ kcal/mole} \qquad (3\text{-}12)$$

obvious that $\Delta G = 0$ at equilibrium (when $Q = K$). When $Q < K$ (the value of Q is smaller than it would be at equilibrium) the reaction will of course tend to proceed, since conversion of A and B to C and D increases the value of Q and moves the system toward equilibrium. Under these circumstances $\Delta G < 0$, and its (negative) value is greater the farther the system is from equilibrium (the smaller the value of Q/K). Thus the reaction will tend to proceed in the direction written whenever $\Delta G < 0$. Conversely, when $Q > K$, the reaction clearly cannot proceed in the direction written, because the resulting increase in the value of Q would take the system away from equilibrium. When $Q > K$, the value of ΔG is of course positive. It follows that a reaction cannot proceed when $\Delta G > 0$. Under those conditions, the reaction must go in the reverse direction. The value of ΔG for the reverse reaction, under any conditions, is equal to that for the forward reaction under the same conditions, but opposite in sign. If we know the value of the equilibrium constant and the effective concentrations of the reactants and products, we know directly from the relative values of Q and K in which direction the reaction must go to approach equilibrium (to bring the value of Q to equal K). Equation 3-12 provides a formal statement of the direction of equilibrium and a quantitative measure of the distance of the system from equilibrium, expressed in the conventional units of kilocalories. The values of ΔG could of course be expressed in any units of energy; for example, replacing the numerical term in equation 3-12 by 5.7 would give ΔG in kilojoules per mole.

Elementary thermodynamics courses stress the fact that ΔG is the measure of the maximum amount of useful work that the system could in principle do on its environment as a consequence of the chemical reaction. Except for muscle contraction, flagellar movement, and similar mechanical motions, a cell rarely if ever does work on its environment, however, and this property of ΔG therefore has very little applicability in metabolic chemistry. (When

ATP serves as an energy-coupling agent between a catabolic sequence and a biosynthetic one, it is not doing work in the thermodynamic sense.)

The first term on the right-hand side of equation 3-10 is defined as the standard free energy change, ΔG^0 (equation 3-13). This relationship is val-

$$\Delta G^0 = -RT \ln K \qquad (3\text{-}13)$$

uable in that it allows calculation of equilibrium constants from tabulated values of free energies of formation of compounds. It has no other significance, being in effect a useful bit of mental scaffolding that is of no interest once it has served its purpose. From the derivation of equation 3-10 in any textbook of physical chemistry or thermodynamics, it can be seen that ΔG^0 is in effect a constant of integration, and that it is a scaling factor relating the equilibrium situation to the arbitrary standard states used in physical chemistry. The standard state used for most solutes is an idealized 1 M solution; that is, one containing effectively 1 gram molecular weight of solute per liter of solution. If instead we took as our standard state a solution that effectively contained 1 ounce molecular weight per gallon, all ΔG^0 values would be different, but the results of all calculations for real situations would of course be unchanged. This illustrates the fact that ΔG^0 values are of no significance in themselves, but are useful only in calculation of K and ΔG.

Some older biochemistry textbooks failed to distinguish between ΔG^0 and ΔG, and consequently contained ambiguous or misleading treatments of metabolic energetics. For example, metabolic reactions were sometimes divided into those that were termed *exergonic* (proceeding with a decrease of free energy) and those termed *endergonic* (proceeding with an increase in free energy). These words are unnecessary, since the distinction is merely between possible and impossible reactions—or, more correctly, between the possible and the impossible directions of each reaction. Under any given set of conditions (except at equilibrium), ΔG will be negative for the reaction in one direction and positive for the reaction in the other. It can proceed only in the direction for which ΔG is negative (the exergonic direction). There are no endergonic real processes, in metabolism or elsewhere. Confusion regarding endergonic reactions often arose in texts from use of ΔG^0 rather than ΔG. There are metabolic reactions for which ΔG^0 in the physiological direction is positive, and these have often been termed endergonic. In view of the arbitrary nature of standard states, it is clear that this usage has no relevance to the understanding of metabolism. All that a positive value of ΔG^0 means is that the reaction would proceed in the reverse direction if all components were at their standard states. Under physiological conditions, ΔG for the physiological direction is, of course, negative and such reactions, like all others, are exergonic.

Since a system can contain chemical potential energy only by virtue of not being at equilibrium, and since all reactions go toward equilibrium, it is clearly impossible to store energy in a system under the same conditions as those in which the system will provide energy. It is not possible to store energy in a system by pushing it farther from equilibrium; reactions do not go away from equilibrium. Charging is possible only by changing conditions so that the system will move toward a different equilibrium; if the movement is away from the equilibrium that applies when the system is to be used, energy is stored with respect to the conditions of use. A lead storage battery may serve to illustrate the point. If the electrodes (terminals) of such a battery are connected by a good conductor, the short-circuited battery will discharge until the electrical potential difference between the electrodes is zero. The battery is then fully discharged, the chemical potentials of electrons at the two terminals are equal, and the cell reaction (equation 3-14) is at

$$Pb + PbO_2 + 2 H_2SO_4 \rightleftharpoons 2 PbSO_4 + 2 H_2O \qquad (3\text{-}14)$$

equilibrium. If an external circuit is attached in such a way as to impose a difference in electrical potential of the correct polarity between the terminals (that is, to cause a difference in the chemical potentials of electrons at the two electrodes), electrons will move through the cell from one electrode to the other, causing reduction of Pb^{2+} to Pb as they enter the cell solution from one electrode and oxidation of Pb^{2+} to PbO_2 as they flow into the other electrode. The cell reaction (equation 3-14) thus proceeds toward the left as written; the cell is being charged. The cell components are moving toward equilibrium with the chemical potentials of electrons that have been established in the two electrodes; thus charging, like any other chemical reaction, is an exergonic reaction running "downhill" toward equilibrium. The flow of electrons and the conversion of Pb^{2+} to Pb and PbO_2 will stop if the cell reaction comes into equilibrium with the potentials of electrons in the electrodes. When the charging circuit is removed, the chemical potentials of electrons in the two electrodes remain at equilibrium with the cell reaction, and thus the electrical potential difference between the electrodes is maintained. If a conductor is now connected between the terminals, however, electrons flow through it in the direction that tends to equalize the chemical potential of electrons in the electrodes. The resulting decrease in potential difference between electrodes brings them out of equilibrium with the cell reaction, which then must proceed toward the right as written, which is the direction toward the new equilibrium. If a motor, rather than a simple conductor, is connected between the terminals, the battery can do work in the course of its reaction toward equilibrium (discharge). If a suitable electrochemical reaction cell is connected instead, the cell reaction in the battery may cause a chemical conversion in the reaction cell—that is, the battery in discharging may in turn cause another chemical system to move toward an equilibrium different from the equilibrium of the isolated system.

Except that it does not function electrochemically, the biological adenylate energy-storage system is closely similar in principle to the lead storage battery. The system is charged (ADP is phosphorylated) in reactions for which the equilibrium ratio of ATP to ADP concentrations is high. For the known reactions by which ATP is regenerated—those catalyzed by phosphoglycerate kinase and pyruvate kinase—the equilibrium constants are known approximately, and are large in the direction of ATP production. Most ATP is regenerated, in aerobic cells, by presently unknown mechanisms in electron-transfer phosphorylation, but here, too, the equilibria must strongly favor ATP production. In contrast, when ATP is consumed in energy-requiring sequences, the equilibrium constants for the reactions in which ATP is used are large in the direction of ADP production. Thus the reactions in which ADP accepts a phosphoryl group (analogous to charging the lead battery) and those in which ATP donates that group (analogous to discharge of the lead battery) are nearly all far from equilibrium. They are, of course, all exergonic reactions going toward equilibrium. The typical relationship of the adenylate system to metabolic reactions is analogous to that described for the lead storage battery and the electrochemical reaction cell. As the adenylate system discharges (by transferring phosphoryl groups) it causes another chemical reaction to proceed farther than would be possible for that reaction in isolation.

Magnitude of the ATP Equivalent

The function of an energy-coupling agent is to cause a chemical reaction to proceed farther than it otherwise would. It cannot "push a reaction past its equilibrium"; it makes possible another pathway, using other reactions, with different overall stoichiometry and hence a different overall equilibrium constant. Assume that the equilibrium of the reaction shown in equation 3-15

$$A + B \rightleftharpoons C + D \qquad (3\text{-}15)$$

is unfavorable, so that at physiological concentrations of A and B only very low concentrations of C and D could be formed. If, by whatever sequence of actual reactions, the conversion can be carried out by a pathway that obligately utilizes ATP and produces ADP and P_i, as indicated by equation 3-16 (for example, A might be phosphorylated and the phosphorylated product might then react with B), the overall equilibrium constant must be the product of the equilibrium constant for equation 3-15 and that for the hydrolysis of ATP (equation 3-17). Therefore $K_{3\text{-}16} = K_{3\text{-}15} \cdot K_{3\text{-}17}$ and

$\Delta G^0{}_{3\text{-}16} = \Delta G^0{}_{3\text{-}15} + \Delta G_{3\text{-}17}$. It should be emphasized that whatever path

$$A + B + ATP + H_2O \rightleftharpoons C + D + ADP + P_i \qquad (3\text{-}16)$$

$$ATP + H_2O \rightleftharpoons ADP + P_i \qquad (3\text{-}17)$$

is taken in the conversion summarized by equation 3-16, the reactions of equations 3-15 and 3-17 are definitely not involved; the steady-state concentration of P_i would be unacceptably large. Those equations merely provide a pathway that is useful for discussion or calculation. For any pathway that can be written for a given conversion, the product of the individual equilibrium constants must be the overall equilibrium constant, and the sum of the individual ΔG^0 values must be the overall value of ΔG^0. When the equilibrium constant for the hydrolysis of ATP to ADP is coupled to the conversion of A and B to C and D, a much higher value of the concentration ratio $(C)(D)/(A)(B)$ can be achieved than is possible from the noncoupled reaction (equation 3-15). Since this difference results from the expenditure of one ATP equivalent, it is of interest to evaluate the effect semiquantitatively. Just how great is the chemical effect when ATP is coupled into a biochemical reaction?

Because the equilibrium constant for the hydrolysis of ATP is so large, it has not been measured accurately by direct analysis of equilibrium mixtures, and because the reaction does not involve oxidation and reduction, it cannot be measured electrochemically. The values of K and ΔG^0 for this reaction are therefore not known precisely. Recent values for $\Delta G'$, the standard free energy of hydrolysis of ATP, with pH 7 designated the standard state of proton concentration (instead of pH 0, as is usual in physical chemistry) and the approximate physiological concentration of Mg^{2+} as the standard state for Mg^{2+}, are generally around -7.5 kcal/mole (54). From that figure, it follows that under physiological conditions the value of the concentration ratio $(ATP)/(ADP)(P_i)$ at equilibrium would be about 4×10^{-6} M^{-1}. More importantly in a metabolic context, if the concentration of orthophosphate is about 10 mM in the cell, the concentration ratio $(ATP)/(ADP)$ at equilibrium would be about 4×10^{-8}. The physiological concentration ratio, $(ATP)/(ADP)$, is held at about 10^8 times as high a value, between 4 and 6, by extremely efficient kinetic controls (discussed in Chapter 4). Of course the ratio $(ATP)/(ADP)(P_i)$ is about 500 when the concentration of P_i is 10 mM, so this ratio also differs from its equilibrium value by a factor of about 10^8.

It is intuitively obvious that, if the physiological $(ATP)/(ADP)$ ratio is 10^8 times as large as the equilibrium ratio, the effective equilibrium ratio for any other conversion will be changed by that same factor if the conversion is coupled to the use of ATP (and, of course, by 10^{-8} if coupled to the regeneration of ATP). This conclusion will, however, be demonstrated algebraically. The reaction parameter Q for the reaction 3-16 is shown in equation 3-18, and the equilibrium constants for reactions 3-15 and 3-17 are shown in equations 3-19 and 3-20. At physiological concentrations, the actual

$$Q_{3-16} = \frac{(\text{ADP})(\text{P}_i)(\text{C})(\text{D})}{(\text{ATP})\ (\text{A})(\text{B})} \tag{3-18}$$

$$K_{3-15} = \frac{(\text{C})_{eq}(\text{D})_{eq}}{(\text{A})_{eq}(\text{B})_{eq}} \tag{3-19}$$

$$K_{3-17} = \frac{(\text{ADP})_{eq}(\text{P}_i)_{eq}}{(\text{ATP})_{eq}} \tag{3-20}$$

value of Q for ATP hydrolysis (equation 3-17) differs from the equilibrium value by a factor of about 10^8 (equation 3-21). The equilibrium constant for

$$Q_{3-17(\text{phys})} = \frac{(\text{ADP})_{\text{phys}}(\text{P}_i)_{\text{phys}}}{(\text{ATP})_{\text{phys}}} = 10^{-8}\ K_{3-17} \tag{3-21}$$

reaction 3-16 is the product of equilibrium constants for reactions 3-15 and

$$K_{3-16} = K_{3-17} \cdot K_{3-15} = \frac{(\text{ADP})_{eq}(\text{P}_i)_{eq}}{(\text{ATP})_{eq}} \cdot \frac{(\text{C})_{eq}(\text{D})_{eq}}{(\text{A})_{eq}(\text{B})_{eq}} \tag{3-22}$$

3-17 (equation 3-22). But in the cell ATP, ADP, and P_i are not at equilibrium with respect to hydrolysis. When the physiological concentrations are substituted into equation 3-22 we obtain equation 3-23, where the primes indicate concentrations of A, B, C, and D that would be at equilibrium with respect to reaction 3-16 when ATP, ADP, and P_i are at their physiological concentrations. Setting the two expressions for K_{3-16} from equations 3-22 and 3-23 equal to each other and solving for $(\text{C})'(\text{D})'/(\text{A})'(\text{B})'$, we obtain equation 3-24, which shows that the equilibrium concentration ratio of the metabolites A, B, C, and D, when the conversion of A and B to C and D is coupled to the use of 1 mole of ATP, is about one hundred million times as large as the same concentration ratio when the uncoupled conversion (reaction 3-15) is at equilibrium. Of course the same reasoning applies when the

$$
\begin{aligned}
K_{3-16} &= Q_{3-17(\text{phys})} \cdot Q'_{3-15} \\
&= 10^{-8}\ K_{3-17} \cdot Q'_{3-15} \\
&= 10^{-8}\ \frac{(\text{ADP})_{eq}(\text{P}_i)_{eq}}{(\text{ATP})_{eq}} \cdot \frac{(\text{C})'(\text{D})'}{(\text{A})'(\text{B})'}
\end{aligned} \tag{3-23}
$$

$$\frac{(\text{C})'(\text{D})'}{(\text{A})'(\text{B})'} = 10^8\ \frac{(\text{C})_{eq}(\text{D})_{eq}}{(\text{A})_{eq}(\text{B})_{eq}} \tag{3-24}$$

reaction coupled to ATP involves fewer or more reactants and products than reaction 3-15. For a simple conversion of A to C, the equilibrium ratio (C)/(A) will be 10^8 times as large if the conversion is coupled to the use of ATP as if it is not.

It hardly need be pointed out that 10^8 is a large number, but the magnitude of the consequences of ATP coupling should be emphasized. For example, if the equilibrium constant for the conversion of A to C is 10^{-4} and the physiological concentration of A is 10 μM, the conversion could occur by way of a noncoupled reaction only if the concentration of C were less than 1 nM, and it would be impossible to maintain a useful concentration of C. When the coupled reaction is used, the conversion of A to C is favored at all concentrations of C up to 100 mM. Thus the utilization of ATP makes any reasonable concentration thermodynamically available, and the cell can set the steady-state physiological concentration range by evolution of suitable kinetic controls.

This section leads us to two of the most fundamental generalizations of energy metabolism. *Maintenance, by kinetic controls, of an ATP/ADP concentration ratio in the cell that is about 10^8 times as great as the equilibrium ratio provides the driving force for nearly all biochemical events. Any useful conversion can be made thermodynamically favorable by coupling it to the utilization of a suitable number of ATP's.* The first of these generalizations will be discussed further in Chapter 4, and the second in later sections of this chapter.

UNIDIRECTIONALITY

Futile Cycles

It follows from the discussion in the preceding section that if two pathways exist for an interconversion, and if their ATP coupling coefficients are different, the two pathways will move toward different equilibrium ratios of A to B. Such pairs of oppositely directed reactions or sequences, which are very common in metabolism, have been termed "futile cycles" by Scrutton and Utter (*106*). They might also be called pseudocycles, because, except perhaps in a few special cases involving heat generation or other such specialized functions, they cannot be expected to occur as cycles; that is, both pathways will not ordinarily proceed at the same time.

One of the most centrally located, and the most frequently discussed, of these futile cycles is that formed by phosphofructokinase and fructose-diphosphate phosphatase. These enzymes (equations 3-25 and 3-26) catalyze the interconversion of fructose 6-phosphate and fructose diphosphate. The phosphofructokinase reaction uses 1 mole of ATP per mole of fructose

6-phosphate; its coupling coefficient is thus -1. The coupling coefficient of the phosphatase reaction is zero, since ATP is neither utilized nor regenerated. Reaction 3-25 can be considered, for purposes of calculation or

$$\text{fructose 6-P} + \text{ATP} \rightarrow \text{fructose diphosphate} + \text{ADP} \qquad (3\text{-}25)$$

$$\text{fructose diphosphate} + \text{H}_2\text{O} \rightarrow \text{fructose 6-P} + \text{P}_i \qquad (3\text{-}26)$$

comparison, to be the sum of reactions 3-27 and 3-28. Since 3-28 is the same reaction as 3-26, but written in the opposite direction, it is clear that reactions

$$\text{ATP} + \text{H}_2\text{O} \rightarrow \text{ADP} + \text{P}_i \qquad (3\text{-}27)$$

$$\text{fructose 6-P} + \text{P}_i \rightarrow \text{fructose diphosphate} + \text{H}_2\text{O} \qquad (3\text{-}28)$$

3-25 and 3-26 supply a specific example of the general case illustrated by equations 3-15, 3-16, and 3-17; that is, they differ by 1 ATP equivalent. Hence, as shown for the general case in equation 3-24, the reactions catalyzed by phosphofructokinase and fructose-diphosphate phosphatase move toward equilibrium concentration ratios of fructose diphosphate to fructose 6-phosphate that differ by a ratio of about 10^8.

If the value of ΔG^0 for the phosphatase reaction is about -2 kcal/mole, the equilibrium constant is about 100. At an orthophosphate concentration of 10 mM, the equilibrium ratio of fructose 6-phosphate to fructose diphosphate is thus about 10^4. For the phosphofructokinase reaction, because of the coupling to ATP, the equilibrium ratio of fructose diphosphate to fructose 6-phosphate is about 10^4. Thus whenever the (FDP)/(F6P) ratio is between 10^{-4} and 10^4, *both* reactions will be thermodynamically favored. Since it is obvious that the ratio of the physiological concentrations will always be in this range, the conversion of fructose 6-phosphate to fructose diphosphate by the phosphofructokinase reaction and the conversion of fructose diphosphate to fructose 6-phosphate by the phosphatase reaction will both always be favored in an intact cell. This is equivalent to the statements that both, in their physiological directions, are exergonic, are proceeding toward equilibrium, and are associated with a decrease in free energy. Of course, if the two reactions occurred at significant rates simultaneously, the only result would be the hydrolysis of ATP, as is seen by adding equations 3-25 and 3-26. It is evident that effective kinetic controls are necessary to avoid a catastrophic wastage of the cell's energy.

Advantages of Unidirectionality

Although the preceding sentence is correct, it misses the point and, in terms of metabolic function, puts the cart before the horse. We should not imagine that oppositely directed reactions, constituting futile cycles, somehow just happened to arise and that kinetic controls then had to be evolved to prevent them from short-circuiting the cell's energy supply. Rather, oppositely directed sequences with different equilibrium constants must have evolved specifically because of the advantages of kinetic control of metabolic direction as well as of rate. Although each "sequence" in this case is only a single reaction, the fructose 6-phosphate/fructose diphosphate futile cycle illustrates clearly the functional advantages of such oppositely directed sequence pairs. Since both are thermodynamically favorable at all times, the evolved control mechanisms that regulate both enzymes can cause either reaction to occur, in response to metabolic needs for glycolysis or glyconeogenesis, while the other proceeds slowly if at all. Various experimental approaches have led to results suggesting that some cycling (simultaneous operation of both reactions) occurs. Confirmation and quantitation of the extent of cycling is desirable, but it is clear that an organism could not survive unless this and all of the many other futile cycles in metabolism were quite effectively regulated to prevent extensive cycling.

   Another very small futile cycle, containing three reactions, is that involving the interconversion of pyruvate and phosphoenolpyruvate. The equilibrium constant for the pyruvate kinase reaction (equation 3-29) is large, so that

$$\text{phosphoenolpyruvate} + \text{ADP} \rightarrow \text{pyruvate} + \text{ATP} \qquad (3\text{-}29)$$

reversal under physiological conditions would not be feasible. In eukaryotic cells the reverse conversion is carried out by way of oxaloacetate (equations 3-30 and 3-31). The overall equation (3-32) differs from the reverse of reaction 3-29 in the use of two nucleoside triphosphates, hence 2 ATP equivalents, whereas only one is involved in the pyruvate kinase reaction. The coupling coefficient for the pyruvate kinase reaction is 1, and that for the

$$\text{pyruvate} + CO_2 + \text{ATP} \rightarrow \text{oxaloacetate} + \text{ADP} + P_i \qquad (3\text{-}30)$$
$$\underline{\text{oxaloacetate} + \text{GTP} \rightarrow \text{phosphoenolpyruvate} + \text{GDP} + CO_2} \qquad (3\text{-}31)$$
$$\text{pyruvate} + \text{ATP} + \text{GTP} \rightarrow \text{phosphoenolpyruvate} + \text{ADP} + \text{GDP} + P_i \quad (3\text{-}32)$$

conversion of pyruvate to phosphoenolpyruvate is -2. Thus the two sequences of this futile cycle, like those of the F6P/FDP futile cycle, differ by 1 ATP equivalent. The pyruvate kinase reaction moves toward a pyruvate/phosphoenolpyruvate ratio that differs by about 10^8 from that toward which the pyruvate carboxylase-phosphoenolpyruvate carboxykinase sequence moves. Thus, again, both conversions are thermodynamically favorable at all times in a living cell.

   In at least some bacteria, the conversion of pyruvate to phosphoenolpyruvate is catalyzed by a single enzyme, phosphoenolpyruvate synthase (equation 3-33). This conversion is thermodynamically equivalent to the

$$\text{pyruvate} + \text{ATP} \rightarrow \text{phosphoenolpyruvate} + \text{AMP} + \text{P}_i \qquad (3\text{-}33)$$

pathway through oxaloacetate used by eukaryotes, however, since ATP is converted to AMP. Two phosphorylations are required to regenerate ATP from AMP so, as noted earlier, the production of AMP from ATP entails the expenditure of 2 ATP equivalents.

These two simple futile cycles illustrate the distinguishing features of all pairs of oppositely directed sequences. The two sequences always differ in ATP coefficients, and it is this difference that allows them to be simultaneously tending at all times, in their opposite physiological directions, toward very different equilibrium ratios of starting materials and products. When the difference in ATP equivalents is 1, these ratios will differ by about 10^8; if the difference is 2 ATP equivalents, the difference will be about 10^{16}, and so on.

Generality of Unidirectionality

It has become evident from work of the past few years that nearly all metabolic sequences are unidirectional, and that their rates are controlled by modulation of regulatory enzymes. In fundamental metabolic terms, these generalizations are equivalent to the statements that the rates of metabolic reactions are not determined by mass action considerations, and the directions of metabolic conversions are not determined by simple equilibrium considerations involving only the compounds directly involved in the conversion. This is one of the fundamental differences between the living and nonliving worlds. Not only the rates of metabolic conversions, but also their directions, are determined by the concentrations of regulatory compounds that need not be directly involved in the reactions that they regulate; in the last analysis, these rates and directions are determined by the needs of the cell. Kinetic control by means of enzyme modulation will be discussed in later chapters. Here we will consider metabolic unidirectionality.

A cell or organism in which conversions in both directions proceeded by the same reversible sequence of reactions, with the direction of conversions being under simple thermodynamic or equilibrium control, would necessarily respond sluggishly to changes in condition or in metabolic needs. For example, fatty acids are made from acetyl-SCoA at the expense of ATP and NADPH. When the supply of food is limited, stored fat can be utilized by reconversion to acetyl-SCoA. ATP is regenerated in the reconversion, and the AcSCoA then serves as a source of further ATP. If the direction of the metabolic conversion between acetyl-SCoA and fat were under simple equilibrium control, fat would be stored whenever the concentrations of acetyl-SCoA, ATP, and NADPH rose above the equilibrium level, and fat could be utilized only when the concentrations of these metabolites fell below their equilibrium values. Furthermore, the rates of the conversions would tend to be low in the vicinity of equilibrium; thus for a reasonable rate of storage or breakdown of fat the concentrations of the soluble metabolites would need to rise or fall considerably above or below the equilibrium point. Similar statements would also apply to the storage of glycogen. Such a situation would have highly undesirable consequences for organisms of any type, which may perhaps be best illustrated in the case of a higher animal. A fox, for example, may prosper and store moderate amounts of glycogen and fat as long as field mice and rabbits are abundant. If, however, because of a scarcity of prey or for any other reason, he is forced to go without food for a day or so he must draw on his stored energy reserves. If his metabolism were equilibrium-controlled, glycogen and fat could be utilized only when the concentrations of ATP, glucose 1-P, and acetyl-SCoA were considerably lower than under normal conditions. Such a deficiency of ATP and of metabolites that can be oxidized to produce ATP would inevitably affect the fox's overall fitness. His speed would be decreased, and his chances of obtaining a meal would decline still further. Unless he had a stroke of unusually good luck, he would be well on the way to starvation. An organism that responded to the first touch of adversity by a decrease in fitness (especially by a decrease in the ability to obtain food) would leave few descendents. Present-day organisms are of necessity those whose ancestors were quite good at leaving descendents; thus it is not surprising that they respond more positively to adversity than our hypothetical equilibrium-controlled fox. A real fox, of course, is quite capable of maintaining the levels of the intermediates in primary metabolic sequences, and especially the ATP supply, in their normal ranges while depleting not only stored glycogen and fat, but considerable amounts of protein as well.

Escape from simple equilibrium control, and acquisition of the ability to control the directions of metabolic conversions on the basis of metabolic need, was possible only by the evolution of oppositely directed pairs of sequences for virtually every metabolic conversion. The overall equations for synthesis of palmityl-SCoA from acetyl-SCoA (equation 3-34) and for production of acetyl-SCoA from palmityl-SCoA (equation 3-35) differ widely in their coupling coefficients. The synthesis requires 14 NADPH, with a metabolic value of 4 ATP equivalents each, and 7 ATP. The cost of

$$8 \text{ AcSCoA} + 7 \text{ ATP} + 14 \text{ NADPH} + 14 \text{ H}^+$$

$$\rightarrow \text{palmSCoA} + 7 \text{ ADP} + 7 \text{ P}_i + 14 \text{ NADP}^+ \quad (3\text{-}34)$$

$$\text{palmSCoA} + 7 \text{ NAD}^+ + 7 \text{ FAD} \rightarrow 8 \text{ AcSCoA} + 7 \text{ NADH} + 7 \text{ FADH}_2 \quad (3\text{-}35)$$

the conversion is $(4 \times 14) + 7 = 63$ ATP equivalents, and its coupling coefficient is thus -63. The breakdown of palmityl-SCoA to acetyl-SCoA yields 7 NADH (each worth 3 ATP equivalents) and 7 $FADH_2$ (each worth 2 ATP equivalents); its coupling coefficient is $(3 \times 7) + (2 \times 7) = 35$. The difference, 28 ATP equivalents, is the cause of irreversibility of the two sequences and the guarantee that both will be strongly favorable thermodynamically at all times, so that whichever is appropriate can be selected by the organism's metabolic regulatory system. A difference of 28 ATP equivalents corresponds to a difference in free energies of the two pathways of about 322 kcal/mole of palmityl-SCoA made or degraded, and thus to a difference by a factor of about 10^{230} in the equilibrium ratios of (palmSCoA)/$(AcSCoA)^8$ toward which the two sequences are tending. Such a factor is inconceivably large, and can be thought of only as an infinitely large barrier to reversal of either sequence.

The most important pair of oppositely directed sequences, in terms of total magnitude of the conversions in the biosphere and in terms of basic biology as well, are photosynthesis and respiration. As discussed in an earlier section, the coupling coefficient, or yield of ATP, for respiration is 38 ATP equivalents per glucose. This number is the sum of 30 from 10 NADH, 4 from 2 $FADH_2$, and 6 from substrate level phosphorylations (2 each from the phosphoglycerate kinase, pyruvate kinase, and succinylthiokinase reactions), minus the 2 ATP's used in phosphorylation of glucose to fructose diphosphate. The overall equilibrium constant for respiration, based on the coupling coefficient of 38 (equation 3-37), is about 10^{170}.

As was emphasized in the earlier discussion, the coupling coefficient for any sequence, and hence the overall equilibrium for the conversion, is a phenotypic characteristic that has evolved, like any other, on the basis of biological advantage. We might imagine coupling coefficients other than 38 for respiration, and three are shown in equations 3-36, 3-38, and 3-39. The subscript "equiv" is used to indicate that the coefficients of the ADP and

$$\text{glucose} + 6\,O_2 + 20\,ADP_{equiv} + 20\,P_i$$
$$\updownarrow \qquad\qquad K = 10^{320} \qquad (3\text{-}36)$$
$$6\,CO_2 + 20\,ATP_{equiv} + 26\,H_2O$$

$$\text{glucose} + 6\,O_2 + 38\,ADP_{equiv} + 38\,P_i$$
$$\updownarrow \qquad\qquad K = 10^{170} \qquad (3\text{-}37)$$
$$6\,CO_2 + 38\,ATP_{equiv} + 44\,H_2O$$

$$\text{glucose} + 6\,O_2 + 59\,ADP_{equiv} + 59\,P_i$$
$$\updownarrow \qquad\qquad K = 1 \qquad (3\text{-}38)$$
$$6\,CO_2 + 59\,ATP_{equiv} + 65\,H_2O$$

$$\text{glucose} + 6\,O_2 + 66\,ADP_{equiv} + 66\,P_i$$
$$\updownarrow \qquad\qquad K = 10^{-60} \qquad (3\text{-}39)$$
$$6\,CO_2 + 66\,ATP_{equiv} + 72\,H_2O$$

ATP terms correspond to the number of ATP equivalents involved, rather than to actual amounts of ATP as such. For comparison with the actual sequence (equation 3-37), the approximate value of the equilibrium constant corresponding to each equation is shown. A decrease in the coupling coefficient (equation 3-36) would increase the equilibrium constant beyond its already inconceivably high value. Conversely, an increase in the coupling coefficient would decrease the overall equilibrium constant. At a coefficient of about 59 the equilibrium constant would be 1, and glucose, O_2, and CO_2 at their standard states would be in equilibrium with physiological concentrations of ATP, ADP, and P_i.

If the atmospheric concentrations of O_2 and CO_2 are taken into account, a coupling coefficient of about 61 would be required to bring glucose at 10 mM into equilibrium with O_2, CO_2, and the other reaction components at physiological concentrations. In view of the approximations involved in the computations, and especially in view of the enormous magnitudes of the energetic differences that have evolved between oppositely directed sequences, it would be pointless to worry about the exact values of coupling coefficients that would correspond to equilibrium for various sequences. For example, if a value of -12 rather than -11.5 kcal/mole were taken for the free energy of hydrolysis of ATP under physiological conditions (this is within the range of uncertainty), the coupling coefficients for equilibrium of respiration would be about 56 under standard conditions and 58 at atmospheric concentrations of O_2 and CO_2. But such uncertainties should not affect our appreciation of the underlying generalizations—that coupling coefficients have evolved so as to cause the overall equilibrium constants of typical metabolic sequences to be very large in the physiological direction and hence unidirectional under any conditions that can arise in the intact cell.

If the coupling coefficient is higher than about 59, the conversion of glucose to CO_2 becomes thermodynamically unfavorable, which is to say that the reverse conversion of CO_2 to glucose becomes favorable. It is not surprising that this is the approach used by autotrophic organisms for the production of carbohydrate from CO_2, since it is hard to see what other means was possible. ATP and NADPH, regenerated photochemically or by the oxidation of inorganic substances, are coupled to the CO_2/carbohydrate system with a coefficient making carbohydrate production the favored (exergonic) direction of reaction. In green plants and in those chemoautotrophs that also use the ribulose diphosphate pathway, the coupling coefficient appears to be -66, as in equation 3-39. The 12 moles of NADPH per mole of hexose produced that are required by the chemistry of the system correspond to 48 ATP equivalents, and at least 18 moles of ATP are used directly (12 in the reduction of 3-phosphoglycerate to 3-phosphoglyceraldehyde, and 6 in the phosphorylation of ribulose 5-phosphate). Thus the reductive fixation of CO_2 into organic compounds, which is the most important conversion in the energy metabolism of the biosphere taken as a whole, and respiration, the most important sequence in the energy metabolism of most aerobic heterotrophs, differ at the level of metabolic thermodynamics only in their ATP coupling coefficients, which are such as to make both sequences unidirectional under physiological conditions.

Numbers such as 10^{60} and 10^{170}, the approximate equilibrium constants for photosynthesis and respiration, are too large for comprehension. If A and C are perfect gases, if the equilibrium constant for the reaction A $\rightleftharpoons$ C is 10^{60}, and if a sphere with radius equal to that of the earth's orbit around the sun were filled with C at the standard temperature of $273°$K and the standard pressure of 1 atmosphere, this enormous quantity of gas would be in equilibrium with one molecule of A inhabiting that same volume. (If the value of K is 10^{60}, the concentration of A at equilibrium must be 10^{-60} that of C. Since 1 mole of C under standard conditions will occupy 22 liters, 1 mole of A at equilibrium will occupy 22×10^{60} liters. Dividing by Avogadro's number, 6×10^{23}, we obtain 4×10^{37} liters, or 4×10^{34} m³, as the volume occupied by one molecule of A. This is the volume of a sphere with radius about 2×10^{8} km. The radius of the earth's orbit is about 1.5×10^{8} km.) If the equilibrium constant were 10^{170}, one molecule of A would be in equilibrium with the amount of C that, at standard temperature and pressure, would occupy a sphere of radius about 10^{32} light years, which is incomparably larger than the known universe. If gas C were hydrogen, its mass would be over 10^{80} times the estimated mass of the universe.

These values are not particularly unusual in themselves. The equilibrium constant for the burning of a match stick (the oxidation of carbohydrate with an ATP coupling coefficient of zero) would be much larger still. The point of biological interest is that a living cell is able, merely by changing the evolved coupling coefficients of sequences (the numbers of molecules of ATP, NAD$^+$, and NADPH that are stoichiometrically involved, and hence the number of ATP equivalents) to establish and to contain simultaneously two such emphatically unidirectional pathways for the same conversion, one with an equilibrium constant of 10^{170} in one direction, and the other with a constant of 10^{60} in the opposite direction. Metabolic unidirectionality is not a mere tendency favoring one direction over the other; it is real and solid. The primary stoichiometric role of ATP is the establishment of pathways with very large overall equilibrium constants; its coordinate and equally important role in the kinetic regulation of these pathways will be discussed in Chapter 4.

In most pairs of oppositely directed sequences, the reactions in the two directions are quite different, and most of the intermediates are usually different as well. In marked contrast, glycolysis and gluconeogenesis, an important pair of reaction sequences in many kinds of cells, share most of their intermediates and enzymes, and hence their reactions. The reactions that are different are only those in small futile cycles, including those that we have already considered—the pyruvate/phosphoenolpyruvate and the fructose 6-phosphate/fructose diphosphate cycles. It is clear that enzymes of these central sequences of carbohydrate metabolism differ only when difference is essential for unidirectionality. Perhaps this unusual situation evolved because of the relatively high concentrations of these enzymes, which must catalyze the highest fluxes that occur in metabolism. Use of the same enzymes for most steps of these two pathways thus effects a very considerable saving in the amount of enzyme protein required. Whatever the reason, it is only in carbohydrate metabolism (in glycolysis and in the pentose phosphate pathway) that many of the same enzymes seem to participate in oppositely directed sequences of considerable length.

Glycolysis and gluconeogenesis are shown in Figure 3-3, with price assignments for the intermediates. The numbers to the right of the names apply to glycolysis, and should be read downward; those on the left apply to gluconeogenesis, and should be read upward. The numbers in circles are the values of the intermediates in terms of the numbers of ATP's to which they can give rise in aerobic metabolism, as in Figure 3-2. The numbers in squares are the corresponding values for anaerobic metabolism. Since there is no

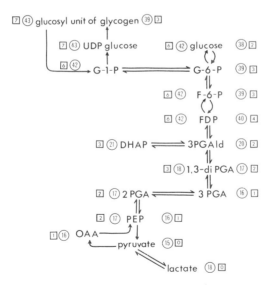

Figure 3-3. Metabolic prices of intermediates of glycolysis and gluconeogenesis. Numbers to the right of the names of the compounds indicate the number of moles of ATP produced on metabolism of the compounds. Numbers in circles apply to oxidative metabolism; thus they are the same as those shown in Figure 3-2. Numbers in squares apply to anaerobic metabolism. Numbers to the left of the names indicate the costs of the intermediates during gluconeogenesis.

net oxidation or reduction in the conversion of glucose to lactate, the differences between the ATP values of glucose and lactate are the same in both cases. The aerobic value of glucose, 38, minus the aerobic value of 2 lactates, 36, gives a net ATP yield of 2, as shown directly by the anaerobic value for glucose. Similarly, for a glucosyl unit of glycogen, the net anaerobic yield of 3 is the same as may be calculated from the aerobic figures, 39 and 36.

Whether the starting point for glycolysis, and the product of gluconeogenesis, is glycogen or glucose, the pathways differ at three places. Each of these points of difference is clearly functional, since each allows for a difference of 1 ATP equivalent in the stoichiometries of the two sequences. Going in the direction of gluconeogenesis, the first of these pseudocycles is that involving pyruvate and phosphoenolpyruvate. Since 2 moles of phosphoenolpyruvate are required to make 1 of hexose, a difference of 1 ATP equivalent per phosphoenolpyruvate is 2 per hexose. The fructose diphosphate/fructose 6-phosphate pseudocycle contributes an additional difference of 1 ATP equivalent per hexose. When the end product is glucose, the glucose 6-phosphate/glucose cycle brings the total difference to 4 ATP equivalents. When glycogen is the product, the glucose 1-phosphate/glycogen cycle similarly adds an ATP equivalent to the difference between the two pathways. Thus in either case the difference between glycolysis and gluconeogenesis is 4 ATP equivalents, and the corresponding ratio of overall equilibrium constants is about 10^{32}. It is noteworthy that this very respectable difference is attained in spite of the fact that nine of the twelve steps in the conversion of glucose to lactate are used also in the reverse conversion.

In terms of effective use of stored energy, the breakdown of glycogen to lactate and resynthesis of glycogen does not rate very highly. When a glucosyl unit is converted to lactate, 3 ATP's are produced, but 7 must be expended to resynthesize a glucosyl unit. These 7 ATP equivalents are obtained, of course, by oxidation of part of the lactate, and hence they constitute a drain on the glycogen stores. Thus if a muscle breaks down glycogen to obtain ATP by lactate production, each ATP that is produced costs 2.3 ATP equivalents during the subsequent aerobic resynthesis of glycogen. This is a quite inefficient use of reserves, but its selective advantage is obvious. An organism that can obtain some additional energy beyond the rate that is made possible by the oxygen supply to its muscles may escape being eaten or, if it is a predator, may capture its prey and thus escape death by starvation, because of the extra ATP made available by lactate fermentation. In either case, he can well afford to "waste" some of the lactate in resynthesizing glycogen, and we can be sure that if he understood the energy balance sheet involved he would not begrudge the inefficiency of the process.

When liver glycogen is the source of muscle lactate, and liver glycogen is resynthesized after the emergency has ended, the process is even more inefficient. Because glucose 1-phosphate obtained from phosphorolysis of glycogen must be hydrolyzed to glucose for transport to the muscle, the yield per glucosyl unit is only 2 ATP equivalents. Resynthesis of glycogen will require 8 ATP equivalents per glucosyl residue (6 to synthesize free glucose, which is transported by the blood to the liver, where 2 more ATP equivalents are required to add the glucosyl unit to glycogen by way of glucose 6-P, glucose 1-P, and UDPglucose). Thus (ignoring any energy requirements of a round trip in the bloodstream from liver to muscle and back and transport across at least four cell membranes) the ultimate cost of each ATP obtained from lactate fermentation is 4 ATP equivalents. But of course the same selective advantages that were discussed above apply here, with the added advantage of a larger storage capacity.

Fat is a major energy store in many organisms, so it is of interest to compare the cost of synthesizing a simple fat with the amount of ATP regenerated when the fat is degraded. Synthesis of 1 mole of tripalmitin (glycerol esterified with three palmityl groups) requires 3 moles of palmityl-ACP and 1 mole of glycerol phosphate. Each mole of palmityl-ACP is made from 8 moles of acetyl-SCoA, and, as seen above, the conversion cost is 63 ATP equivalents. Thus the cost of each palmityl ACP is $(8 \times 12) + 63 = 159$ ATP equivalents. If glycerol phosphate is made by reduction of dihydroxyacetone phosphate (20 ATP equivalents) with NADH, its value is 23 ATP equivalents. The cost of 1 mole of tripalmitin is then $(3 \times 159) + 23 = 500$ ATP equivalents. Degradation of a mole of tripalmitin presumably begins with hydrolysis to 3 moles of palmitate and 1 mole of glycerol. One mole of ATP is required for the conversion of glycerol to glycerol phosphate, with a value of 23; thus the metabolic value of glycerol is 22 ATP equivalents. When palmitate is activated by conversion to palmityl-SCoA, 1 mole of ATP is converted to AMP, so 2 ATP equivalents are expended. The yield of ATP in the conversion of palmityl-SCoA has been seen earlier to be 35. Thus the net coupling coefficient for the reaction sequence that takes palmitate to acetyl-SCoA is $+33$, and the yield from 3 palmitates is 99 ATP equivalents. The 24 moles of acetyl-SCoA produced have a value of $24 \times 12 = 288$ ATP equivalents. Hence the total oxidation of a mole of tripalmitin should yield $22 + 99 + 288 = 409$ ATP equivalents (10). Nearly identical results for the cost and value of tripalmitin, based on a different but essentially equivalent approach, have been calculated by Milligan (84).

Comparison of the production cost of tripalmitin, 500 ATP equivalents per mole, with the selling price, 409 ATP equivalents, might suggest that fat is not a very economically useful compound. Fat storage, within limits, is in fact biologically very useful, and the difference between a cost of 500 and a selling price of 409 does not indicate inefficiency but rather illustrates our earlier comments concerning the advantages gained by irreversibility of biological conversions. Because of this difference in coupling coefficients, both the synthesis and breakdown of fat are simultaneously thermodynamically feasible. This allows an organism, like the fox that we discussed earlier, to maintain as high levels of intermediates when utilizing fat as when storing it. The difference of about 90 ATP equivalents, or 19% of the metabolic energy that is devoted to fat storage at a time when energy is abundant, is the price that the organism pays to have the remaining 81% stored in a form that is thermodynamically available, with an extremely high equilibrium constant, when energy is needed.

When excess hexose is available in the diet of a heterotroph, either directly as glucose or fructose or in the form of other carbohydrates such as sucrose, lactose, starch, or glycogen, it may be added to the organism's glycogen stores and recovered with remarkably little loss. The conversion of glucose to a glycosyl residue in glycogen costs 2 ATP equivalents. The pathway proceeds through phosphorylation to glucose 6-phosphate with a coupling coefficient of −1, isomerization to glucose 1-phosphate, reaction with UTP to form UDPglucose, and transfer of the glucosyl unit to glycogen, with UDP as the other product. These last two steps taken together have a coupling coefficient of −1, since they convert UTP to UDP, and ATP must be used for the regeneration of UTP. The cost of a glucosyl residue in glycogen, obtained from free glucose, is thus 38 + 2 = 40 ATP equivalents. On phosphorolysis, glucose 1-phosphate, with a metabolic value of 39 ATP equivalents, is produced. Thus the loss in storage and recovery of hexose is only 1 ATP equivalent, or 2.5% of the total cost of 40. If the glycogen is stored in the liver and the glucose is to be used in muscle or other tissues, the glucose phosphate must be hydrolyzed to glucose for transport in the bloodstream. In this case, glucose with a value of 38 is obtained from a glucosyl unit that cost 40 ATP equivalents, which is a 95% recovery of the stored metabolic energy.

A plant is similarly efficient in storage and mobilization of energy, since polysaccharides are the primary storage forms. Hexose phosphate formed by photosynthesis can be converted to starch through production of ADP-glucose. On transfer of the glucosyl unit to starch, ADP is released, so the energy expenditure is 1 ATP equivalent. When the product is mobilized for transport to roots, tubers, or other storage sites, 1 ATP equivalent, in the form of UTP, is required in production of sucrose, the transport sugar of plants. Reconversion of sucrose to starch in the storage tissue presumably requires 3 ATP equivalents if the sucrose is split phosphorolytically, yielding fructose and glucose 1-phosphate. Since two glucosyl units of starch are produced from each molecule of sucrose, the total cost of such a unit in starch of a potato tuber, for example, appears to be 40 + 1/2(1 + 3), or 42 ATP equivalents. On phosphorolysis, glucose 1-phosphate, worth 39 equivalents, is produced. However, if carbohydrate is to be transported from the storage tissue to regions of the plant where growth is occurring, an additional ATP equivalent is required for reconversion of the two hexose phosphates to sucrose. The average cost of each hexose unit in sucrose being sent back to points of use in the plant is thus 42.5 ATP equivalents. On arrival at its destination, the sucrose will be phosphorolyzed, and the resultant fructose and glucose 1-phosphate have an average value of 38.5. It thus appears that a plant can store hexose temporarily as starch in the leaf, transport it to sites of long-term storage, and months or years later be able to mobilize about 90% of the total energy expended, ignoring any energy component of transport. (Of course the actual metabolic cost of the original hexose phosphate to the plant was 66 ATP equivalents, the coupling coefficient of photosynthesis, but we have arbitrarily revalued it at its metabolic price as soon as it was produced, for the sake of comparison with energy storage in heterotrophs.)

It may seem strange that plants store and mobilize energy more efficiently, in terms of the percentage of the ATP equivalents expended in storage that can be recovered, than do animals. Since energy is frequently a limiting factor in heterotrophic metabolism, but relatively seldom is in plants, we might have expected greater selective pressure on animals for efficient energy storage. The answer to this apparent paradox is simple. We have seen that a mole of tripalmitin yields 409 ATP equivalents when it is oxidized. The molecular weight of tripalmitin is 806, so 1.97 g of this fat is required for regeneration of 1 mole of ATP. Each glucosyl residue in starch or glycogen, with a molecular weight of 162, yields 39 ATP equivalents on oxidation. Thus 4.15 g of polysaccharide is required per mole of ATP regenerated. The number of ATP equivalents, which is to say the amount of metabolic energy, stored in a gram of fat is slightly more than twice the number stored in a gram of polysaccharide. This is unimportant to a plant which, having produced storage polysaccharide, leaves it in the same place for weeks, years, or even centuries before using it. An animal, having produced an energy-storage compound, must carry it with him wherever he goes, even when running for his life or for his dinner.

In typical higher animals, energy storage is of two types. Because most animals are periodic feeders, they must have enough short-term energy storage to tide them over between meals—probably usually a matter of hours. To provide for more extended periods when food is not available at maintenance levels, there must also be a long-term storage of energy. In nature, as a function of the annual cycle in food availability, the interval between storage and use will frequently be several months. The two types of storage compounds that have evolved are ideally suited to the relative amounts of material stored by the two systems and the relative durations of storage. A major part of an animal's total metabolic energy must be stored for a short period (the interval between meals), but the amount stored at any one time is small (sufficient to maintain the animal for a few hours). By use of glycogen for short-term storage, the animal can reclaim stored energy with high efficiency. This is important because of the large portion of the dietary energy that is stored temporarily; a 19% loss of ATP equivalents in short-term storage would significantly affect the animal's overall metabolic energy efficiency. The extra weight per ATP equivalent is not important because of the small amount of short-term storage material that exists at any time.

In long-term storage, the relative importance of the two factors (efficiency of energy recovery and weight per ATP equivalent) is reversed. Since only a small amount of the animal's dietary energy goes into long-term storage, and since long-term storage compounds turn over infrequently, 19% of the ATP equivalents used in long-term storage is very small compared to total dietary intake, and averaged over a year is probably insignificant. But the amount of energy that accumulates in long-term storage must be very much greater than the amount needed in short-term pool, so weight becomes an important factor. Thus the use of glycogen for short-term storage and of fat for long-term storage is clearly a design feature of advantage to the animal.

Even in plants, fat storage is an adaptation for mobility, and it has long been recognized that the common occurrence of fats and oils in seeds has evolved as an aid to dispersal; lighter seeds will tend to travel farther. In this case the lower density of fats may also be a factor—in addition to having a lower total mass, a seed containing much fat or oil will be more buoyant than one containing the same amount of stored energy as starch, and so can probably sail farther in the air or be moved more easily by surface water.

1-Carbon Metabolism

Because the generalization that NADPH is used in biosynthetic reductions and NAD^+ in substrate oxidation is so well established, systems that do not fit this general pattern are of special interest. The most obvious exception (aside from such $NADP^+$-coupled oxidations as those catalyzed by glucose-6-phosphate dehydrogenase and 6-phosphogluconate dehydrogenase, which presumably serve to regenerate NADPH and thus are not really exceptions at all) involves the interconversion of the 1-carbon intermediates bound to tetrahydrofolate. The main pathway by which these intermediates are generated is shown in Figure 3-4. Transfer of the terminal C of serine to H_4-folate yields the hydroxymethyl derivative I, in which the C atom of metabolic interest is at the oxidation level of formaldehyde. This intermediate may be reduced to the amine II, in which the C atom is at the oxidation level of methanol, or oxidized to the amide III, at the oxidation level of formic acid.

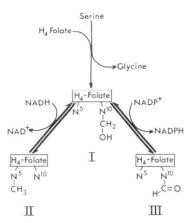

Figure 3-4. Metabolic relationships among the activated 1-carbon metabolic intermediates. I, active formaldehyde, N^{10}-hydroxymethyl H_4-folate; II, active methyl, N^5-methyl H_4-folate; III, active formyl, N^{10}-formyl H_4-folate.

To clarify the assignment of oxidation levels, all three compounds are written with a single attachment of the 1-carbon fragment to H_4-folate, although compounds I and III exist primarily as cyclic anhydrides with the carbon bridging between N-5 and N-10. The point of interest in the context of our present discussion is that $NADP^+$ is used as the oxidizing agent in production of the active formate, and NADH as the reducing agent in the production of the methyl derivative. This is opposite to the usual pattern of use of these compounds, in which NAD^+ is the oxidizing agent and NADPH the reducing agent. However, consideration of the system and its metabolic roles supplies a simple functional rationale for the reversal of roles of the two cofactors. Compounds at the aldehyde level of oxidation are relatively unstable. For example, the equilibrium constant for the dismutation of two molecules of an aldehyde to one each of the corresponding acid and alcohol is large, as are the equilibrium constants for the reduction of an aldehyde to an alcohol by a reduced pyridine nucleotide or the oxidation of an aldehyde to an acid by a pyridine nucleotide in its oxidized state. Therefore the reactions shown in Figure 3-4 tend to go far toward compounds II and III. But it is necessary that compound I be present at a reasonable concentration in the metabolic steady state, both because this compound serves as the source of 1-carbon groups, for example in the syntheses of thymine and hydroxymethylcytosine, and because interconversion of compounds III and II by way of I is probably sometimes necessary. Thus the "reverse" use of the pyridine nucleotide is a means of maintaining a higher level of compound I than would be possible if NAD^+ were used for the oxidation of I to III and NADPH for the reduction of I to II. In other words, the usual generalization

with regard to NAD and NADP should be broadened to the statement that
NAD^+ is used when it is advantageous for oxidation to be facilitated, and
NADPH when reduction is to be facilitated. Therefore NAD^+ is used in
most oxidations and NADPH in most reductions because in nearly every
metabolic sequence it is advantageous to facilitate the sequence in the physiological direction, as we have discussed in terms of oppositely directed
sequences and coupling coefficients. When, as in 1-carbon metabolism, the
unusual situation arises of reactions that must proceed but that would be
deleterious if they proceeded too far, use of NADH for reduction and
$NADP^+$ for oxidation is an obviously useful expedient.

METABOLIC COSTS OF GROWTH

Since the intermediates of glycolysis and the citrate cycle are the starting
materials used in most biosynthetic sequences, the prices of such building
blocks as amino acids and nucleotides can be obtained by adding the costs
of the starting materials and the conversion costs of the coupling factors
used in the conversions. These prices, together with the known or estimated
ATP costs of incorporating each building block, can be used in estimating
the costs of synthesis of biological macromolecules. These costs may then
serve as the basis for discussion of the minimal energy cost of growth.

Prices of Starting Materials

The primary inputs into any calculation of biosynthetic costs must be the
prices of the basic biosynthetic starting materials listed in Figure 3-1 and the
conversion costs of the major coupling agents. These conversion costs were
listed in Table 3-2, and the prices of the starting materials are given in Table
3-3. These are taken from Figure 3-2, except for the two pentose phosphate
shunt intermediates, ribose 5-phosphate and erythrose 4-phosphate. Assignment of prices to these two compounds involves some ambiguity. The method
that was used is illustrated in Figure 3-5. Since three molecules of pentose
phosphate lead to the production of two molecules of hexose phosphate,
with a value of 78 ATP equivalents, and one molecule of triose phosphate,
with a value of 20, the value assigned to pentose phosphate is 98/3 or 32.7
ATP equivalents. This assignment leads to prices for sedoheptulose 7-phos-
phate and erythrose 4-phosphate of 45.3 and 26.3, respectively. The prices
of ribose 5-phosphate and erythrose 4-phosphate are rounded to the nearest
whole number for tabulation in Table 3-3. The same prices, within half an
ATP equivalent in each case, would be obtained from the simple assumption
that each carbon atom in a sugar phosphate corresponds to 6.5 ATP equiva-

TABLE 3-3

Metabolic Prices of Biosynthetic Starting Materials

Compound	Price (ATP equivalents)
Triose phosphate	20
Erythrose 4-P	26
Ribose 5-P	33
Hexose phosphate	39
Pyruvate	15
Oxaloacetate	16
α-Ketoglutarate	25
Succinyl coenzyme A	22
Acetyl coenzyme A	12
Phosphoenolpyruvate	16

lents. Price assignments for sugar phosphates of different sizes would then be 7-carbon, 45.5; 6-carbon, 39; 5-carbon, 32.5; 4-carbon, 26; and 3-carbon, 19.5.

It will be noted that assignment of prices on the basis of the pentose phosphate shunt leads to some disagreement with the standard prices based on glycolysis. Two molecules of NADPH are produced in the conversion of a molecule of hexose phosphate to pentose phosphate. Since the price of NADPH has been taken as 4, this means that the value of each glucose 6-phosphate metabolized through the pentose phosphate shunt is 32.7 + 8, or 40.7. The corresponding full accounting is 3 glucose 6-phosphate yield 2 fructose 6-phosphate (78), 1 triose phosphate (20), and 6 NADPH (24). The sum of the values of the products (78 + 20 + 24) is 122, so the value of each glucose 6-phosphate is 122/3, or 40.7.

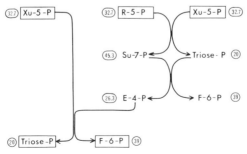

Figure 3-5. Prices of intermediates in the pentose phosphate pathway. Abbreviations are Xu-5-P, xylulose 5-P; R-5-P, ribose 5-P; Su-7-P, sedoheptulose 7-P; E-4-P, erythrose 4-P.

It should not be surprising that metabolic yields, in terms of ATP equivalents, can be different even for closely related pathways. The overall equilibrium constant for oxidation of glucose was seen earlier to be so enormously large that there would be room for even extensive differences in overall coupling coefficients. The difference here is relatively small. The coupling coefficient for the oxidation of glucose 6-phosphate to CO_2 by way of the glycolytic path is 39, whereas the same conversion by way of the pentose phosphate shunt has a coupling coefficient of 40.7. It seems best to use 39 as the price of hexose phosphate in all calculations dealing with the utilization of carbohydrate. In effect, this amounts to saying that the pentose phosphate shunt is a more economical source of NADPH than is the ATP-driven transhydrogenase reaction discussed earlier. If 3 molecules of glucose 6-phosphate, with an assigned value of $3 \times 39 = 117$ ATP equivalents, produce 2 molecules of fructose 6-phosphate and 1 of triose phosphate, with a total value of $2 \times 39 + 20 = 98$ ATP equivalents, the metabolic cost of the 6 molecules of NADPH that are also produced must be $117 - 98 = 19$ ATP equivalents. Each NADPH then costs 3.3 ATP equivalents. We will retain the assigned price of 4 ATP equivalents for NADPH, and consider the pentose phosphate shunt to be a way of obtaining extra value from hexose phosphate beyond its normal assigned value of 39 ATP equivalents.

Prices of Building Blocks

Amino Acids

In Table 3-4 the costs of synthesizing the 20 protein amino acids are tabulated. This table is modified from an earlier paper (10). More extensive tables of conversion requirements in biosynthesis, but without reduction of these requirements to a common energy currency, were later published by Penning de Vries et al. (91).

The assignments of costs to syntheses of amino acids are in the main definite and straightforward, but there are a few points of ambiguity. The only one affecting several amino acids is the question of the cost of transamination. Incorporation of inorganic nitrogen from ammonia has been thought to proceed by way of the glutamate dehydrogenase reaction (equation 3-40), so that the cost assigned in the earlier publication (10) was the conversion cost of NADPH, 4 ATP equivalents. It is now known that, at least in some prokaryotes, ammonia is incorporated by a different pathway

$$\alpha\text{-ketoglutarate} + NH_3 + NADPH \rightarrow glutamate + NADP^+ \qquad (3\text{-}40)$$

that is facilitated by the use of ATP, and that can utilize ammonia at lower concentrations because of a much lower effective Michaelis constant for ammonia. This pathway, shown in equations 3-41 and 3-42, consumes one molecule each of NADPH and ATP, and so has a conversion cost of 5 ATP equivalents (equation 3-43). Although we do not yet know how general this pathway is, a cost of 5 ATP equivalents has been assigned to transamination in Table 3-4.

$$\alpha\text{-ketoglutarate} + \text{glutamine} + \text{NADPH} \rightarrow 2\ \text{glutamate} + \text{NADP}^+ \tag{3-41}$$

$$\underline{\text{glutamate} + \text{NH}_3 + \text{ATP} \rightarrow \text{glutamine} + \text{ADP} + \text{P}_i} \tag{3-42}$$

$$\alpha\text{-ketoglutarate} + \text{NH}_3 + \text{ATP} + \text{NADPH} \rightarrow \text{glutamate} + \text{ADP} + \text{P}_i + \text{NADP}^+ \tag{3-43}$$

The other ambiguity involves only glycine and methionine; it arises from uncertainty in the apportionment of costs in the serine hydroxymethyltransferase reaction (equation 3-44). The metabolic price of serine, 18 ATP equiva-

$$\text{serine} + \text{H}_4\text{-folate} \rightarrow \text{glycine} + \text{hydroxymethyl H}_4\text{-folate} \tag{3-44}$$

lents, must be divided between glycine and the active formaldehyde moiety of the other product, but there is no clear and obvious basis for this division. The figures in the table were obtained by assigning a cost to glycine on the basis of a possible alternative route of synthesis through the isocitritase reaction followed by transamination (equations 3-45 and 3-46). From the

$$\text{isocitrate} \rightarrow \text{glyoxylate} + \text{succinate} \tag{3-45}$$

$$\text{glyoxylate} + \text{glutamate} \rightarrow \text{glycine} + \alpha\text{-ketoglutarate} \tag{3-46}$$

metabolic prices of isocitrate (28) and of succinate (21) given in Figure 3-2, it follows that the cost of glyoxylate is 7 ATP equivalents. If the cost of transamination is taken to be 5, the cost of synthesizing glycine by this route would be 12 ATP equivalents. This somewhat arbitrary assignment leads to the values for the activated 1-carbon tetrahydrofolate derivatives shown in Figure 3-6.

Compounds I and III (or the anhydride forms in which the carbon atom bridges between N-5 and N-10) are used directly as sources of 1-carbon groups at the aldehyde and acyl levels when these are needed in metabolism. Compound II, however, is merely an amine, and not sufficiently activated to provide large equilibrium constants if it served as a methyl donor to other metabolic intermediates. This compound is therefore not used generally as the primary methyl donor. Its primary role is in the production of *S*-adenosylmethionine (equations 3-47 to 3-49). When *S*-adenosylmethionine serves as methyl donor in a metabolic reaction (equation 3-50), the *S*-adenosylhomocysteine that is produced is converted back to homocysteine (equations 3-51 and 3-52). The overall equation (3-53) shows that the transfer of the methyl

TABLE 3-4

Cost, in ATP Equivalents, of Synthesizing Amino Acids[a,b]

Amino acid product	Starting materials	Conversion requirements	Cost
Glutamate	α-Ketoglutarate $(25)^c$	NADPH $(4)^c$; ATP (1)	30
Aspartate	Oxaloacetate (16)	trans-NH$_2$ $(5)^d$	21
Glutamine	Glutamate (30)	ATP (1)	31
Asparagine	Aspartate (21)	ATP (1)	22
Alanine	Pyruvate (15)	trans-NH$_2$ (5)	20
Serine	3-P-glycerate (16)	NAD$^+$ → NADH (-3); trans-NH$_2$ (5)	18
Glycine	Serine (18)	H$_4$-folate → methylene H$_4$-folate (-6)	12
Cysteine	Serine (18)	AcSCoA → AcOH (1)	19
Threonine	Aspartate (21)	2 NADPH (8); 2 ATP (2)	31
Isoleucine	Threonine (31); pyruvate (15)	NADPH (4); trans-NH$_2$ (5)	55
Valine	2 Pyruvate (30)	NADPH (4); trans-NH$_2$ (5)	39
Leucine	2 Pyruvate (30); AcSCoA (12)	trans-NH$_2$ (5)	47
Proline	Glutamate (30)	2 NADPH (8); ATP (1)	39
Arginine	Glutamate (30); carbamyl-P (2)	ATP (1); NADPH (4); trans-NH$_2$ (5); aspartate → fumarate (2)	44
Histidine	P-ribosyl-PP (35)	ATP → AICAR (7); trans-NH$_2$ (5); 2 NAD$^+$ → 2 NADH (-6); glutamine → glutamate (1)	42
[Chorismate]^e	2 P-enolpyruvate (32); erythrose 4-P (26)	NAD$^+$ → NADH (-3); ATP (1); NADPH (4)	60
Phenylalanine	Chorismate (60)	trans-NH$_2$ (5)	65
Tyrosine	Chorismate (60)	NAD$^+$ → NADH (-3); trans-NH$_2$ (5)	62
Tryptophan	Chorismate (60); P-ribosyl-PP (35) $-$Pyruvate (-15)	Glutamine → glutamate (1); serine → 3 P GAld (-3)	78
[Homocysteine]	Aspartate (21)	Cysteine → pyruvate (4); 2 NADPH (8); SuccSCoA → succinate (1); ATP (1)	35
Methionine	Homocysteine (35)	Me H$_4$-folate → H$_4$-folate (9)	44
Lysine (diaminopimelate pathway)	Pyruvate (15); aspartate (21)	ATP (1); 2 NADPH (8); SuccSCoA → succ (1); trans-NH$_2$ (5)	51
Lysine (aminoadipate pathway)	α-Ketoglutarate (25); AcSCoA (12)	2 NAD$^+$ → 2 NADH (-6); 2 NADPH (8); 2 trans-NH$_2$ (10); ATP (1)	50

[a] Calculations are based on metabolic relationships in typical aerobic eukaryotic cells.

[b] A similar table, with some differences in assignments, was presented in Atkinson (*10*).

[c] Numbers in parentheses are the costs of starting materials or the costs of regenerating the coupling agents used in the conversion.

[d] Transamination involves the conversion of glutamate to α-ketoglutarate; therefore, the cost of transamination is taken as 5 ATP equivalents (see text).

[e] Products in brackets are intermediates for which the synthetic cost must be calculated.

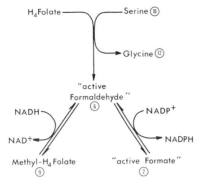

Figure 3-6. Metabolic conversion costs of the 1-carbon tetrahydrofolate derivatives.

group from the amine linkage in the H_4-folate derivative to a methylated product, by way of the highly activated sulfonium methyl group in S-adeno-

$$\text{methyl } H_4\text{-folate} + \text{homocysteine} \rightleftharpoons \text{methionine } + H_4\text{-folate} \tag{3-47}$$

$$\text{methionine} + \text{ATP} \rightleftharpoons S\text{-adenosylmethionine} + \text{POP}_i + \text{P}_i \tag{3-48}$$

$$\text{POP}_i + \text{H}_2\text{O} \rightleftharpoons 2 \text{ P}_i \tag{3-49}$$

$$S\text{-adenosylmethionine} + \text{substrate} \rightleftharpoons \text{methylated substrate} + S\text{-adenosylhomocysteine} \tag{3-50}$$

$$S\text{-adenosylhomocysteine} + \text{H}_2\text{O} \rightleftharpoons \text{homocysteine} + \text{adenosine} \tag{3-51}$$

$$\underline{\text{adenosine} + 2 \text{ ATP} \rightleftharpoons 3 \text{ ADP}} \tag{3-52}$$

$$\text{methyl } H_4\text{-folate} + 3 \text{ ATP}_{\text{equiv}} + \text{substrate} \rightleftharpoons H_4\text{-folate} + 3 \text{ ADP}_{\text{equiv}} + 3 \text{ P}_i + \text{methylated substrate} \tag{3-53}$$

sylmethionine, costs the cell an additional 3 ATP equivalents, making the total cost of a biological methylation 12 ATP equivalents. Thus in being reduced and activated to form the methyl group of S-adenosylmethionine, a carbon atom from glucose is promoted from an average value of 6.3 equivalents (38/6) to a cost of 12 equivalents. Active methyl is probably the most expensive metabolic compound or group on a per-carbon basis.

Nucleotides

The costs of synthesizing the nucleotide building blocks for nucleic acid synthesis can be calculated by the same approach used for the amino acids. These calculations are summarized in Table 3-5.

Costs of Synthesizing Macromolecules

The amino acids vary rather widely in cost of synthesis per gram, depending mainly on their relative degrees of reduction. The cost in ATP equivalents per gram of each type of amino acid residue is given in Table 3-6. The

TABLE 3-5

Cost, in ATP Equivalents, of Synthesizing Nucleotides

Product[a]	Starting materials	Conversion requirements	Cost
[IMP][b]	PRPP (35); glycine (12)	2 Glutamine → 2 glutamate (2); 4 ATP → 4 ADP (4); 2 formyl H_4-folate → 2 H_4-folate (4); aspartate → fumarate (2)	59
AMP	IMP (59)	GTP → GDP (1); aspartate → fumarate (2)	62
GMP	IMP (59)	NAD^+ → NADH (−3); ATP → AMP (2); glutamine → glutamate (1)	59
[OMP]	Aspartate (21); carbamyl-P (2) PRPP (35)	NAD^+ → NADH (−3)	55
CTP	OMP (55)	Glutamine → glutamate (1); 3 ATP → 3 ADP (3)	59
UMP	OMP (55)		55
dADP	AMP (62)	NADPH → $NADP^+$ (4); ATP → ADP (1)	67
dGDP	GMP (59)	NADPH → NAD^+ (4); ATP → ADP (1)	64
dCDP	CTP (59)	NADPH → NAD^+ (4); ADP → ATP (−1)	62
dTDP	UMP (55)	NADPH → $NADP^+$ (4); ATP → ADP (1); $HOCH_2 \cdot H_4$-folate → H_2-folate (6)	66

[a] This table lists the ribonucleoside monophosphates and the deoxyribonucleoside diphosphates because these are the first products, except that CTP appears to be the first cytosine nucleotide produced. Triphosphates obviously cost 2 ATP equivalents more than monophosphates and 1 equivalent more than diphosphates.

[b] Products in brackets are intermediates for which the synthesis cost must be calculated.

cost of synthesizing a gram of any protein must of course lie within the range spanned by the individual residues, and will in most cases probably be between 0.3 and 0.4. If the cost of a protein of specified composition were desired, it could easily be calculated from the figures in Table 3-6. Thus for a hypothetical protein containing equal numbers of all 20 amino acid residues, the mass of a 20-amino-acid portion would be 2,375 g and the total cost of synthesis of the 20 amino acids would be 769 ATP equivalents. The average cost per gram of constituent amino acid residues would then be 769/2375, or 0.324 ATP equivalents. The average mass of an amino acid residue is 118.8 daltons, so if 4 ATP equivalents are required in the production of a peptide bond (1 ATP converted to AMP in the activation of the amino acid and 2 GTP's used in chain elongation), the average cost is 4/118.8, or 0.034 ATP equivalents per gram. The total direct cost of synthesizing this hypothetical protein is thus 0.324 + 0.034 = 0.358 ATP equivalents per gram. This calculation ignores overhead and indirect costs such as the cost of synthesis of the messenger RNA and the ribosomes that are required for protein synthesis.

TABLE 3-6

Costs per Gram of Amino Acid Residues[a]

Residue	Mass (daltons)	Cost (ATP equiv.)	Cost/g
Alanine	71	20	0.282
Arginine	156	44	0.282
Asparagine	114	22	0.193
Aspartic acid	115	21	0.183
Cysteine	103	19	0.184
Glutamic acid	129	30	0.233
Glutamine	128	31	0.242
Glycine	57	12	0.211
Histidine	137	42	0.307
Isoleucine	113	55	0.487
Leucine	113	47	0.416
Lysine	128	50	0.391
Methionine	131	44	0.336
Phenylalanine	147	65	0.442
Proline	97	39	0.402
Serine	87	18	0.207
Threonine	101	31	0.307
Tryptophan	186	78	0.419
Tyrosine	163	62	0.380
Valine	99	39	0.394

[a] Costs are from Table 3-4. Masses are those of the residues in proteins, which are the masses of the free amino acids minus 18.

By means of calculations similar to those outlined for proteins, the minimal or direct cost of synthesis of macromolecules of any type may be estimated. Table 3-7 presents such estimates for the hypothetical protein described above, for nucleic acid, assuming equal concentrations of the nucleotides, and for simple storage polysaccharides such as starch or glycogen, and storage fats such as tripalmitin. The costs of synthesis of a glucosyl residue in polysaccharide and of tripalmitin were discussed earlier in this chapter.

Estimates of Costs of Growth

Numbers such as those in Table 3-7, and similar values for other types of macromolecules such as structural phospholipids or for proteins of known overall amino acid composition, could be used in conjunction with information on composition of organisms for the estimation of the direct cost of growth. Since protein is the major class of macromolecules in typical cells,

TABLE 3-7

Costs of Synthesis of Some Macromolecules

	g/ATP (equiv)	ATP (equiv/g)
Protein (see text)		
(equal numbers of all amino acids)	2.79	0.358
769 ATP equiv/2,375 g = 0.324		
4 ATP equiv/118.8 g = 0.034		
0.358		
Nucleic acid		
(equal amounts of component nucleotides)		
RNA 241 ATP equiv/1,150 g	4.77	0.210
DNA 263 ATP equiv/1,100 g	4.18	0.239
Polysaccharide		
(storage polyglucose: starch or glycogen)		
43 ATP equiv/162 g	3.77	0.265
Lipid		
(storage fat: tripalmitin)		
500 ATP equiv/804 g	1.61	0.622

it is evident that the maximal possible growth yield, on a dry weight basis, per mole of ATP equivalent would be somewhat less than 3 g. A real organism could not be expected to approach this value at all closely because the estimate ignores all other uses of energy, such as active transport, motility, breakdown and resynthesis of macromolecules, and whatever wasteful operation of futile cycles occurs. These other uses in the aggregate are probably greater than the direct costs of synthesis, so the value of 3 g is by no means a realistic estimate of growth costs.

It should be kept in mind that the estimates described here relate to the total costs of synthesis; that is, costs of all of the components that are incorporated into the organism are taken into account as if they had been synthesized from glucose. Thus these estimates apply most directly to an organism that is growing with glucose as the sole carbon source. Other situations or other assumptions would of course lead to different estimates. Thus if all amino acids were present in the environment and were considered to be free, the only cost of synthesizing proteins would be the cost of producing peptide bonds. As the numbers in Table 3-7 show, on this basis the cost of making a gram of protein would be only about 1/10 as great as that estimated when the costs of the amino acids are taken into account.

Gunsalus and Shuster (53) were the first workers to predict maximal growth yields on the basis of known biosynthetic pathways. They estimated a yield of about 30 g (dry weight) per mole of ATP, taking only conversion costs into account.

Perhaps the most painstaking and thorough analysis of the direct requirements for growth was supplied by Hommes *et al.* (*58*) for a human infant. On the basis of the gross chemical composition of the major organs and tissues in an average 3-week-old baby and the rate of growth of each, these workers calculated the total amount of each class of macromolecule synthesized daily and the corresponding metabolic cost. Amino acids and fatty acids were assumed to be available as needed in the diet, and no cost was assigned to them. For materials assumed to be made from glucose, such as cholesterol, only conversion costs were counted. The total conversion costs associated with the biosyntheses required for normal growth were estimated by this approach to be 2.2% of the energy content of the normal diet. Hommes *et al.* noted that if the caloric equivalents of the nutrients that are incorporated were added to the conversion costs, 13.4% of the caloric value of the diet would be accounted for in growth.

Many workers have treated the energy requirements for growth in various ways. Most of these studies have dealt either with bacteria or with animals domesticated for food production. A few of these papers will be mentioned, mainly to illustrate the diversity of approaches. Many earlier papers had reported ratios of dry weight of organism formed to amount of substrate consumed. Beyond demonstrating that the amount of growth of a given organism under specified conditions could be predicted from the amount of substrates supplied, this approach could contribute little to understanding of growth. Attempts to relate growth yield to metabolic processes and parameters date from the 1960 paper of Bauchop and Elsden (*21*), who calculated the amount of ATP that should be produced from the substrate utilized, and related the result to the gain in dry weight of the organism. For microorganisms grown anaerobically in a rich medium containing all of the protein amino acids, the observed value was about 10.5 g of dry weight per mole of ATP. (This value is not in conflict with our calculation above that the maximal yield is about 3 g, because the experimental approach of Bauchop and Elsden corresponds to taking only conversion costs into account, since only the ATP expected from the amount of substrate observed to be fermented is used in the calculation.) A number of papers have reported values remarkably close to 10.5, but some later measurements have deviated considerably, as is to be expected since the ratio of direct conversion costs to other types of energy expenditure must vary with conditions. Several other parameters, including notably the yield per mole (or faraday) of available electrons in aerobes, have been suggested. The relevant literature up to 1970 was reviewed in an excellent article by Payne (*90*).

Related Nutritional Concepts

We have discussed prices of metabolites in terms of ATP equivalents per molecule (or per mole) because that seems to be the most useful basis for general metabolic considerations. However, prices could be expressed in many other ways; for instance, as ATP equivalents per carbon atom or per electron available for transfer to oxygen. These alternative bases for pricing will probably not be directly useful in metabolic calculations of most types, but they are of some interest in themselves, and they may also facilitate comparison with some results and concepts from the field of nutrition. In Table 3-8, ATP yields per carbon atom and per available electron are tabulated for several metabolites, assuming normal aerobic heterotrophic metabolism. The compounds are arranged in order of the formal oxidation number, or "valence," of carbon calculated by assigning a value of -2 to oxygen and $+1$ to hydrogen. The steady decrease in the yields of ATP per carbon atom as the oxidation number increases reflects the overriding importance of oxidation in the production of ATP in aerobic organisms. The more reduced a compound, the greater its potential ATP yield.

If all ATP were produced by electron transfer phosphorylation, and if all electrons lost by the substrate were transferred to NAD^+, the yield of ATP would be 3 per electron pair, or 1.5 per electron. The values in the last column of Table 3-8 show how closely this proportionality applies. The basic figure is 1.5. Slightly higher values for sugars and compounds, such as glycerol, that are converted to sugars reflect the substrate-level phosphorylations in glycolysis. Slightly lower values for fats and fatty acids result from the fact that half of the electrons liberated in the conversion of a long-chain fatty acid to acetyl-SCoA are transferred directly to FAD, with an ATP yield of 2 per electron pair, instead of to NAD^+. But these divergences are minor, and the figures in the last column serve mainly to illustrate the obvious fact that aerobic organisms obtain their energy primarily from electron transport phosphorylation.

The heat of combustion of organic materials is closely correlated with the number of electrons that are transferred to oxygen in the combustion. Therefore, since they are both correlated with the number of electrons transferred, the heat of combustion and the ATP yield must be correlated with each other. As early as 1962 Blaxter (24) suggested that ". . . it should be possible to deduce calorimetric efficiencies for oxidative processes solely from a knowledge of intermediary-energy transfers." By dividing the heat of combustion of a nutrient by the number of moles of ATP produced when the nutrient is oxidized to CO_2, he related the customary energy parameter of nutrition, the caloric value expressed in kilocalories, to the energy quantum of metabolism, the ATP equivalent. Such ratios as 18 for glucose (673 kcal/

TABLE 3-8

Yields of ATP from Selected Metabolites[a]

Compound or group	Oxid. No.	ATP/mole	ATP/C	ATP/e^-
Palmityl group of palmSCoA	−1.75	131	8.2	1.4
Tripalmitin	−1.69	409	8.0	1.4
Glycerol	−0.67	22	7.3	1.6
Glucose	0	38	6.3	1.6
Glucosyl in polysaccharide	0	39	6.5	1.6
Hexose phosphate	0	39	6.5	1.6
Triose phosphate	0	20	6.7	1.7
Acetyl group of AcSCoA	0	12	6.0	1.5
Lactate	0	18	6.0	1.5
Succinate[b]	+0.5	20	5.0	1.4
Pyruvate	+0.67	15	5.0	1.5
α-Ketoglutarate[b]	+0.8	24	4.8	1.5
Citrate[b]	+1.0	27	4.5	1.5
Fumarate[b]	+1.0	18	4.5	1.5
Malate[b]	+1.0	18	4.5	1.5
Oxaloacetate[b]	+1.5	15	3.75	1.5

[a] The metabolites are listed in the order of increasing average formal oxidation number of carbon (see text), and ATP yields per molecule, per carbon atom, and per electrons lost during oxidation are tabulated.

[b] The values for citrate cycle intermediates in this table are less by 1 ATP equivalent per mole than those shown in Figure 3-2. This reflects the fact that when oxaloacetate is to be oxidized as a primary fuel, rather than merely used as a catalytic intermediate in the cycle, it must be converted to acetyl-SCoA by way of pyruvate. The conversion of oxaloacetate to pyruvate entails no net gain or loss of ATP, so the value of oxaloacetate under such conditions is the same as that of pyruvate, or 15 ATP equivalents. Similarly, the value of each of the other intermediates in the cycle as a fuel is less by one equivalent than the price assigned in Figure 3-2, because they all lead to oxaloacetate, and must pass through pyruvate and acetyl-SCoA for complete oxidation.

38 ATP) and 21 for acetate were obtained. The clustering of the ratios around 18 is of course a consequence of the fact, noted above, that both the heat of combustion and the number of moles of ATP produced are correlated with the number of electrons transferred during the oxidation of the nutrient. This ratio of about 18 kcal (heat of combustion) of feed per mole of ATP regenerated has been found useful by others working on the nutrition and energy metabolism of domestic animals (14, 84). The similar near-constancy of the ratio between the free energy of combustion and the amount of ATP regenerated has been unfortunately misinterpreted as showing that the yield of ATP follows from the fundamental thermodynamic features of the oxidation rather than from the details of the metabolic pathways (85). As was empha-

sized earlier in this chapter, the ATP yield is in fact dependent entirely on the pathway and is an evolved property that is independent, to a first approximation, of thermodynamics. (Thermodynamic considerations would set limits on the ATP yield, but, as was pointed out in the earlier discussion, the actual yields observed are enormously far from the region of thermodynamic constraints.) The near-identity of the ratio of ΔG^0_{comb} to ATP yield for different metabolites thus is not an indication that the amount of ATP regenerated is independent of the path; on the contrary, it follows entirely from the properties of catabolic pathways—specifically from the fact that in aerobic cells most ATP is regenerated by a common pathway that yields 1.5 molecules of ATP for each electron transferred to oxygen.

SUMMARY

Any metabolic reaction or sequence may be characterized by its ATP coupling coefficient—the number of ATP molecules produced per molecule of substrate converted to product. The coupling coefficient is negative for reactions or sequences that consume ATP. These coupling coefficients determine the stoichiometric relationships between metabolic sequences.

Although they are stoichiometric quantities, metabolic coupling coefficients differ from other stoichiometric parameters in that they do not depend on, and are not predictable from, the chemical properties of the reactants, intermediates, or products. They depend on the properties of the enzymes that participate in the various sequences, and they have been fixed, like any other phenotypic characteristics of organisms, by mutation and selection.

The most important consequence of the coupling coefficient of a sequence is that it determines the direction of flow through the sequence. Any sequence could be made more thermodynamically favorable by a decrease in the value of its ATP coupling coefficient or less favorable by an increase. Nearly every metabolic sequence is paired with a sequence that carries out the same conversion in the opposite direction. Each sequence has an ATP coupling coefficient of an appropriate size to insure that the sequence will be thermodynamically feasible in its physiological direction under essentially all possible conditions in the cell. Each pair of oppositely directed sequences together comprise a futile cycle, or pseudocycle; if they functioned simultaneously the only result would be the hydrolysis of ATP. But by providing at all times a thermodynamically feasible pathway in each direction, such pairs of sequences make possible the kinetic control, reflecting metabolic needs, that is essential for life and is perhaps its chief distinguishing chemical characteristic.

Assignment of prices to metabolic intermediates and of costs to metabolic conversions, both in terms of ATP equivalents, allows us to deal with metabolic relationships semiquantitatively. These prices and costs may be of value in the estimation of minimal costs of syntheses of macromolecules, or even in estimation of the direct costs of growth.

4

Adenylate Control and the
Adenylate Energy Charge

KINETIC CONTROL OF METABOLISM

Need for Kinetic Control

Living organisms differ from the inanimate world in many ways, but perhaps most strikingly in the close functional correlation between a large number of chemical reaction sequences. This correlation is based on the evolved stoichiometric relationships discussed in Chapter 3, but is equally dependent on precise and fast-acting control of the rates of key reactions in each sequence. The unique metabolic significance of the adenylate system in stoichiometric coupling and in metabolic energy transduction was illustrated schematically in the functional diagram of Figure 3-1 and discussed in Chapter 3. Energy transduction and energy storage, involving ATP, ADP, and AMP, are at the heart of metabolism. But an energy-transducing and energy-storing system could not function without regulation of the rate of energy deposit and energy withdrawal. An automobile storage battery soon ceases to perform its intended function if the voltage regulator fails. Similarly, the adenylate energy storage system can serve the function outlined in the preceding two chapters only if the ratios of its component compounds are held within the functional range. The more complex the interactions within any device, the more rigorous is the necessity for stabilization. The adenine nucleotides interact with all sequences in a living cell, which is incomparably the most complex chemical system known. Uncontrolled changes in the relative concentrations of ATP, ADP, and AMP would affect the rates of all metabolic reactions and be highly disruptive. Close control of the relative concentrations of ATP, ADP, and AMP is thus evidently essential to correlation of the fluxes through these sequences. Therefore the kinetic aspects of adenylate metabolism are as essential as the thermodynamic aspects to cell function. Indeed, as noted in Chapter 3, the primary advantage of the pairs of unidirectional oppositely directed sequences that are found throughout metabolism is that they allow for kinetic regulation, based on metabolic needs, of metabolic conversions.

Results of analyses and of experiments with intact cells that establish directly the existence of tight control of adenine nucleotide concentration ratios and mole fractions will be discussed in Chapter 7. Here we merely note that it seems impossible that the complex pattern of interactions among metabolic sequences could be maintained unless the concentration ratios of these compounds, which stoichiometrically couple all sequences, were held nearly constant. This, in turn, requires that metabolism be regulated largely on the basis of the relative concentrations of ATP, ADP, and AMP. A designer, desiring to add automatic control to a system in which all processes are stoichiometrically coupled by the adenine nucleotides, would undoubtedly use those same nucleotides as the basis for kinetic control. It would be very difficult, if not logically impossible, to design a system that would stabilize the concentrations of the adenine nucleotides unless these concentrations, or some quantities directly dependent on them, were among the variables sensed by the control system. In somewhat more general terms: ATP is consumed or regenerated in every metabolic sequence. Thus the level of energy storage in the adenylate system can be controlled only by controlling the rates of all metabolic sequences, and only by sensing the energy level of the adenylate system and using this information as a basis of control. It would, I think, be impossible to design a homeostatic system having any significant resemblance to metabolism that did not contain this feature of universal kinetic control by the universal stoichiometric coupling agent. In this respect, as in so many others, evolutionary design has hit upon the same solution as would have been used by a conscious designer.

From the steady-state concentration of ATP and some measure of the metabolic rate (for example, the rate of oxygen uptake in the case of aerobic cells), it is possible to calculate that the turnover time for ATP is typically of the order of 1 second or less. That is, the amount of ATP used per second is usually about equal to the steady-state amount of ATP in the cell. This fact emphasizes the precision and speed of response required in metabolic regulation, since a relatively small imbalance between the rates of use and of regeneration of ATP would cause a drastic change in its concentration within a very short time. The time scale may be compared with that for regulation of the charge of an automobile storage battery. If the charging system fails totally, the capacity of the battery is such that it can continue to provide electricity to the ignition system for many hours. Even if the failure occurs at night, when the headlights are needed, the battery can meet the energy demands for a considerable time. In contrast, the capacity of the adenylate "battery" is so small that it would be totally discharged in about a second if charging were to stop and energy use to continue at the normal rate. The observation that the energy level of the system in all kinds of actively metabolizing cells that have been studied is remarkably constant, regardless of changes of external conditions and of very large changes in overall metabolic rates (Chapter 7), supplies convincing evidence for operation *in vivo* of an effective and fast-acting ATP-sensing regulatory mechanism.

Recognition of Adenylate Control

Although it may seem that the logical necessity of regulation of ATP-regenerating and ATP-utilizing sequences should have led to a search for general metabolic regulatory mechanisms based on the adenylates, this was not the case. Adenylate control, like most other scientific generalizations, was recognized only after the essentially accidental accumulation of relevant experimental results. Stimulation of phosphorylase activity by AMP was observed in the Coris' laboratory in 1938 (*40, 41*). The possibility of some regulatory significance was suggested at that time, but because the role of the adenine nucleotides in metabolism was then only beginning to be appreciated, no specific proposal was possible. By 1962 the participation of ATP in metabolism was known to be general, and evidence of various sorts had suggested that phosphofructokinase might be an especially important control point in glycolysis. Thus Mansour's discovery of nucleotide control of phosphofructokinase activity (*80, 81*) was immediately assumed to be of regulatory importance. Passonneau and Lowry (*89*) suggested that stimulation of phosphofructokinase by AMP might explain the Pasteur effect. At about the same time, on the basis of other experimental evidence largely from his own laboratory, Krebs proposed that the concentration of AMP might be a primary determinant of the direction of metabolic conversions between carbohydrate and pyruvate, with a high level of AMP favoring glycolysis and a low level favoring gluconeogenesis (*68*). He pointed out that, at physiological ratios of ATP, ADP, and AMP, and assuming near equilibrium of the adenylate kinase reaction, when the concentration of ATP falls and those of ADP and AMP rise the percent change in concentration will be greatest for AMP because its absolute concentration is by far the lowest of the three nucleotides. Thus response to AMP might be considered an amplification of response to ATP.

With the finding in 1963 of AMP stimulation of isocitrate dehydrogenase (*56*), it became clear that adenylate control must be a widespread phenomenon. Phosphorolysis of an acetal bond in polysaccharide (catalyzed by phosphorylase), phosphorylation of a hydroxyl group in fructose 6-P (catalyzed by phosphofructokinase), and oxidation of the hydroxyl group of isocitrate to a ketone, followed by decarboxylation (catalyzed by isocitrate dehydrogenase), have nothing in common chemically, and there is no chemical reason why AMP should be involved with any of these three reactions. Thus the facilitation of these disparate reactions by AMP must have evolved because of selective advantage to the organism, that is, it must have a biological function. From the fact that the three reactions are, respectively, the first step in the metabolism of stored polysaccharide, a reaction that was already thought to be involved in the regulation of glycolysis, and the first oxidative step in the citrate cycle, it seemed likely that the biological function of AMP stimulation might be acceleration of the rate of ATP regeneration. Since the level of AMP will rise when the ATP concentration falls, an increase in the rate of ATP regeneration in response to an increase in AMP concentration would obviously be a type of feedback control, and would tend to stabilize the concentrations of ATP and AMP. It was accordingly proposed that AMP might exert a regulatory effect at every branch point where a metabolite must be partitioned between ATP regeneration and other metabolic functions (4, 97).

THE ADENYLATE ENERGY CHARGE

As further experimental results accumulated, it became clear that this initial adenylate control hypothesis was inadequate. ADP and ATP, as well as AMP, modulate the activities of a number of regulatory enzymes. Thus citrate synthase from yeast and pig heart was shown to be very little affected by AMP, but strongly inhibited by ATP (57). ADP, rather than AMP, is the activator for isocitrate dehydrogenase from mammalian tissues (32) and for phosphofructokinase from Escherichia coli (6). In all of these cases the effect is in the same direction, in terms of metabolic consequences, as AMP stimulation. However, such effects are not covered by the simple statement that the level of AMP should control the use of metabolites for ATP regeneration. Clearly a broader generalization was needed to allow comparison of the effects of different adenine nucleotides and especially to facilitate relating the results obtained in vitro to the metabolic situation in the intact cell. Observations of effects of adenine nucleotides on individual enzymes were beginning to accumulate in a formless and chaotic way, and they could be related to conditions in vivo only in vague and qualitative terms. A unifying conceptual approach was suggested by the analogy between the adenine nucleotide pool and a chemical storage battery or accumulator cell. The

adenine nucleotide pool has in common with a storage battery the fundamental properties that the total amount of material in the system typically
remains constant but chemical potential energy can be stored or recovered
by alteration in the ratio of the components. In the lead cell, for example
(equation 4-1), maximal energy is stored when the lead sulfate is converted

$$2Pb(SO_4) + 2\,H_2O = Pb + PbO_2 + 2\,H_2SO_4 \qquad (4\text{-}1)$$

to an equimolar mixture of free lead and lead dioxide; in this condition the
cell is fully charged. A condition of full discharge, or zero stored energy,
corresponds to complete conversion to lead sulfate. In an ideally functioning
cell, the amount of stored energy is a stoichiometric function of the amount
of lead sulfate that has been converted. Because all three of the participating
lead compounds are insoluble, the charge of a lead cell is easily measured
by the concentration of sulfuric acid in the electrolyte, and this can be estimated simply by determining the density of the electrolyte.

Equation 4-2 represents the adenylate storage system. Unlike the equation
for the lead storage cell, however, this equation does not correspond to an

$$AMP + 2\,P_i \rightleftharpoons ATP + 2\,H_2O \qquad (4\text{-}2)$$

actual reaction. Rather it is the sum of the reactions shown in equations 4-3
and 4-4. Equation 4-3 represents interconversions between ADP and ATP, as

$$2\,ADP + 2\,P_i \rightleftharpoons 2\,ATP + H_2O \qquad (4\text{-}3)$$

$$AMP + ATP \rightleftharpoons 2\,ADP \qquad (4\text{-}4)$$

in kinase reactions, electron transfer phosphorylation, and the like. Equation
4-4 shows the reaction catalyzed by adenylate kinase. It is clear that if the
adenylate-orthophosphate system were closed—that is, if the sum of the
phosphate occurring in the adenine nucleotides and as free inorganic phosphate were constant—the concentration of free phosphate would, like the
concentration of H_2SO_4 in the lead cell, serve as a measure of the charge of
the system. A decrease in concentration of phosphate would correspond to
an increase in stored energy. However, the system is not closed in this sense.
There are many other phosphorylated compounds in the cell; thus the total
phosphate content of a living system is partitioned between many compounds
whose concentrations vary in complex ways, and the concentration of free
phosphate cannot be expected to bear any meaningful relationship to the
balance among the adenine nucleotides. In order to have a measure of the
degree of energy charge of the adenine nucleotide system it is therefore necessary to use the concentrations of the nucleotides themselves.

Energy is put into any chemical system by displacing it from the equilibrium that will apply under the conditions of use. The lead cell is charged

by supplying electrons, at what amounts to a high chemical potential (98), to the appropriate electrode. Similarly, the adenylate energy storage system is charged by supplying a phosphoryl group at effectively high chemical potential (that is, from a compound with a large negative free energy of hydrolysis) to ADP. The system is fully charged when all of the adenylate present is converted to ATP, and fully discharged when only AMP is present. Thus, as indicated by equation 4-5, in a system containing only AMP and ATP the charge would be simply the mole fraction of ATP. But the real adenylate pool also contains ADP. By the action of adenylate kinase (equation 4-4), 1 mole of ADP can be used for the production of $\frac{1}{2}$ mole of ATP.

$$\text{charge} = \frac{(\text{ATP})}{(\text{ATP}) + (\text{AMP})} \tag{4-5}$$

Thus ADP contributes half as much, on a molar basis, to the amount of energy stored in the adenylate system as does ATP. This fact must lead to a second term in the parameter that is to express the energy state, or degree of charge, of the system. Thus the charge of the three-component adenine nucleotide system must be the mole fraction of ATP plus half the mole fraction of ADP (equation 4-6).

$$\text{energy charge} = \frac{(\text{ATP}) + \frac{1}{2}(\text{ADP})}{(\text{ATP}) + (\text{ADP}) + (\text{AMP})} \tag{4-6}$$

The charge as defined in Equation 4-6 is a linear measure of the metabolic energy stored in the adenine nucleotide system. It is a stoichiometric quantity; a given amount of phosphorylation of ADP, or of use of ATP, will cause the same change in charge at any point along the scale. It is thus closely analogous to the charge of an electric storage cell. In contrast, the "phosphate potential," or free energy of hydrolysis of ATP, varies in a nonstoichiometric way with charge, and is closely analogous to the electrical potential of an electric storage cell. The relation between the energy charge and the phosphoryl potential will be discussed later in this chapter.

At the extremes of the charge scale the composition of the adenine nucleotide pool is fixed, since only AMP is present at a charge of 0 and only ATP at a charge of 1. At any intermediate value of charge, there is a range of possible compositions. If, for the sake of simplicity in the present discussion, we assume that the adenylate kinase reaction (equation 4-4) is at equilibrium, the relative amounts of the three adenine nucleotides will be fixed at any specified value of charge, as seen in Figure 4-1. The concentrations of ATP and AMP vary between 0 and 100%, but the ADP concentration rises to a maximum at 0.5 charge and falls symmetrically as the charge increases to 1.

Because ATP binds Mg^{2+} more firmly than do ADP and AMP, the apparent equilibrium constant for the adenylate kinase reaction varies with the

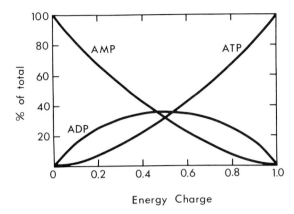

Figure 4-1.   Relative concentrations of ATP, ADP, and AMP as a function of the adenylate energy charge. The adenylate kinase reaction was assumed to be at equilibrium, and a value of 1.2 was used for its effective equilibrium constant, in the direction shown in equation 4-4.

concentration of Mg^{2+}. This point is discussed, with references to earlier work, by Alberty (3). Because of its dependence on Mg^{2+} and because of the difficulty of determining the chemical potential of Mg^{2+} in an intact cell, the value of the apparent equilibrium constant for the adenylate kinase reaction *in vivo* is uncertain. The value is probably never far from 1, and the general shapes of the curves in Figure 4-1 are not changed by small changes in the concentration of Mg^{2+}. As is evident from equation 4-4, a change in the value assumed for the apparent equilibrium constant will change the value calculated for the maximal concentration of ADP. If $K_{app} = 1$, for example, all three curves will intersect at a charge of 0.5, and at this charge each nucleotide will constitute 33% of the total pool. Because of these uncertainties, it should be recognized that Figure 4-1 cannot be a strictly quantitative representation of adenylate kinase equilibrium conditions *in vivo*.

Responses of Enzymes *in Vitro* to the Adenylate Energy Charge

The hypothesis that every metabolic sequence is regulated by the adenylate energy charge in such a way as to contribute to stabilization of the charge has received strong support from studies of enzyme responses *in vitro*. In these studies, a series of tubes containing ATP, ADP, and AMP is prepared in such a way that they represent the desired range of energy charge values and each contains the same adenylate pool level (total concentration of the three nucleotides). The components of the assay mixture are then added and the reaction rate is determined. In the absence of evolutionary design, response curves of many types, rising or falling in different energy charge ranges, would seem equally likely. The curves actually observed show re-markable uniformity. Enzymes that respond to variation in the energy charge fall cleanly into two types corresponding to the two generalized response curves shown in Figure 4-2. This figure was presented in 1968 on the basis of the first such observations (5). Later work has confirmed the expectation that the pattern represented by the figure should be general.

Regulatory enzymes that participate in sequences in which ATP is regen-erated respond to variation in the value of the adenylate energy charge in the general way shown by curve R (Figure 4-2). This is true even when the reac-tion itself consumes ATP. Thus ATP is a substrate for the reaction catalyzed by phosphofructokinase, but that reaction is one of the steps in the degrada-tion of hexose, which leads to the regeneration of many molecules of ATP for each one used in the phosphofructokinase reaction. Evolved regulatory responses reflect metabolic functions of reactions rather than their chemical characteristics; thus phosphofructokinase gives an R-type response. Regu-latory properties of phosphofructokinase will be discussed further in Chap-ter 5.

Regulatory enzymes that participate in sequences in which ATP is utilized respond to variation in the value of the adenylate energy charge in the general way shown by curve U (Figure 4-2). Such sequences usually lead to biosyn-thesis of cell components or to production of storage compounds.

It is clear that the responses generalized in Figure 4-2, with the steep regions of curves of both types in the same range of energy charge, are evolved char-acteristics that contribute to stabilization of the adenylate energy charge. Any tendency for the charge to fall would be resisted by the resulting increase in the fluxes through ATP-regenerating sequences (curve R) and by the de-crease in fluxes through sequences that consume ATP (curve U). By holding

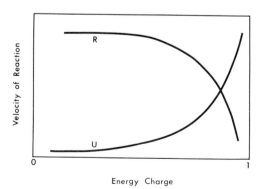

Figure 4-2.   Responses to the energy charge of regulatory enzymes in sequences in which ATP is regenerated (R) and in which it is used (U). From Atkinson (5). Reprinted with per-mission from *Biochemistry* **7**, 4030 (1968). Copyright by the American Chemical Society.

variation in the energy charge within very narrow limits, the types of interactions seen in the figure supply the stable background for operation of all
other types of regulatory effects. Response curves for individual enzymes
are modified and modulated in specific ways by other metabolic inputs, such
the concentration of the end product of a synthetic sequence. Some types of
modulations that have been observed are discussed in Chapter 6. But the
interactions illustrated in Figure 4-2 remain in effect for what may be termed
the weighted average of ATP-regenerating and ATP-utilizing sequences,
and the energy charge remains within the same narrow range in actively
metabolizing cells, whether aerobic or anaerobic, in a rich medium or a
minimal medium, and indeed under any conditions compatible with normal
metabolism, whether rapid or severely limited (Chapter 7).

ROLES OF ADENYLATES IN METABOLISM

Graphical Representation of the Adenylate System

As noted earlier in this chapter in connection with the derivation of the
energy charge concept, the fact that the adenylate system has three components requires somewhat different treatment than would be adequate if only
two compounds were involved. Similar problems arise in connection with
graphical representation. It is of course impossible to represent all possible
states of a three-component system on a two-dimensional graph. However,
a three-component system in which the total concentration is constant has
only two degrees of freedom—that is, specification of any two concentrations
fixes the third. This is also true, of course, for mole fractions even if the total
is not constant; the composition of the mixture is known when any two mole
fractions are determined. Thus, compositions of such systems can be represented on two-dimensional graphs. For this purpose, triangular coordinates,
as illustrated in Figure 4-3, are convenient. On such a graph, each corner
corresponds to a pure compound and the amount of that component in a
mixture is indicated by a linear scale from that corner (100% or a mole fraction of 1.0) to the midpoint of the opposite side (0% or a mole fraction of
0.0). Any point within the triangle specifies the relative concentrations of all
three components. Thus in the figure, point a corresponds to a mixture in
which the mole fractions of A, B, and C are 0.1, 0.1, and 0.8. Corresponding
values for point b are 0.75, 0.1, and 0.15, and for point c, 0.15, 0.6, and 0.25.
The midpoint, where the three axes cross, represents an equimolar mixture
of the three components. Plots of this type are commonly used in physical
chemistry, and were first applied to the adenine nucleotide system by Garland (47).

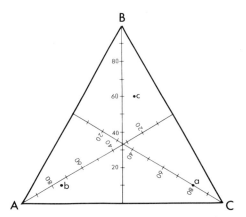

Figure 4-3. Illustration of the triangular composition graph for a three-component system.

Figure 4-4 is a triangular composition plot of the adenine nucleotide system. If the adenylate kinase reaction (equation 4-4) is assumed to be at equilibrium, only one degree of freedom remains, and specification of any one of the three mole fractions fixes the system; thus the locus of possible points becomes a curve rather than an area. This locus is shown in Figure 4-4 by the curve connecting the AMP and ATP corners. This single curve corresponds to all three curves of Figure 4-1, and contains all of the information of that figure.

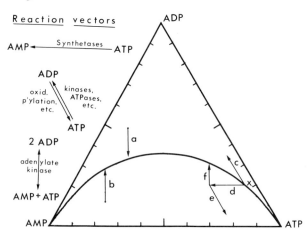

Figure 4-4. Triangular composition graph for the adenine nucleotide system. The curve is the locus of all compositions that are in equilibrium with respect to the adenylate kinase reaction (calculated on the basis of an effective equilibrium constant of 1.2). The vectors to the left of the graph show the effects of different kinds of adenylate interconversions. Vectors inside the triangle are discussed in the text.

Since any possible composition of the adenine nucleotide pool is represented by a point inside the triangle of Figure 4-4, it follows that any reaction involving interconversion of these nucleotides will be represented by a vector on that graph. Orientations of vectors for the major conversions are shown to the left of the triangle. The quantitatively most important group of interconversions, those between ADP and ATP, are represented by vectors parallel to the ADP-ATP side of the triangle. The length of the vector is proportional to the amount of chemical reaction, and the direction, of course, depends on the direction of chemical conversion—ADP to ATP or the reverse. The class of enzymes traditionally termed pyrophosphorylases, which catalyze reactions in which ATP is converted to AMP, are represented by vectors parallel to the base of the triangle as drawn (the AMP-ATP side). As Kornberg pointed out (62), these enzymes should more properly be termed synthetases because they participate in metabolism in a synthetic direction (that is, in the direction indicated by the vector shown in Figure 4-4, with production of AMP), rather than in the direction of pyrophosphorolysis. Because of their ATP coupling coefficient of -2 as compared to -1 for kinases, these reactions contribute strongly to the unidirectionality of biosynthetic sequences. The adenylate kinase reaction is represented by a vector perpendicular to the base of the graph. On the addition of adenylate kinase a composition represented by any point on the graph will be converted to the composition represented by the point at which the adenylate kinase equilibrium curve intersects a vertical line through the initial point. Such reactions are shown in Figure 4-4 by vector **a**, for which the initial mixture was rich in ADP with respect to the equilibrium composition, and vector **b**, for which the initial mixture was poor in ADP.

Interactions among reactions involving adenine nucleotides are conveniently indicated vectorially on the triangular plot, as illustrated by the other vectors in Figure 4-4. Point x represents approximate physiological conditions; an energy charge of 0.85 and equilibrium of the adenylate kinase reaction. Beginning at this point, vector **c** represents the utilization of an amount of ATP equal to 15% of the total adenylate pool in a kinase reaction (or in muscular work, etc.). Phosphorylation of ADP could move the system back along the same vector to the initial point x. Use of the same amount of ATP in a synthetase ("pyrophosphorylase") reaction is represented by vector **d**. The obvious fact that this loss of ATP cannot be made good by electron transport phosphorylation alone is shown graphically by the addition of vector **e** to vector **d**. This graph illustrates the fact that any cell using ATP in reactions that produce AMP (as all cells do) has an absolute dependence on the adenylate kinase reaction (vector **f**) for regeneration of ATP.

The triangular plot is useful in comparison of the free energy of hydrolysis of ATP (often termed the phosphoryl potential) and the energy charge, as shown in Figure 4-5. The base of the triangle represents two-component mixtures of AMP and ATP. In such mixtures, the energy charge is a simple mole fraction of ATP; thus the base of the triangle is a linear energy charge scale. Changes in composition that can be represented by vertical vectors, such as **a** and **b**, do not change the energy charge. In moving vertically upward, 2 moles of ADP are produced for each mole of ATP used, and of course downward movement on the figure corresponds to the opposite conversion; the value of energy charge is not altered by such changes. This is metabolically appropriate, since in the presence of adenylate kinase all compositions corresponding to points on the same vertical line will be converted to the composition corresponding to the intersection of that vertical line with the adenylate kinase curve, as previously discussed in connection with vectors **a** and **b**. Thus pure ADP (represented by the ADP corner of the graph) and an equimolar mixture of ATP and AMP (represented by the midpoint of the base of the graph) will both be converted to the same three-component mixture through the action of adenylate kinase. The resulting mixture will be that represented by the intersection of the adenylate kinase curve with the vertical line connecting points corresponding to the initial conditions. At those initial points, at the final equilibrium point, and at every other point on the same vertical line, the energy charge of the mixture is 0.5.

In a triangular composition plot the three component axes are perpendicular to the three sides, and in most applications of such plots there is no reason

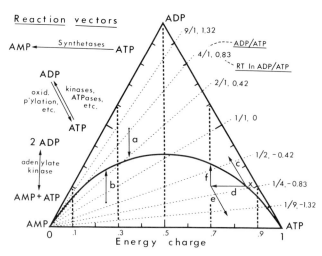

Figure 4-5. Same as Figure 4-4, with addition of lines of constant energy charge and of constant phosphoryl potential.

to indicate a scale along any of the sides. The fact that vertical lines are loci of points of equal energy charge value shows, however, that the base of the triangular plot for the adenine nucleotide system has an important meaning, and a scale along it indicates the energy charge value for any point within the triangle. This is illustrated by the heavy broken lines for energy charge values of 0.1, 0.3, 0.5, 0.7, and 0.9 in the figure. Reaction vectors thus indicate directly the changes in energy charge that result from the corresponding reactions, as well as changes in relative concentrations of the three component nucleotides.

The free energy of hydrolysis, or phosphoryl potential, has been suggested as a parameter for use in study of metabolic regulation. It is evident that, since the triangular plot represents all compositions of the three-component adenylate system, it should be possible to construct loci of constant phosphoryl potential. This is in fact easily done.

During hydrolysis of ATP (equation 4-7), the free energy change is given by equation 4-8. The situation is more complex than might appear from that

$$ATP + H_2O \rightarrow ADP + P_i \qquad\qquad (4\text{-}7)$$

$$\Delta G_h = \Delta G_h{}^0 + RT \ln \frac{(ADP)(P_i)}{(ATP)} \qquad\qquad (4\text{-}8)$$

simple equation, since ATP, ADP, and P_i will all be ionized to an extent depending on the pH, and in the cell will be complexed with cations, especially Mg^{2+}, and bound to proteins and other cell components to varying and generally unknown degrees. The standard free energy term, ΔG^0, corresponds to a specified set of standard conditions. In conventional physical chemical practice, the standard pH is 0, and the standard states of ATP, ADP, and AMP are the un-ionized and uncomplexed molecules at an activity (idealized molarity) of unity.

The value of ΔG_h under specified conditions is of course a fixed and definite value, but it can be partitioned in any of an infinite number of ways for calculation. None of these, including the traditional physical chemical way, is superior to any other; the effective criterion is convenience. It would be inconvenient to use a different set of standard states every time a different situation was considered, because agreement on standard states leads to uniformity of approach and facilitates the storage of data in handbooks. On the other hand, such conventions as standard states are not features of the real world, but only man-made aids to computation, and they may be changed when it seems advantageous to do so. Biochemists almost unanimously have adopted a pH of 7, rather than 0, as the standard state. The standard free energies corresponding to this convention are not the same as ΔG^0, which is referred to pH 0; thus a different symbol is required. There is no uniformity as yet in usage, but $\Delta G'$ is perhaps the most widely used (equation 4-9). In addition, because in biochemical systems it is usually impossible

$$\Delta G_h = \Delta G_h' + RT \ln \frac{(ADP)(P_i)}{(ATP)} \qquad (4\text{-}9)$$

to measure the free and un-ionized forms of reactants or products, it is customary but not universal practice, in biochemical thermodynamic equations such as equation 4-9, to base standard states on total concentrations rather than concentrations of free and uncharged parent molecules. Lack of uniformity in this regard sometimes leads to ambiguity if the conventions used are not specified, but the ambiguity is probably less in most cases than other uncertainties in the systems under consideration.

In comparing equations 4-8 and 4-9 as they might be applied to the same system, it should be emphasized that the two merely represent alternate ways of partitioning the free energy change that accompanies hydrolysis. ΔG_h^0 and $\Delta G_h'$ have different numerical values because they refer to different standard states; (ADP), (P$_i$), and (ATP), although they describe the same situations in the two equations, have different numerical values because they are based on different standard states (the concentration—strictly speaking, the activity—has a value of 1.0 at the standard state by definition). But the value of ΔG_h as calculated from both equations must be identical if the assumptions and measurements are accurate.

Other ways of partitioning ΔG_h between the standard term and the term containing variable concentrations may be useful in specific cases. Many biochemists go a step farther, as described above, and lump the constants for formation of complexes, such as the complexes of phosphate-containing compounds with magnesium ion, into the $\Delta G'$ term. In that case, the concentration terms in equation 4-9 would refer to total concentrations of ADP, P$_i$, and ATP, whether or not complexed with Mg^{2+}, and the value of $\Delta G_h'$ would vary with the concentration of Mg^{2+}. When conventions of this kind are used, the "standard" free energy term is usually called the "apparent standard free energy."

For use with the triangular plot, we will go one step farther yet in lumping terms into the "standard" term. Equation 4-9 can be rewritten as equation

$$\Delta G_h = \Delta G_h' + RT \ln(P_i) + RT \ln \frac{(ADP)}{(ATP)} \qquad (4\text{-}10)$$

4-10 in which the concentration of phosphate has been taken out of the concentration ratio term. On the assumption that the concentration of phosphate is relatively constant, the $RT \ln (P_i)$ term can be added to $\Delta G_h'$. The sum will be symbolized by $\Delta G_h''$, and the resulting expression (4-11) allows us, if we

$$\Delta G_h = \Delta G_h'' + RT \ln \frac{(ADP)}{(ATP)} \tag{4-11}$$

ignore fluctuations in (P_i), to plot lines of constant phosphoryl potential on the triangular composition graph.

From equation 4-11 it is seen that, at constant concentrations of Mg^{2+} and P_i, the phosphoryl potential depends on the ratio of concentrations of ADP and ATP. Thus lines along which that ratio is constant will be loci of constant phosphoryl potential. Such lines radiate from the AMP corner of the plot, and a few are shown in Figure 4-5. Each is labeled with the (ADP)/(ATP) ratio and the value of the term $RT \ln$ (ADP)/(ATP). The values of ΔG_h, the phosphoryl potential, will of course be the values shown on the graph plus $\Delta G_h''$. If, for example, $\Delta G_h''$ at a phosphate concentration of 10 mM is assumed to be -10 kcal/mole, the lines in the figure correspond to ΔG_h values ranging from -11.32 to -8.68 kcal/mole.

In the region of physiological significance, near point x in the figure, lines of constant energy charge and lines of constant phosphoryl potential are nearly perpendicular to each other. Thus, although they depend on some of the same concentrations and can be used in discussion of the same processes, they are far from equivalent. Comparison of vectors **c** and **d** illustrate this lack of equivalence. For the sake of this comparison, $\Delta G_h''$ is taken as -10.0 kcal/mole, but the relationships to be discussed are independent of the value of $\Delta G_h''$. Vectors **c** and **d** represent the utilization of the same amount of ATP. At point x, the charge is 0.85 and $\Delta G_h = -10.77$ kcal/mole. The kinase reaction changes these values to 0.775 and -10.31 (the tip of vector **c**). Use of the same amount of ATP in a synthetase reaction (vector **d**) changes the charge by twice as much (to 0.70), but causes a much smaller change in ΔG_h (to -10.63). This comparison is illustrative only; it seems probable that in the intact cell the action of adenylate kinase simultaneously with kinases or synthetases would cause the composition of a system to move along (or near) the curve representing equilibrium of the adenylate kinase reaction. It is clear, however, that the energy charge, rather than the phosphoryl potential, is the relevant parameter in terms of metabolic stoichiometry; as a consequence of a synthetase reaction, twice as much phosphate must be transferred to the adenylate pool to restore initial conditions as would be needed if the same amount of ATP had been used in a kinase reaction. This is reflected in the relative changes in energy charge values corresponding to the synthetase and kinase reactions. Changes in the phosphoryl potential, however, are not related in any simple or straightforward way to changes in the amount of energy stored in the adenylate system or to the amount of phosphorylation required to restore initial conditions.

Thermodynamic and Kinetic Roles of Adenylates

A dynamic and intricately interrelated chemical system such as a living cell could not exist if it were not specifically organized for stability. Some part of the system must serve as a primary stabilizing entity. In metabolism the adenylates play that stabilizing role, and metabolism is organized around the adenine nucleotides to a remarkable degree.

We considered in Chapters 2 and 3 various related aspects of the thermodynamic involvement of the adenylates. They provide for stoichiometric coupling of all metabolic sequences. They are often involved in production of the activated metabolites that contribute to the conservation of solvent capacity. Most dramatically in terms of the overall organization of metabolism, it is different stoichiometries of use or regeneration of ATP (and of the pyridine nucleotide electron-transfer agents) that lead to the fundamental metabolic pattern of oppositely directed unidirectional pathways. It is this pattern, in turn, that makes kinetic control of metabolism possible, and thus allows for dynamic regulation on the basis of metabolic need. Not only do the adenine nucleotides provide the thermodynamic pattern that makes kinetic regulation possible, but they are also the basis of kinetic control. We have seen in this chapter some of the enzyme responses that underlie kinetic control, and this will be discussed further in the following three chapters.

Because of this evolved pattern of metabolic organization, we must deal with the adenine nucleotides when considering any aspect of metabolic correlation, whether thermodynamic or kinetic. The validity and cogency of our considerations must depend to a considerable degree on the relevance of the parameters that we use. It is thus a matter of more than trivial importance to attempt to choose the most appropriate and useful parameters.

The most obvious parameters, and those that were quite naturally first used in the study of metabolic energetics, are the concentrations of the individual nucleotides, especially ATP. In view of the functions of the adenylate system in stoichiometric coupling of metabolic sequences and in energy transduction, however, it is clear that concentrations of individual components are not relevant. It is the adenylate system as a whole, not one component of it, that couples sequences. And in metabolic energy transduction, as in any other context involving chemical energy, it is concentration ratios, rather than individual concentrations, that are important. We may safely conclude that the concentrations of individual adenine nucleotides (and similarly individual concentrations of the oxidized and reduced forms of the pyridine nucleotides) have little if any applicability to the attempt to understand metabolism. Reports of increases or decreases in the level of ATP *in vivo*, for example, provide little information. Direct experimental observations have confirmed the prediction, based on the functional interrelationships of the adenylate system, that such integrated processes as protein synthesis and growth are much more sensitive to changes in energy charge than to changes in the concentration of ATP (Chapter 7). Similarly, the demonstration *in vitro* that the activity of an enzyme is increased or decreased by changes in the concentration of ATP, ADP, or AMP tells us almost nothing. Enzymes have evolved in the milieu of the living cell, where all three adenine nucleotides are continuously present. It would be difficult to devise an experiment less relevant to the physiological function and the possible regulatory interactions of an enzyme than to test its response *in vitro* to graded levels of ATP, for example, in the absence of ADP and AMP. ATP is never encountered alone in nature; for functional reasons enzymes have evolved responses to ratios of adenine nucleotides; and thus the results of an experiment of the type described are fortuitous responses to totally artificial conditions, and can tell us little or nothing about the responses of the enzyme to changing conditions *in vivo*.

We may thus say definitely that measurements of individual concentrations *in vivo* of adenine or pyridine nucleotides, or observations of the effects of variation of individual concentrations of these coupling agents *in vitro*, are not relevant to the study of metabolic function or metabolic regulation, and that such experiments have no useful place in metabolic enzymology. (They may, of course, be valuable in studies on enzyme-ligand interactions and on mechanisms of modulation of enzymic activity.) In order to have possible relevance to physiological function, experiments dealing with the effects of coupling agents must deal with ratios or mole fractions. Either ratios and related parameters, such as the phosphoryl potential, or mole fractions and related parameters, such as the energy charge, could in principle be used. Neither type of parameter can be said to be entirely inapplicable, as are absolute concentrations, but they differ in degree of relevance in different contexts. The choice between them must depend on convenience, on degree of relevance, and on how well the chosen parameter facilitates consideration of the broader metabolic implications of the enzymic reaction or reaction sequence under study.

We must therefore compare the relative utility of the ATP/ADP ratio, the phosphoryl potential, and the energy charge as aids in the understanding of metabolic energy relationships. The energy charge has the primary advantage that, like other parameters based on mole fractions, it is stoichiometric and thus linear with nearly all conversions of chemical (or metabolic) interest. The value of the energy charge indicates directly the amount of metabolically available energy in the adenylate system, and changes in the energy charge are directly proportional to the net amount of energy that has been put into or removed from the system. The energy charge is compatible with discussions of metabolic stoichiometry in terms of ATP equivalents (Chapter 3). In contrast, a concentration ratio or the phosphoryl potential (which is the logarithm of a concentration ratio plus a constant) is not linear with any measure of extent of chemical change, as was illustrated graphically in the preceding section.

Probably few enzymes interact directly, in their regulatory responses, with all three adenine nucleotides. It has been recognized from the first that most energy charge responses are, at the molecular level, responses to either the ATP/ADP or the ATP/AMP ratio (5). Indeed, the energy charge was first conceived as a framework for comparison of the physiological roles of enzymes that respond to the ATP/ADP ratio with those that respond to ATP/AMP, and for consideration of interactions between enzymes of those two types. It was immediately seen to have broader potentialities. At no time has the energy charge concept implied that individual enzymes must establish meaningful relationships with each of the three adenine nucleotides. Thus, if a worker studied an enzyme "for its own sake" with no interest in its biological function, there would be no reason for him to invoke the adenylate energy charge concept, and the ATP/ADP ratio, for example, might well be an appropriate parameter. If he had no interest in the physiological functioning of his enzyme, however, it is not clear why he should bother with regulatory responses at all. If he is interested in the function of his enzyme *in vivo*, a mole-fraction-based parameter like the energy charge allows much greater opportunity for relating his results to the energy status of the cell, and to the stoichiometric relationships in the cell, than is possible with any other type of parameter.

It is sometimes objected that the energy charge is not a thermodynamic parameter, and that the phosphoryl potential, or free energy of hydrolysis of ATP, is preferable for that reason. This is a dangerous type of argument—a syllogism with one premise stated and the second implied. In one sense the stated premise—that the energy charge is not a thermodynamic parameter—might be disputed. Chemical thermodynamics deals quantitatively with heat, energy, and chemical conversions, and any stoichiometric parameter is at least indirectly thermodynamic. But it is true that the free energy of hydrolysis is a standard thermodynamic quantity, and so is closer to the standard equations of elementary thermodynamics than are parameters based on mole fractions. It does not appear, however, that this point has any bearing on study of the metabolic roles of the adenylate nucleotides or on the study of kinetic regulation of metabolic fluxes. It is the implied premise—the assumption that kinetic regulation can and should be discussed in thermodynamic terms—that is in error. To clarify this point we must recapitulate some aspects of our earlier discussion of metabolic thermodynamics.

The fundamental thermodynamic roles of the adenine nucleotide system were discussed in Chapters 2 and 3. They relate to provision of activated molecules, so that high concentrations can be avoided, and to adjustment of overall equilibrium constants, so that metabolic sequences will be uni-directional and kinetic control will be possible. As we saw in Chapter 3, for each conversion of ATP to ADP that is coupled to a metabolic sequence, the equilibrium ratio of product to reactant concentrations is increased by a factor of about 10^8. Equilibrium constants for most metabolic sequences are extremely large, and the precise value of that factor of about 10^8 can seldom be important. This comment seems to apply even to the simplest type of metabolic pseudocycle, in which each "unidirectional sequence" is a single reaction, and the difference between the two reactions is a single ATP equiva-lent. The phosphofructokinase/fructose diphosphatase pseudocycle may be used again to illustrate this point. We saw in Chapter 3 that under physio-logical conditions the equilibrium ratio of fructose 6-phosphate to fructose diphosphate for the fructose diphosphatase reaction is about 10^4, whereas the equilibrium ratio of fructose diphosphate to fructose 6-phosphate is about 10^4 for the phosphofructokinase reaction. If the equilibrium ratio of ATP to ADP were to be different from the value we assumed by a factor of 10, the phosphoryl potential would increase or decrease by 1.4 kcal/mole, and the difference between the physiological equilibrium ratios of fructose 6-phosphate to fructose diphosphate for the two reactions would increase to about 10^9 or decrease to about 10^7. It is hard to believe that any serious effects would follow directly from that change. The magnitude of the free energy of hydrolysis of ATP and the evolved ATP coupling coefficients of metabolic sequences are such that equilibrium constants are very large, and most sequences are very far from equilibrium. Mass action or "thermody-namic" control of reaction rates could be exerted only in a system very close to equilibrium; thus only in such cases could phosphoryl potential be a direct factor in metabolic regulation. And in addition, in many or most metabolic uses of ATP, orthophosphate is not a direct product. Even if such reactions were at equilibrium and subject to thermodynamic or equilibrium control, the concentration of phosphate would not be directly involved and thus neither would the phosphoryl potential.

The control of metabolic fluxes is in fact kinetic rather than thermody-namic. As we have noted several times in this and the preceding chapter, oppositely directed pairs of reaction sequences, both far from equilibrium, are characteristic of metabolic organization. Thermodynamic control, whether by the phosphoryl potential or by any other similar parameter, is impossible in such cases. Thermodynamic or equilibrium control must by its nature be exerted on a sequence as a whole (a segment of a sequence that is isolated from the remainder of the sequence by kinetic controls may be locally near equilibrium, but this cannot regulate the flux through the sequence). When a sequence is far from equilibrium it cannot be under equilibrium control. Kinetic controls, in contrast, act on specific reactions. Kinetic regulation of the first reaction in a sequence controls the flux through the entire sequence. It is thus no accident that kinetic control of first reactions in sequences ("first committed steps") is a widely observed feature of metabolic regulation. To speak of regulation of a sequence that is far from equilibrium by thermodynamic control of its first step would be to use words without meaning; no actual chemical situation that would fit that description can be imagined.

In summary, individual concentrations of adenine nucleotides are not relevant to the study of metabolic regulation. (This is in contrast to concentrations of individual end products, which are important regulatory parameters affecting biosynthetic rates. The functional and operational differences between these two types of regulation will be considered in Chapter 6.) Concentration ratios, such as ATP/ADP, are involved in regulation of enzymes in probably all metabolic sequences, but this is *kinetic* regulation, acting through effects on the activity of an enzyme or, usually, on its affinity for substrates, and is not mass action, equilibrium, or thermodynamic regulation. Such thermodynamic parameters as the phosphoryl potential are directly related to the evolution of oppositely directed pathways, because the number of ATP equivalents used in a sequence (the summation of the phosphoryl potentials) is one of the factors that determine the overall equilibrium constant. But such parameters have no direct relation to rates, which depend on kinetic controls. When the kinetic effects, which usually depend on ATP/ADP or ATP/AMP concentration ratios, are referred to the adenylate energy charge, a framework is provided for comparison of responses of different enzymes, for relating enzyme responses to the energy state of the cell, and for understanding how the energy charge can be so strongly stabilized in metabolizing cells.

I suggested above that changes of considerable magnitude in the ATP/ADP ratio, and thus in the phosphoryl potential, could hardly lead to drastic thermodynamic effects in metabolism because most sequences are so far from equilibrium. If that suggestion is correct, it follows that strong stabilization of the energy charge (and the ATP/ADP ratio) has not evolved because of thermodynamic advantage. The evolutionary advantage is kinetic. I proposed at the beginning of this chapter that a stable dynamic system containing many interrelated sequences of chemical reactions could exist only if all sequences were regulated by the same central signal. But regulation is necessarily circular in operation, and the other aspect of the situation is that the more complex the system and its interactions, the more important it is that the central signal be stable. Since this signal (the adenylate energy charge) can be stabilized only by its regulation of the balance among all metabolic sequences (each of which, by using or by regenerating ATP, tends either to lower or raise the energy charge), we have come full circle in considering the circular regulatory logic of the cell. Thus a brief recapitulation of some aspects of the mutual interactions between thermodynamic and kinetic aspects of metabolism may be appropriate at this point.

In any regulated system the cause and effect relationships are necessarily circular, so that each feature of the system both controls and is controlled by each other feature. Thus the evolution of metabolic ATP coupling coefficients that provide oppositely directed pairs of unidirectional sequences is a necessary condition for kinetic control, as discussed in the preceding chapter. But the ATP coupling coefficients can determine the direction of each sequence only if the ATP/ADP ratio under physiological conditions is maintained far from its equilibrium value. This ratio can be held far from equilibrium only by kinetic control of each sequence. Thus the central thermodynamic feature of metabolic organization—paired unidirectional sequences—is an absolutely necessary basis for effective kinetic control, but at the same time it is possible only as a consequence of kinetic control. Looking at the same relationships from the other side, we see that effective functional control of all sequences is possible only if they are all thermodynamically favorable at all times, but sequences can be thermodynamically favorable at all times only as a consequence of the kinetic controls that maintain the ATP/ADP ratio. The thermodynamic feature, unidirectional paired pathways, and the kinetic feature, correlated control, are each simultaneously required for and caused by the other. We must be careful, however, not to allow this mutual interdependence, or the fact that the adenine nucleotides are central to both, to confuse our thinking or to blur the very real distinction between the thermodynamic and the kinetic aspects of metabolic organization.

In order that all sequences can be correlated there must be many refinements and secondary controls. For example, different control curves must differ in steepness of response to variation of energy charge, and perhaps slightly in the midpoint of the response, in order that there may be a hierarchy of regulatory responses (reflecting, for example, whether an ATP-consuming sequence is used only to store excess energy, is needed for growth, or is essential for survival). Some experimental evidence for such differences exists (Chapter 6), but they would appear to be logically necessary even if no evidence for them had yet been obtained. Presumably such differential responses can be evolved relatively easily within a narrow range of energy charge values. Storage sequences should be active only at the upper end of the range, and only essential sequences should operate when the charge is at the lower end of its range. It would be much more difficult to evolve or design a system in which many sequences responded to the value of the energy charge with different sensitivities, and maintained the same relative sensitivities over a wide range of energy charge values. In fact, it would probably be impossible, since the steeper the response the narrower the energy charge range over which it can be exerted. Thus the evolutionary advantage of stabilization of concentration ratios and mole fractions of the adenine nucleotides seems clearly to be that such stabilization is essential to functional kinetic correlation of the diverse metabolic activities of a living cell.

SUMMARY

In a complex and dynamic system like a living cell, stabilization of concentrations is essential, and homeostasis has been recognized for years to be an important characteristic of life. When its component parts are far from equilibrium, such a system can be stabilized only by kinetic controls. The adenine nucleotides, since they are operationally linked with all metabolic sequences, are ideally situated to be the agents of this control, and the responses of enzymes *in vitro* lend strong support to the assumption that these nucleotides do in fact serve that function *in vivo*.

Mole fractions, being linearly related to extent of chemical change, are more convenient for use in a metabolic context than are concentration ratios. The effective mole fraction of ATP in the adenine nucleotide pool (the energy charge; the actual mole fraction of ATP plus half the mole fraction of ADP) is the stoichiometric measure of the amount of metabolically available energy stored in the adenylate system. Hence it is a convenient parameter for use in the study of metabolic regulation.

The thermodynamic and kinetic aspects of the participation of the adenine nucleotides in metabolism should be clearly distinguished. Metabolic reactions are made physiologically unidirectional by the thermodynamic effect of the number of ATP-to-ADP or of ADP-to-ATP conversions to which they are stoichiometrically coupled; because the ATP/ADP concentration ratio is far from equilibrium in the cell, the overall equilibrium constant of a metabolic sequence can be set at any useful value by evolution of an appropriate number of interactions with ATP. Two oppositely directed sequences, coupled to different numbers of ATP-to-ADP conversions, make up the basic unit of metabolic organization. Each sequence is always thermodynamically favorable because of differences in ATP coupling. This thermodynamic feature allows for kinetic controls which determine what conversions will actually occur. The ATP/ADP and ATP/AMP ratios, most conveniently expressed in terms of the adenylate energy charge, are among the most important kinetic regulatory inputs. It is these kinetic effects of the adenine nucleotides that modulate the rates of ATP-regenerating and ATP-utilizing sequences so as to maintain the essential and basic thermodynamic feature of an ATP/ADP concentration ratio far from equilibrium. Thus the thermodynamic and kinetic roles of the adenylates, although conceptually quite distinct, are totally interdependent functionally. Neither could exist, nor would serve any purpose if it did exist, without the other.

5

Enzymes as Control Elements

Metabolism is the sum of a large number of reactions, all of which are catalyzed by enzymes. It is obvious, however, that no mixture of catalysts with fixed properties could possibly result in a complex regulated system of the type that we know metabolism to be. Many of the catalysts must be control elements as well—that is, their catalytic properties must vary in response to the momentary needs of the cell. I have previously compared enzymes to vacuum tubes or transistors (8). The vacuum tube is primarily a device for conducting electricity, just as the enzyme is a device for catalyzing reactions. But mere conduction is not enough. Bits of copper wire are cheaper than tubes and much better conductors, but one cannot replace the vacuum tubes or transistors by copper wires and expect a television set to continue to function. It is not enough that currents flow; their magnitudes must be precisely modulated if a picture, changing with time, is to be produced. Similarly, the regulatory properties of enzymes are fully as important as their catalytic properties. Mere catalysis of reactions would lead to nothing resembling a living cell; the rates of the reactions must be very precisely modulated if a functional and homeostatically stable cell is to result. The common definition of an enzyme as a protein catalyst is thus as incomplete as would be the definition of a vacuum tube or transistor as a current-carrying device. Both definitions are true as far as they go, but both miss the main point.

In the most fundamental sense, the great selectivity of enzymes, together with their enormous catalytic power, has regulatory consequences of the greatest significance. As was discussed in Chapter 2, the presence of specific enzymes results in selection, for each metabolite, of one or a few reactions from among several that are chemically possible. The consequence of these many selections is an orderly metabolic system with discrete pathways (although they branch and anastomose freely) rather than a formless and

109

chaotic muddle of random reactions. But, although we are probably justified in considering the great catalytic effectiveness and high selectivity of enzymes to be their primary regulatory characteristics, more specific regulatory properties, involving modulation of catalytic activity, are also essential to life. Regulation is not a later development superposed on metabolism after catalysis had become well-established—a mere refinement added to an already functioning system. Regulation is the most fundamental difference between living and nonliving systems, and it must have coevolved with other properties of life from the beginning.

This chapter deals in an elementary way with some aspects of enzyme behavior that appear to be related to metabolic control. We will not discuss the purportedly more sophisticated approaches to enzyme kinetics, because those approaches have been well reviewed elsewhere and because little, if any, contact between the parameters and equations of that type of enzyme kinetics and the study of metabolism and its control is yet apparent. At the present stage of development of our understanding of enzyme kinetics and of metabolic regulation, a modified Michaelis approach seems to supply the best basis for discussion of regulatory properties of enzymes. We will therefore consider this approach and some of its consequences.

The most fundamental characteristic of enzyme catalysis is that it occurs at a surface. Although an enzyme solution can be considered by some criteria to be a true solution, and thus a single phase, an enzyme-catalyzed reaction is in its essential features a heterogeneous reaction (one catalyzed at a phase boundary) rather than a homogeneous reaction (one occurring in a single phase, usually in solution in a liquid). Whether an enzyme is to be considered a protein molecule in true solution or a small solid particle in suspension (thus a separate phase) depends on the context. In any consideration of enzyme-catalyzed reactions the latter is the valid approach. Many features of enzyme-catalyzed reactions are attributable to the fact that they occur at discrete and specific sites at what is in effect a solid-liquid phase boundary.

SINGLE OR NONINTERACTING SITES

The rates of first-order homogeneous reactions typically increase linearly with the concentration of substrates (Figure 5-1A). The maximal rate of a heterogeneous reaction may, in contrast, be limited by the number of catalytic sites available (Figure 5-1B). The observation that rates of enzyme-catalyzed reactions depend on substrate concentration as indicated in Figure 5-1B, with the maximal rate being proportional to the amount of enzyme present, led Brown to suggest that such reactions are catalyzed at

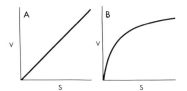

Figure 5-1. Dependence of reaction velocity (v) on reactant concentration (S) for a typical first-order homogeneous reaction (A) and for a reaction catalyzed at a limited number of non-interacting sites (B).

discrete sites and Henri to derive the corresponding equation [see Segal (*107*) for a brief discussion of the early development of concepts regarding enzyme action]. Michaelis and Menten applied Henri's equation to the reaction catalyzed by sucrose hydrolase. Curves like that of Figure 5-1B have since been known as Michaelis curves, and the corresponding equation as the Michaelis equation. In spite of its familiarity, we will briefly review the derivation of the Michaelis equation because of its importance to our consideration of regulatory enzyme activity.

A simple one-substrate, one-product enzyme-catalyzed reaction may be represented by equation 5-1. (This equation and our derivation are slightly

$$E + S \underset{k_2}{\overset{k_1}{\rightleftharpoons}} ES \underset{k_4}{\overset{k_3}{\rightleftharpoons}} EP \underset{k_6}{\overset{k_5}{\rightleftharpoons}} E + P \qquad (5\text{-}1)$$

generalized from the original.) We begin with the reasonable assumption that k_3 and k_4, the constants for the actual reaction, are small in comparison with k_1, k_2, k_5, and k_6, the constants for binding and dissociation. If this assumption is valid, the enzyme, the substrate, and the enzyme-substrate complex will remain nearly at equilibrium during the course of the reaction, since the relatively slow draining off of ES by conversion to EP will not significantly perturb the mobile binding equilibrium. Enzyme, product, and the enzyme-product complex will also be at virtual equilibrium. Since the Michaelis treatment deals only with initial conditions, the concentration of product is considered to be effectively zero. From the equilibrium assumption, it follows that the concentration of the complex EP is also close to zero. The premise that the chemical reaction is slow relative to the association and dissociation steps has two consequences that are the heart of the Michaelis treatment:

(1) The rate of the overall reaction is proportional to the concentration of the enzyme-substrate complex (equation 5-2). This statement that

$$\text{velocity} = k_3(\text{ES}) \qquad (5\text{-}2)$$

the net reaction is equal to the forward reaction is based, of course, on the assumption that the concentration of EP can be taken to be zero. Otherwise, the reverse reaction, with a velocity of k_4(EP), would be subtracted from k_3(ES) to obtain the net reaction rate.

(2) The enzyme is partitioned between free enzyme and the ES complex (equation (5-3). This equation explicitly states that (EP) = 0.

$$(E)_T = (E) + (ES) \qquad (5\text{-}3)$$

It is important to emphasize that the basic assumption of the Michaelis treatment is that association-dissociation steps are fast in comparison with the chemical reaction itself; that as a consequence the concentration of EP during the initial stages of the reaction is zero; and that the two other statements that are sometimes termed assumptions of the treatment [$v = k_3$(ES) and $(E)_T = (E) + (ES)$] are not in fact assumptions, but consequences of the primary assumption. This is important because failure to appreciate the logical basis of the Michaelis treatment led Briggs and Haldane to accept the two consequences while rejecting the assumption on which they are based, and to suggest a supposed generalization of the Michaelis treatment that is not generally valid, but that is still widely encountered (see Appendix C).

If the Michaelis assumption is accepted, the rate constants for association and dissociation (k_1, k_2, k_5, and k_6) can be replaced by equilibrium constants. That is, if ES is virtually in equilibrium with E and S, the absolute values of k_1 and k_2 will have no effect on the velocity of the overall reaction; only their ratio, the association constant, will be relevant. Because the association constant has the dimensions of reciprocal concentration, Michaelis used its inverse, the dissociation constant $K = k_2/k_1$, in his derivation. This constant conveniently has the dimensions of concentration.

From the defining equation 5-4 we obtain equation 5-5. The term (S)/K

$$K = (E)(S)/(ES) \qquad (5\text{-}4)$$

$$(ES)/(E) = (S)/K \qquad (5\text{-}5)$$

was termed the "reduced substrate concentration" by Straus and Goldstein in a perceptive discussion of the consequences of Michaelis kinetics (*113*). It is substrate concentration normalized to take the affinity of the enzyme for the substrate into account.

Using equation 5-3, the left-hand side of equation 5-5 may be converted to (ES)/[(E)$_T$ − (ES)]. We assume (equation 5-2) that v = k_3(ES). Then when the catalytic sites are saturated with substrate, so that (ES) = (E)$_T$, we will observe the maximal velocity V_m.

$$V_m = k_3(E)_T \qquad (5\text{-}6)$$

By substitution, equation 5-5 becomes equation 5-7. The two terms in

$$\frac{v}{V_m - v} = \frac{(S)}{K} \equiv \phi \qquad (5\text{-}7)$$

this form of the Michaelis equation, $v/(V_m - v)$ and $(S)/K$ (which we will term ϕ) are the fundamental parameters in the Michaelis treatment. The equation illustrates that, for any enzyme for which the Michaelis assumption applies, the velocity relative to maximal velocity is fixed by the value of ϕ. This is the generalized form of the equation, in which velocities are normalized relative to maximal or saturation velocity and substrate concentrations are normalized relative to the Michaelis constant, giving a linear equation in dimensionless terms that allows direct comparison between enzymes, or between two or more ligands competing for the same catalytic site.

From equation 5-7 we may obtain an expression for K in terms of substrate concentration and reaction velocity (equation 5-8), from which follows

$$K = (S)[(V_m - v)/v] \qquad (5\text{-}8)$$

the operational definition of the Michaelis constant as the substrate concentration at which the reaction velocity is half of the maximal velocity.

Although the expression $v/(V_m - v)$ is in a sense the most fundamental normalized velocity parameter in the Michaelis treatment, since it is linearly proportional to substrate concentration, with the Michaelis constant as the proportionality factor (equation 5-8), it is sometimes more convenient to use the simple fraction of maximal velocity, v/V_m. Solving equation 5-8 for v/V_m gives equation 5-9. This is the form of the relationship

$$\frac{v}{V_m} = \frac{(S)}{K + (S)} = \frac{\phi}{\phi + 1} \qquad (5\text{-}9)$$

that is usually referred to as the Michaelis equation by biochemists. If this fraction is defined as θ, equation 5-7 becomes equation 5-10. Equation 5-9

$$\phi = \frac{\theta}{1 - \theta} \qquad (5\text{-}10)$$

similarly is converted to equation 5-11.

$$\theta = \frac{\phi}{1 + \phi} \qquad (5\text{-}11)$$

Since 1956 many regulatory enzymes, which respond to changes in the concentrations of modifier metabolites by changes in the kinetic Michaelis constant with little or no change in the maximal velocity observed when the substrate is present at saturating concentrations, have been discovered. The existence of enzymes with such properties is a strong argument for quasiequilibrium between enzyme, substrate, and enzyme-substrate complex, as is assumed in the Michaelis approach. When the kinetic Michaelis constant changes, the relation between free substrate and the ES complex must be altered; since the maximal velocity is unchanged, it follows that association between enzyme and substrate must not be a rate-determining step; that is, substrate binding is so fast that changes in its rate have no effect on the velocity of the overall reaction. If that is true, k_1 and k_2 (and their ratio) can be modulated by the concentrations of metabolite modifiers with the result that, as is observed for most regulatory enzymes, the Michaelis constant is affected and the maximal velocity is not. If we assumed that the Michaelis concept did not hold, and that the rate of association contributed to determination of the overall reaction velocity, we could explain the observed results only by highly unlikely *ad hoc* assumptions involving changes in velocity constants that, under a wide variety of conditions, exactly counter each other and lead to constant maximal velocity. The Razor of Occam (the concept that simple explanations are to be preferred to complex ones) must be used with care in biology. Nevertheless, in this case its use seems justified. Interactions between enzymes, substrates, and modifiers are extremely complex in detail, but for many enzymes their general aspects fit much more easily into the simple Michaelis framework than into any other.

Metabolic Significance of Michaelis Constants*

During the past 20 years, primarily as a result of work on regulatory enzymes, the affinity of an enzyme for its substrate has come to be recognized as one of its most important functional characteristics. Michaelis constants had earlier been determined as part of the routine characterization of newly discovered enzymes, but they were not recognized to have any special functional significance. Indeed, for a number of years (about 1955 to 1970) it was rather widely believed that the Michaelis assumption is seldom if ever valid, and some textbooks and other discussions still deprecate the Michaelis approach. The statement ". . . there is no validity whatsoever for the widely held notion that K_s, determined from steady-state kinetics, is necessarily even a distant approximation of the enzyme-substrate affinity constant. Nor is it possible to decide even the relative affinities of different substrates for an enzyme from steady-state determinations of k_3 and K_s . . . . The term K_s can be considered only a constant characteristic of the particular enzyme-

---

* Some of the concepts in this section have been discussed in earlier papers (*7, 12*).

substrate system, which sets an upper limit to the enzyme-substrate affinity constant and is useful for the determination of the degree of saturation of the enzyme at various substrate concentrations but is of no further signfi-cance . . ." (*107*) probably expresses the view of most enzyme kineticists (and of a smaller fraction of metabolic biochemists) in the period around 1960. This viewpoint seems to have been based to a large degree on the demonstration that when peroxidases interact with the substrate hydrogen peroxide the absorption spectrum of the heme group changes. The new spectra were taken to be those of enzyme-peroxide complexes. This assump-tion allowed calculation of purported velocity constants for all steps in the reaction pathway from spectrophotometric observations coupled with fast-reaction techniques. The calculated ratio k_2/k_1 differed from the kinetic Michaelis constant by a large factor, and this was thought to show that the Michaelis assumption was not valid (*27*).

If Complex (or Compound) I, the species responsible for the changed spectrum, had been an enzyme-substrate complex, the abandonment of the Michaelis assumption, at least for peroxidases, would have been warranted. However, George showed in 1953 (*48*) that Compound I is an oxidized form of the enzyme rather than an enzyme-peroxide complex. This demonstra-tion seems now to be generally accepted (*104*). There is no evidence as to whether peroxidases form enzyme-substrate complexes in the usual sense; their lack of specificity for electron donors (phenols, aromatic amines, alcohols, and many other organic compounds as well as some inorganic ions such as nitrite will serve) suggests that peroxidases may be designed for efficient acquisition and donation of electrons on collision, and may differ significantly in catalytic mechanism from typical enzymes.

In any case, the spectrophotometric observations on peroxidases are now seen to be irrelevant to the question of the general validity of the Michaelis assumption. We are probably justified in assuming that for the enzymes with which we are interested in the study of metabolic regulation, the catalytic step is the slow step, and the (variable) affinities of an enzyme for its various substrates and modifiers are among its most biologically important features.

The Symbol $(S)_{0.5}$

At this point, we will discontinue use of the term Michaelis constant and substitute the symbol $(S)_{0.5}$ (*66*). This symbol represents the concentration of substrate at which the reaction velocity is half of the velocity at saturating levels of substrate; thus for an enzyme catalyzing a simple first-order reac-tion, $(S)_{0.5}$ is identical with the (kinetic) Michaelis constant. The symbol $(S)_{0.5}$ will be used instead of K_m for two reasons: (a) The symbol has great flexibility. $(S)_{0.5}$ is one member of a family of symbols (*4*) that can be used to express a number of related and useful parameters. For example, $(S)_{0.25}$

represents the concentration of substrate at which the reaction velocity is 0.25 times that at substrate saturation; $(M)_{0.5}$ is the concentration of a modifier at which the effect on the enzyme is half of that at a saturating concentration of the modifier, and so on. This notation lends itself readily to explicit specification of the ligand involved; such terms as $(\text{pyruvate})_{0.5}$ or $(NAD^+)_{0.5}$ are self-explanatory. (b) The use of $(S)_{0.5}$ avoids the implication that this parameter is a constant. The most common effect of metabolite modifiers on regulatory enzymes is change of affinity for substrate. It seems undesirable to use K, the universal symbol for a constant (and to use the name "Michaelis constant") for a variable parameter.

For a simple first-order enzyme with no known modifiers $(S)_{0.5}$ is constant and is identical with the Michaelis constant, but it should be emphasized that $(S)_{0.5}$ is variable for most regulatory enzymes. In these cases, one therefore cannot speak of *the* $(S)_{0.5}$, but must specify the reaction conditions. Further, $(S)_{0.5}$ is the substrate concentration at which the reaction rate is half that at substrate saturation, with all other conditions unchanged—not half of a "maximal V_m" observed under ideal conditions.

Relation between $(S)_{0.5}$ *and Physiological Concentration*

Trevelyan in 1958 (*117*) seems to have been the first to suggest that Michaelis constants usually approximate the physiological levels of the corresponding substrates. Further work has confirmed this prediction. Cause-and-effect relationships are circular in metabolism, and the relationship is equally meaningful if stated in reverse—the physiological steady-state levels of metabolites usually approximate the $(S)_{0.5}$ values of the enzymes for which they serve as substrates. Probably the generalization should be modified slightly—it seems likely that these concentrations are usually somewhat below the corresponding $(S)_{0.5}$ values. This is equivalent to saying that enzymes, under usual conditions *in vivo*, probably catalyze reactions at less than 50% of their maximal velocities. An apparent advantage of this situation is illustrated in Figure 5-2. For a typical first-order homogeneous reaction, the reaction velocity is a linear function of reactant concentration (Figure 5-2A and B). Thus an increase in reactant concentration would result in a proportional increase in the rate at which the reactant was consumed and a new steady state would be established. The situation is quite different when enzymic catalysis is involved. As discussed earlier, the catalytic specificity and the regulation of catalytic activity that are characteristic of living systems could be achieved only by heterogeneous catalysis. But the evolution of surface catalysts with a limited number of discrete and specific catalytic sites led to a problem that would not arise with homogeneous reactions. As also discussed earlier, such catalysts can be saturated with substrate; consequently, curves of reaction velocity as a function of

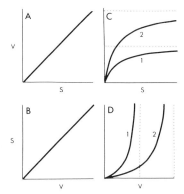

Figure 5-2. Dependence of reaction velocity (v) on reactant concentration (S) for a first-order homogeneous reaction (A and B) and for a typical enzymic reaction following simple Michaelis kinetics (C and D). The two curves in panels C and D represent amounts of enzyme differing by a factor of 2, and the broken lines show the value of V_{max} for each level of enzyme.

substrate concentration will asymptotically approach a maximal value (Figure 5-2C, curve 1). The same relationship is shown, with exchange of coordinates, in Figure 5-2D. As the reaction velocity approaches V_m, increasingly large increases in substrate concentration are needed for each further increment of velocity. The potential danger of this situation is evident when we remember that in the cell the substrate is not furnished in an initial batch amount, as is usual when enzymes catalyze reactions in the laboratory, but is supplied continually through the action of other enzymes. Thus for many enzymes *in vivo* it is appropriate to consider v to be the independent variable, with (S) dependent on it, as is implied by Figure 5-2D. In the metabolic sequence of equation 5-12, if the rate of conversion of R

$$\cdots \rightarrow R \rightarrow S \overset{E}{\rightarrow} T \rightarrow \cdots \qquad (5\text{-}12)$$

to S should approach V_m for enzyme E, the concentration of substrate S would rise to a very high level before a steady state could be established in which S would be used as rapidly as it was produced. If the rate of production of substrate should exceed V_m for enzyme E, a steady state would be impossible and the concentration of substrate would rise catastrophically. The consequences of high concentrations have been discussed earlier; a large increase in the concentration of one or more metabolites would be deleterious and, depending on the reactivity of the metabolite and other factors, could easily be lethal.

Several prerequisites for a stable metabolic sequence are evident from the simple relationships shown in Figure 5-2C and D. (a) The amount of each enzyme must be sufficient to deal with its substrate at the maximal rate at which it will be supplied. In Figure 5-2C and D, curve 2 represents the same situation as curve 1, but with the enzyme at twice the concentration. It is obvious that a rate of supply of substrate that would be disastrous at the lower enzyme level would pose no problems if the enzyme concentration were doubled. (b) As a corollary to (a), the enzymes in a sequence should be present at concentrations causing them to have approximately equal V_m values (or the later enzymes in a sequence should be present at higher activities than the earlier ones). This will minimize the danger that any metabolite will be produced at a rate greater than that at which it can react. (c) The concentration of substrates should be low enough (probably somewhat below the $(S)_{0.5}$ values of the corresponding enzymes) to allow for a reasonable range within which the concentration can fluctuate safely. The margin of safety would increase with each increase in the value of $(S)_{0.5}$, assuming that the concentration of substrate remained constant. But an increase in $(S)_{0.5}$ is a decrease in the affinity of the enzyme for substrate; if $(S)_{0.5}$ increases, the fraction of catalytic sites that bind substrate will decrease. Then reaction velocity will be a smaller fraction of V_m and more enzyme will be necessary if the concentration of substrate is not to rise. Thus an increase in the value of $(S)_{0.5}$ relative to the steady-state concentration of substrate can be achieved only if the amount of enzyme is increased (unless the value of V_m also increases). Increase in the amount of protein committed to a given reaction must in general be detrimental to the organism, as we discussed in Chapter 2. Thus, the relation between $(S)_{0.5}$ and the steady-state level of substrate, like any other feature of a cell, will result from a design compromise. This relationship must be expected to vary between enzymes, depending on such factors as the activity of the metabolite in question, the toxicity of products of its side reactions, the extent to which the metabolic flux through a sequence fluctuates, and the like. It may be safe to guess that the concentration of substrates in the unstressed cell at steady state will often be between 20 and 100% of the corresponding $(S)_{0.5}$ values. If so, the reaction velocity will be between about 15 and 50% of the saturation velocity.

Relation between $(S)_{0.5}$ and $(P)_{0.5}$

A catalytic site necessarily has some affinity for the product of the reaction that is catalyzed at that site and can catalyze the reverse reaction if it becomes thermodynamically favorable. Most enzymes catalyze reactions in only one direction in the intact cell, however. The reasons for expecting that $(S)_{0.5}$ for the substrate should be close to or somewhat greater than the physiological concentration of substrate have just been discussed. In general, there will be no such evolutionary pressure to cause the dissociation constant for product, $(P)_{0.5}$, to approximate the physiological steady-state concentration of product. On the contrary, we may predict that $(P)_{0.5}$ values should generally be considerably larger than the concentration of product. Because P is formed at the catalytic site from S, its binding site is the same, in whole or part, as that of S; thus P must always be a competitive inhibitor of S. A value of $(P)_{0.5}$ that is large in relation to the physiological concentration of P will reduce the degree of competition and presumably will generally have selective advantage. When a given reaction $(A \rightleftharpoons B)$ is known to proceed in either direction *in vivo*, depending on need, and two isozymes capable of catalyzing the reaction are found, it may thus be reasonable to assume that the enzyme with the lower value of $(A)_{0.5}$ will catalyze the conversion of A to B *in vivo* and the enzyme with the lower $(B)_{0.5}$ will catalyze the reverse reaction. This interpretation of such differences is rather widely accepted and seems to be supported by the limited amount of relevant experimental evidence that is available. The opposite suggestion—that the affinity of enzymes for product should exceed that for substrate for kinetic reasons—has been proposed (*38*) but the rationale offered for it seems unconvincing (*8*).

Relation between $(S)_{0.5}$ and $(P)_{0.5}$ for Coupling Agents

The foregoing discussion of reasons why we may expect the $(S)_{0.5}$ value for a substrate of an enzyme reaction to be smaller than that for the product applies to substrates of the ordinary kind; that is, to intermediates in metabolic sequences. The situation is different when we consider metabolic coupling agents such as the adenine and pyridine nucleotides. We discussed in Chapter 3 the need for the ratios of the different forms of the coupling agents to be protected against wide fluctuations, and in Chapter 4 the types of responses to variation in adenylate energy charge that appear to participate in stabilizing the ratio in the case of the adenylates. We will now consider how such responses may be obtained by simple interactions at the catalytic site, without any need for a separate regulatory site.

The general reaction catalyzed by a dehydrogenase is represented by equation 5-13. Just as for other substrate-product pairs, NAD^+ and NADH

$$SH + NAD^+ \rightleftharpoons S + NADH + H^+ \qquad (5\text{-}13)$$

must bind at the same site; thus, as discussed above for substrates generally, NADH is necessarily a competitive inhibitor for NAD^+. In the case of metabolic intermediates it seems desirable that the extent of this competition should be minimized by evolution of a site with greater affinity for substrate than for product, but in the case of cyclically acting coupling agents competition between product and substrate has been put to very important use in regulation.

The effect of variation in the relative affinities for NAD^+ and NADH at the catalytic site of a dehydrogenase is shown in Figure 5-3. Each curve

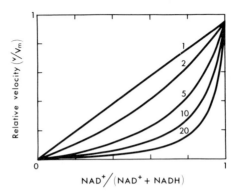

Figure 5-3. Fraction of dehydrogenase catalytic sites at which NAD^+ is bound (and therefore relative reaction velocity) as a function of the mole fraction of NAD^+; effect of relative affinities of the site for NAD^+ and NADH. The figures identifying the curves indicate the affinity ratio by which binding of NADH is favored. The Michaelis constant for NAD^+ was held constant at 0.05 times the pyridine nucleotide pool (NAD^+ + NADH) and curves were calculated for Michaelis constants for NADH of 0.05, 0.025, 0.01, 0.005, and 0.0025 times the pool size.

shows the percent of the catalytic sites that would bind NAD^+ as a function of the mole fraction of NAD^+ in a NAD^+-NADH mixture. Since only sites bearing NAD^+ can catalyze the oxidation of a substrate, the vertical coordinate should be proportional to reaction velocity, assuming the concentration of the substrate to be constant. When the two nucleotides are bound with equal affinity, the NAD^+-binding curve is a linear function of NAD^+ mole fraction. When the affinities differ, the curves are nonlinear. When the affinity for NADH is about three to four times that for NAD^+ [that is, when $(NAD^+)_{0.5}$ is three or four times as large as $(NADH)_{0.5}$] the calculated curves closely resemble those obtained experimentally for the enzymes with which experiments of this type have been done: isocitrate dehydrogenase from yeast (*20*) and pyruvate dehydrogenase from *E. coli* (*109*).

When the fraction of kinase catalytic sites binding ATP is plotted against the adenylate energy charge (Figure 5-4), the family of curves obtained is nearly identical to that of Figure 5-3. Because of the third component, AMP, the plot for equal affinities is not quite linear, and the shapes of the other curves are slightly different. Either figure illustrates the types of regulatory response that can be obtained by simple competition at the catalytic site of an enzyme following ordinary first-order Michaelis kinetics.

It is immediately obvious from Figure 5-4 that when the affinity for ADP is about five times that for ATP the calculated curve resembles the curves of response to adenylate energy charge that have been observed for enzymes of ATP-utilizing sequences (Chapter 4). This resemblance is not accidental;

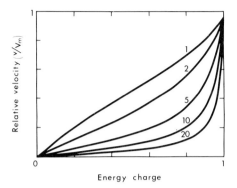

Figure 5-4. Fraction of kinase catalytic sites at which ATP is bound (and hence relative reaction velocity) as a function of the adenylate energy charge; effect of relative affinities of the site for ATP and ADP. The figures identifying the curves indicate the affinity ratio by which binding of ADP is favored. The Michaelis constant for ATP was fixed at 0.05 times the adenine nucleotide pool (ATP + ADP + AMP) and curves were calculated for Michaelis constants for ADP of 0.05, 0.025, 0.01, 0.005, and 0.0025 times the pool size.

evolutionary adjustment of relative affinities at kinase active sites is probably the most common way that U-type responses to energy charge have been produced. Kinase reactions consume ATP, and the great majority of kinases participate in sequences with an overall requirement for ATP, for which a U-type response is therefore appropriate.

The term "regulatory enzyme" is sometimes taken to imply the existence of one or more regulatory sites at which molecules of modifier bind. Figures 5-3 and 5-4 show clearly that this usage is not justified. A U-type response is necessary for proper regulation of sequences that utilize ATP; such a response has regulatory significance no matter how it is obtained. Indeed, it seems quite evident on evolutionary grounds that regulation is likely to be exerted by direct effects at the catalytic site whenever the type of regulation that is metabolically advantageous can be obtained in this way. New functions, sites, or interactions are very much less likely to be evolved than are modifications of existing ones. When a site necessarily binds ATP and ADP, for example, the relative affinities for the two ligands will be subject to modification by random mutation, and the most advantageous ratio will be selected. Thus, response curves like any of those in Figures 5-3 and 5-4 could be evolved without any need for the relatively very unlikely development of a separate site on the enzyme capable of binding a modifier and interacting in the appropriate way with the catalytic site.

Early experimental evidence for saturation of the adenine nucleotide site and for a higher affinity for ADP than for ATP is shown in Figure 5-5. For both phosphoribosyl pyrophosphate synthase (*61*) and ADP-glucose syn-

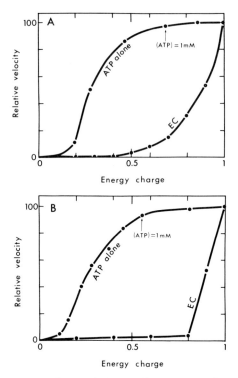

Figure 5-5.   Comparison, for two ATP-requiring enzymes, of response to variation in the value of the adenylate energy charge with response to the concentration of ATP in the absence of ADP and AMP. A: Phosphoribosyl pyrophosphate synthase from *Escherichia coli*. The reaction mixture (1.0 ml) contained 60 mM potassium phosphate buffer (pH 7.5), 6mM MgCl$_2$, 0.5 mM ribose 5-P, enzyme, and (lower curve) a total adenylate pool (AMP + ADP + ATP) of 2 mM, at the energy charge values indicated on the abscissa. The upper curve shows the velocity observed when ATP was added in the absence of ADP and AMP, with each point plotted at the energy charge value at which the amount of ATP in the 2 mM pool would equal the amount used in the "ATP alone" assays. Modified from Klungsøyr *et al.* (*61*). B: Adenosine diphosphate glucose synthase from *E. coli*. The reaction mixture (0.2 ml) contained 0.3 mM glucose 1-P, 7.5 mM MgCl$_2$, 50 mM Tris-Cl (pH 8.0), 50 μg of bovine serum albumin, 0.5 μg of yeast pyrophosphatase, enzyme, and (lower curve) a total adenylate pool (AMP + ADP + ATP) of 3 mM, at the energy charge values indicated on the abscissa. The upper curve shows velocity observed with ATP alone, as explained for A. Modified from Shen and Atkinson (*108*). The shapes of the "ATP only" curves do not reflect cooperative binding of ATP; they result only from the nonlinear increase of ATP concentration with increase in energy charge.

thase (*108*), the reaction velocity has nearly its maximal value, indicating that the catalytic site is nearly saturated, at an ATP concentration of 1 mM. Since this is well below the physiological concentration of ATP, it is clear that the adenine nucleotide binding site will be virtually saturated *in vivo*.

The shape of the energy charge response curves can be seen, by comparison with Figure 5-4, to result from a considerably higher affinity for ADP than for ATP. Alternatively, the relative affinities may also be deduced qualitatively from Figure 5-5 without reference to Figure 5-4. At an energy charge of 0.5 the concentrations of ADP and ATP are approximately equal, yet in both cases the velocity of the reaction at a charge of 0.5 was much less than half of the velocity observed when the same amount of ATP was present as the only adenine nucleotide. That fact alone shows that ADP is bound much more strongly than is ATP. The shape of the response curve for phosphoribosyl pyrophosphate synthase (Figure 5-4A) is reasonably typical of those for biosynthetic enzymes with which such experiments have been done; the response of ADP-glucose synthase is the steepest yet seen. In both cases the adenine nucleotide pools used (2 and 3 mM) were somewhat below the probable concentrations *in vivo*. If a more physiological concentration of 4 or 5 mM had been used, the difference between the two curves would have been about twice as great in each case. That difference would represent the true physiological situation more accurately, but the relationships involved—high affinity for adenine nucleotides relative to physiological concentrations and higher affinity for ADP than for ATP— are clearly evident even from the curves of Figure 5-5.

Regulatory Sites for Coupling Agents

When regulation on the basis of the concentration of a metabolite that is not a substrate or product is necessary, regulatory sites that interact with the catalytic site, usually by altering its affinity for substrate, have evolved. The evolutionary design problem in these cases must have required much more time for solution than did simple adjustment of affinities at the catalytic site. Enzymes of this type will be discussed in the next section.

A third type of control is occasionally necessary—sometimes the activity of an enzyme must be modulated by substrate or product, but with the control acting in the direction opposite to that which could be obtained by direct competition at the catalytic site. The most obvious and perhaps the most important such enzyme is phosphofructokinase. This enzyme has been believed for many years to play an important role in regulation of glycolysis, and observations reported during the past 15 years have confirmed that belief. Glycolysis is an ATP-yielding sequence, so that response to the adenylate energy charge must be of the R type: the reaction velocity must decrease as the charge, and hence the concentration of ATP, increases. But the phosphofructokinase reaction, although a component of this ATP-regenerating sequence, itself consumes ATP (equation 5-14). Thus the R-type response that is required for appropriate metabolic control, and is observed

$$ATP + \text{fructose 6-phosphate} \rightleftharpoons ADP + \text{fructose 1,6-diphosphate} \qquad (5\text{-}14)$$

experimentally, is a response in direct opposition to ordinary mass-action considerations. In fact, a curve showing the velocity of the phosphofructo-kinase reaction as a function of the concentration of ATP has a negative slope in the physiologically important region (Figure 5-6). Thus the order of this reaction with regard to one of its substrates is negative. We must consider how this chemically unexpected behavior arises.*

The negative slope of the curve of Figure 5-6 in the region above an ATP concentration of about 0.1 mM is caused by a decrease in the affinity at the catalytic site for the other substrate, fructose 6-P. This is shown by the fact that when the concentration of fructose 6-P is increased, the extent of in-hibition at any concentration of ATP is decreased. It appears that ATP can bind at a regulatory site, and that the presence of ATP at this site leads, presumably through a change in the conformation of the enzyme, to an increase in $(F6P)_{0.5}$ at the catalytic site.

It seems logically impossible that the regulatory site, at which binding of ATP decreases the affinity of the enzyme for fructose 6-P, could be the same as the catalytic site at which ATP is bound for reaction with fructose 6-P. The distinction between regulatory and catalytic sites is confirmed by the response of the enzyme to other nucleoside triphosphates. Most kinases are specific for ATP as a phosphoryl donor. This specificity appears to be necessary for efficient operation of adenylate energy charge regulation of metabolism. But phosphofructokinase is unusual in accepting any of the common nucleoside triphosphates as phosphoryl donor. This lack of spec-ificity can hardly be accidental, since the pyrimidine nucleotides CTP and UTP are used approximately as readily as the purine nucleotides GTP and ITP, which are much more closely related to ATP. Nonspecificity for the phosphoryl donor must have evolved on the basis of selective advantage. Probably the explanation for this unusual, if not unique, lack of specificity is to be found in the metabolic function of phosphofructokinase. Unlike other kinases, which participate in the utilization of ATP in sequences or processes leading to a metabolically useful result such as synthesis of an intermediate, phosphofructokinase catalyzes what may be thought of as a pump-priming reaction—1 ATP equivalent is consumed in this reaction in order that 38 can be regenerated. Thus the ability, in an emergency, to use any available nucleoside triphosphate as phosphoryl donor might well be advantageous.

* This discussion of phosphofructokinase kinetics is based directly on the properties of the yeast enzyme (97), but phosphofructokinase from a variety of other organisms has been shown to behave in a generally similar manner.

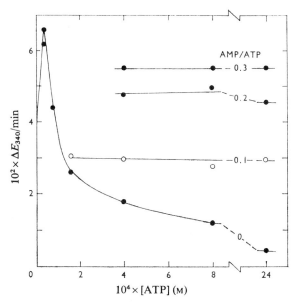

Figure 5-6. Rate of the reaction catalyzed by yeast phosphofructokinase as a function of the concentration of ATP in the absence of AMP and at three constant values of the AMP/ATP concentration ratio. The assay mixture contained 33 mM Tris-HCl, pH 7.5; 0.28 mM fructose 6-P; 3.3 mM MgCl$_2$; 2.3 mM glutathione; 0.1 mM NADH; 0.2 mM ATP, excess of aldolase, triosephosphate isomerase, and α-glycerophosphate dehydrogenase; and ATP at concentrations shown on the abscissa. Where indicated, AMP was added to provide a molar ratio of AMP to ATP as shown on the corresponding curves. From Ramaiah *et al.* (*97*).

The regulatory site, in contrast to the catalytic site, is highly specific for ATP. This is shown by the fact that high concentrations of other nucleoside triphosphates do not inhibit and that when mixtures of ATP and another nucleoside triphosphate at high concentrations are present, the properties of the enzyme are identical with those seen when the same amount of ATP is present alone. Thus, the other triphosphates not only do not inhibit; they also do not compete with ATP for the regulatory site. Phosphofructokinase was the first enzyme for which a regulatory site was observed to exhibit markedly greater specificity than the catalytic site. This observation was useful, since it came at a time when the existence of distinct regulatory sites and of regulatory conformation changes was still under dispute.

The effect of ATP is decreased competitively by AMP. When the concentration of ATP is in the inhibitory range (as is probably always the case *in vivo*), the affinity of the catalytic site for fructose 6-P depends on the ATP/AMP concentration ratio (Figure 5-6). Other nucleoside mono- or diphosphates have no effect on ATP inhibition. This observation indicates that the enzyme's behavior is regulated specifically by the charge of the adenine nucleotide system. This specificity is to be expected in view of the discussion in Chapter 4; even if the ability to use other nucleoside triphosphates as pump-priming phosphoryl donors is occasionally desirable, it is the primary energy state of the cell, as indicated by the charge of the adenylate system, to which energy-transducing (ATP-regenerating) sequences like glycolysis must respond.

AMP has little effect on the phosphofructokinase reaction when phosphoryl donors other than ATP are used. Thus, it appears that binding of AMP does not in itself cause a kinetically significant change in the conformation of the enzyme, but that binding of AMP prevents the conformational change due to ATP binding. The simplest rationalization of this competitive interaction would be postulation of a regulatory site for which ATP and AMP compete, with binding of ATP causing a regulatory change in conformation and binding of AMP being effective merely by exclusion of ATP. However, it seems unlikely that this explanation is correct, because ADP has no effect—it neither inhibits the reaction nor decreases the ATP effect. It is difficult to imagine a site for which ATP and AMP compete, but which does not bind ADP. Thus it may be more likely that ATP and AMP are bound at separate sites that are specific for these individual compounds, and that presence of AMP at its site either (1) causes a conformational change that prevents ATP binding or (2) allows ATP to bind but prevents the kinetically important conformational change that otherwise results from ATP binding. Regardless of the mechanism by which the effects are attained, interaction of sites in such a way as to produce a negative effective kinetic order of reaction with regard to a substrate is both metabolically important and conceptually interesting.

INTERACTING SITES AND COOPERATIVITY

We have dealt thus far only with what is usually termed first-order Michaelis kinetics, in which the formal kinetic order of reaction varies from one to zero, depending on the substrate concentration. For many regulatory enzymes, the velocity is a higher-order function of substrate concentration, with second-order and fourth-order dependency being probably the most common. Although the fact did not affect our discussion of other properties of the enzyme, phosphofructokinase from most sources catalyzes a reaction that is second-order with respect to fructose 6-P.

Higher-order dependency on substrate concentration and the existence of regulatory sites are so generally found together that it seems reasonable to assume that they result from similar interactions. This association is so frequently observed, in fact, that higher-order kinetics is sometimes thought of as the defining characteristic of regulatory enzymes. As our discussion in the previous section emphasized, this assumption is not valid. An enzyme may have important regulatory characteristics as a result of the properties of the catalytic sites, although it catalyzes a first-order reaction and possesses no separate regulatory sites. But the association between regulatory sites and higher-order kinetics seems to be general. Nearly all enzymes for which kinetic studies suggest the existence of regulatory sites catalyze reactions that are of second or higher order with respect to substrate.

Advantages of Cooperative Binding

Hemoglobin

Because it binds oxygen cooperatively but does not catalyze a reaction, hemoglobin is often used as an illustration of some aspects of cooperative binding. The hemoglobin-oxygen interaction also illustrates physiological advantages of cooperativity in binding. The ratio between the ligand concentration required for 10% saturation of binding sites and the concentration required for 90% saturation is a convenient parameter by which the degree of cooperativity may be expressed (66). It is also a parameter with direct functional connotations. For simple (first-order) Michaelis or Langmuir binding, equation 5-15 applies. This is identical with equation 5-7

$$\frac{y}{x - y} = \phi \tag{5-15}$$

except that binding rather than velocity terms are used [x is the number of binding sites, y is the number of filled sites, and ϕ, as before, is $(S)/(S)_{0.5}$]. Thus 10% of the sites will be filled when the substrate concentration is 0.11 $(S)_{0.5}$ and 90% will be filled when the substrate concentration is 9 $(S)_{0.5}$. The ratio between these concentrations, 81, is a characteristic of noncooperative binding. If binding of oxygen by hemoglobin were noncooperative, the concentration of oxygen in the plasma within lung capillaries would need to be 81 times that within capillaries in the tissues if hemoglobin were to be loaded to 90% of capacity in the lungs and unloaded to 10% in the tissues, even if kinetic factors are ignored and it is assumed that equilibrium is attained both in loading and in unloading. A primary characteristic of cooperative binding is steeper binding curves and thus a smaller concentration ratio between the 10% and 90% saturation points. If oxygen binding were fourth order, for example, an oxygen concentration differential of only threefold would allow for loading to 90% and unloading to 10%, making the same assumptions as above. The enormous increase in transport efficiency that is gained by cooperative binding is obvious.

Hemoglobin has four subunits, and fourth-order binding would thus be theoretically possible. The actual degree of cooperativity exhibited by hemoglobin, however, is somewhat lower than third-order, and the oxygen concentration ratio between the 10% and 90% saturation points is about 5. Although less than infinitely cooperative, this behavior permits much more efficient transport than would be possible if binding were noncooperative. The magnitude of the oxygen concentration difference required is further reduced by effects of pH and CO_2 (the Bohr effect). These modifiers, in exact analogy with the effects of modifiers on regulatory enzymes, cause the affinity of hemoglobin for its "substrate," oxygen, to change in response to physiological need. The end result, as discussed in most elementary textbooks of biochemistry or physiology, is that the affinity of hemoglobin for oxygen is enhanced in the lungs and decreased in the tissues.

The properties of hemoglobin illustrate how cooperative binding and change of affinity for ligand as a consequence of binding of specific modifier molecules, both of which were long-established characteristics of regulatory enzymes, were at a comparatively late date in evolutionary history utilized in solving the simpler problem of efficient ligand transport in a liquid circulatory system. Except that no chemical reaction is catalyzed, the behavior of hemoglobin is fully analogous to that of a typical regulatory enzyme.

Modulation of Activity of Cooperative Enzymes

Generalized response curves for a regulatory enzyme that exhibits higher-order kinetics and whose activity is modulated by a modifier are shown in Figure 5-7. The advantages of modulation of enzyme activity by changes in concentrations of appropriate metabolites are obvious. In a very common pattern, the modifier is the end product of a biosynthetic sequence, and the target enzyme catalyzes the first step specific to the synthesis. This is classical

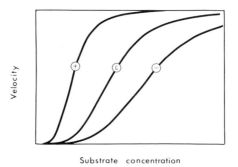

Substrate concentration

Figure 5-7. Generalized effect of modifier on the response curve of a typical regulatory enzyme: c, no modifier; +, positive modifier; −, negative modifier.

end-product negative feedback regulation of the type recognized by Umbarger (*118*) and Yates and Pardee (*128*) in 1956. It is now recognized to be a typical feature of biosynthetic sequences, and is discussed in most elemental biochemistry textbooks. Such feedback appears to be the primary means by which the concentrations of end-product metabolites are stabilized. A tendency for the concentration of such a compound to increase would be countered by the resulting decrease in activity of the enzyme catalyzing the first reaction in the biosynthetic sequence, and a tendency for the concentration to decrease would lead to an increase in the rate of synthesis.

Metabolism contains many branchpoints, at each of which a metabolite must be partitioned between two or more pathways. The first enzyme in each pathway generally has regulatory properties. It is evident that when two enzymes compete for the same substrate, the outcome of the competition (the partition ratio between the two reactions) can be controlled sensitively by changes in affinities of the enzymes for their common substrates. This is illustrated in Figure 5-8. Enzymes A and B are assumed to compete for the same substrate. At the substrate concentration indicated as *a* on the abscissa, most of the branchpoint metabolite molecules will undergo the reaction catalyzed by enzyme A (curve 1) and thus will become committed to the corresponding pathway. If, because of an increase in concentration of the end product of the sequence in which enzyme A catalyzes the first step, the affinity of enzyme A for the common substrate is decreased by a factor of 2 [the value of $(S)_{0.5}$ is doubled], this enzyme (curve 2) will now compete poorly with enzyme B (curve 4), and most of the branchpoint metabolite will now be directed into the pathway for which enzyme B

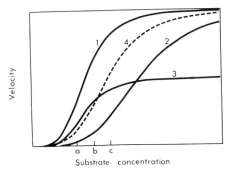

Figure 5-8. Velocity of the reaction catalyzed by a cooperative enzyme as a function of substrate concentration; effect of changes in parameters. For curves 1, 4, and 2, the maximal velocities are equal, and the relative values of $(S)_{0.5}$ are 1, $2^{1/2}$, and 2, respectively. For curve 3 the maximal velocity is half of that for the other curves and the relative value of $(S)_{0.5}$ is 1. The calculations were done for a highly cooperative enzyme with four substrate-binding sites. See text for discussion.

catalyzes the first reaction. The concentration of the branchpoint metabolite will probably rise somewhat because of the decreased rate at which it is utilized by enzyme A (for example, to point *b* on the abscissa), but the size of this increase will have a relatively small effect on the partition ratio.

Now consider the consequences that would follow if the increase in the concentration of end product, instead of causing the $(S)_{0.5}$ of enzyme A to increase by a factor of two, caused the maximal velocity to decrease by the same factor (curve 3). At any substrate concentration in the vicinity of *a* and *b* the reaction catalyzed by enzyme A would still proceed more rapidly than that catalyzed by enzyme B, and most of the branchpoint metabolite would still enter the corresponding pathway. This simple graphical comparison illustrates the generalization that the partition ratio is much less sensitive to changes in maximal velocities than to changes in affinities. A second important advantage of modulation of $(S)_{0.5}$ values, rather than maximal velocities, is also seen in Figure 5-8. If the maximal velocity were the enzyme property that was modulated in response to modifier concentration, the partition ratio would be highly sensitive to changes in the concentration of the common substrate. At the concentration indicated by *b*, for example, the reaction catalyzed by enzyme A would still go faster than that catalyzed by enzyme B, but at concentration *c* the reverse would be true (comparison of curves 3 and 4). There would be a further large shift in favor of the reaction catalyzed by enzyme B if the substrate concentration rose slightly beyond *c*. In contrast, with modulation of the $(S)_{0.5}$ value, the partition ratio is determined primarily by the concentration of regulatory metabolites and is relatively insensitive to the concentration of substrate. This is illustrated by comparison of curves 1 and 4 or of 2 and 4. In the former case the partition strongly favors the reaction catalyzed by enzyme A and does not change markedly when the substrate concentration changes by a reasonable amount; in the latter case the other reaction is favored, and the partition ratio is again relatively independent of substrate concentration.

Figure 5-9 illustrates competition between two enzymes with no cooperative interactions, one of which has a variable affinity for the substrate. The relative $(S)_{0.5}$ and V_m values are the same as in Figure 5-8. This situation is much less favorable for sharp and effective control than is that illustrated in Figure 5-8, mainly because of the relatively low slopes of the lines in Figure 5-9 in the region of the $(S)_{0.5}$ value. As in Figure 5-8, the affinity of enzyme A for substrate is greater than that of enzyme B, so that the reaction catalyzed by enzyme A (curve 1) goes more rapidly than that catalyzed by enzyme B (curve 4). The twofold change in affinity for substrate that is illustrated by the change from curve 1 to curve 2 will, as before, cause the reaction catalyzed by enzyme A (reaction A) to proceed more slowly than

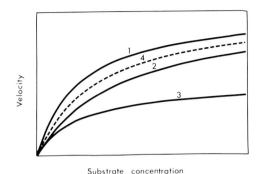

Figure 5-9. Same as Figure 5-8, except for a noncooperative enzyme.

that catalyzed by enzyme B (reaction B). The relative changes are, however, much less in this case than when substrates are bound cooperatively. At the substrate concentration that allows reaction B to go at 10% of its maximal velocity, the rate of reaction A will initially be 136% that of reaction B in the first-order case (Figure 5-9). After the $(S)_{0.5}$ value of enzyme A was doubled, reaction A would proceed at 73% of the rate of reaction B (assuming no change in the concentration of substrate). Corresponding figures for the cooperative four-site enzymes of Figure 5-8 are 308% before and 27% after the change in affinity. Thus the rates of the two reactions would be within 40% of each other both before and after the regulatory modulation in the first-order case. Neither reaction would predominate, and the change in affinity of enzyme A would not cause a sharp change in the partition ratio. In contrast, in the case of the cooperative enzymes, reaction A would be more than three times as fast as reaction B before the modulation, and less than one-third as fast after. The advantage conferred by the steep response curves that are characteristic of cooperative enzymes is obvious. Competition between enzymes that exhibit higher-order responses to changes in substrate concentration (Figure 5-8) allows for larger changes in partition ratio in response to regulatory modulation of the properties of either or both enzymes, while requiring smaller changes in substrate concentration, than does competition between enzymes following first-order Michaelis kinetics. That is, the partition ratio is much more sensitive to changes in enzyme properties when the competing enzymes are characterized by higher-order kinetics than would be possible with first-order enzymes.

Figure 5-8 understates the sensitivity of partition ratios to regulatory modulation of enzyme properties in at least two important ways. First, the affinity of enzyme A for substrate is shown as changing by a factor of only two. Much larger ranges of $(S)_{0.5}$ values have been observed in most kinetic experiments with regulatory enzymes *in vitro*. Second, it is to be expected that in many cases the properties of the two competing enzymes would change reciprocally, so that the effects of an increase in the $(S)_{0.5}$ value of enzyme A would be reinforced by a simultaneous decrease in the $(S)_{0.5}$ of enzyme B for the common substrate.

As was discussed in connection with equation 5-7, the parameter ϕ, or $(S)/(S)_{0.5}$, is the normalized function on which the velocity of an enzyme-catalyzed reaction depends. In classical kinetic experiments *in vitro*, $(S)_{0.5}$ (or the Michaelis constant) was always assumed to be constant, so we are accustomed to thinking of kinetic response curves in terms of velocity as a function of substrate concentration. It is important to keep in mind that for regulatory enzymes $(S)_{0.5}$ is not a constant, and that in an intact functioning cell variations in the parameter ϕ may be at least as likely to arise from changes in the value of $(S)_{0.5}$ (changes in the affinity of the enzyme for substrate) as from changes in the actual concentration of the substrate.

Interactions between Substrate and Modifier

Modifiers may affect the behavior of an enzyme in many ways, but the most common effect is an increase or a decrease in the affinity of the enzyme for one or more substrates. In such cases, as the concentration of the modifier increases, the resulting increase in the fraction of enzyme molecules that bear modifiers causes a progressive change in the effective or average substrate affinity of the enzyme, from that characteristic of the absence of modifier to that characteristic of enzyme saturated with modifier. Some aspects of this type of interaction are represented schematically in Figures 5-10 through 5-12. In these representations of three-dimensional graphs, the concentrations of substrate and of modifier are plotted on logarithmic scales along the two horizontal axes, and reaction velocity on the vertical axis. The grid spacing (the distance between adjacent curves) corresponds to a ratio of $10^{1/2}$ in concentration. The figures show calculated responses for the simple case of an enzyme with two catalytic sites and two sites that bind a negative modifier. In all cases the binding of substrate is rather weakly cooperative; when one site is filled the free energy of binding at the other site is made more negative by 1.4 kcal/mole. This corresponds to a tenfold increase in the affinity of the enzyme for substrate. The modifier is assumed to bind with the same degree of cooperativity. The three figures differ in the extent of interaction between modifier and substrate binding sites.

In Figure 5-10, the binding of modifier does not affect substrate binding. This figure is shown only for comparison; the "modifier" is not in fact a modifier in this case. Each curve running from the front left side to the

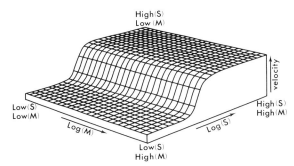

Figure 5-10. Velocity of an enzyme-catalyzed reaction (vertical scale) as a function of the concentrations of substrate and modifier. The figure was calculated for an enzyme with two catalytic sites and two sites at which a negative modifier is bound. Binding of a molecule of substrate or of modifier increases the affinity at the other similar site by a factor of 10 (makes the free energy of binding more negative by 1.4 kcal/mole). For this figure, there is no interaction between the "modifier" and the catalytic sites. The concentration scales are logarithmic, with the distance from one line to the next corresponding to a change in concentration by a factor of $10^{1/2}$. For most viewers, the illusion of three-dimensionality will be enhanced by closing one eye.

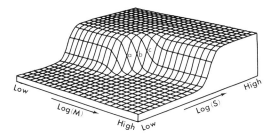

Figure 5-11. Same as Figure 5-10, except that each modifier molecule bound makes the free energy of binding at each substrate site more positive by 1.4 kcal/mole, and each substrate molecule bound has the same effect at each modifier-binding site.

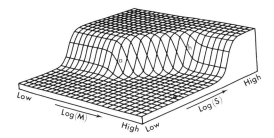

Figure 5-12. Same as Figure 5-11, except that the mutual interaction between modifier and substrate binding sites leads to a change of 2.8 kcal/mole for each ligand of the other type bound.

right rear is a plot of velocity as a function of substrate concentration; since the modifier has no effect, these curves are all identical in Figure 5-10. Each line running from the left rear to the right front side is a plot of velocity as a function of modifier concentration; since the modifier has no effect, the velocity is constant for each line.

In Figure 5-11, the degree of cooperativity of binding of substrate and modifier is the same as in Figure 5-10, but each molecule of modifier bound decreases the affinity at each substrate site by a factor of 10 (or makes the free energy of binding more positive by 1.4 kcal/mole). At low concentrations of modifier the curves showing velocity as a function of substrate concentration are the same as in Figure 5-10, but they are offset as the modifier concentration increases to the range where a significant fraction of the modifier sites are bound. When the modifier sites are saturated (toward the right front side of the graph), the concentration of substrate required for any given velocity is 100 times as high as in the absence of modifier. The operational interaction between modifier and substrate is seen on the face of the rise in the region of the offset. In going from point a to point b, we increase the concentration of substrate by the grid factor, $10^{1/2}$, and increase the concentration of the negative modifier by the same factor. The resulting velocity is nearly unchanged from that at point a. In going from a to c each concentration is increased by a factor of 10, but still the velocity is nearly unchanged. Thus within the concentration range in which the modifier is effective, the velocity of the reaction is as sensitive to changes in the concentration of modifier as to changes in concentration of substrate.

The situation represented by Figure 5-12 is identical to that of Figure 5-11, except that each molecule of modifier bound decreases the affinity of each substrate-binding site by a factor of 100 (makes the free energy of binding more positive by 2.8 kcal/mole). Now the velocity-substrate curves are offset by a factor of 10^4, and the region of modifier effectiveness (the area of the face of the rise in the region of the offset) is much larger than before. In going from point a to point h we have an increase in the substrate concentration of over 3000-fold ($1000 \times 10^{1/2}$), but because the concentration of the negative modifier increases by the same factor the velocity hardly changes. In this whole region, the velocity responds to changes in concentration of modifier or of substrate with almost equal sensitivity.

Figures 5-11 and 5-12 would represent the action of a positive modifier equally well; all that is required is to change the direction of the $\log(M)$ scale. Besides illustrating the interaction of modifier and substrate concentrations in determining reaction velocity, the figures show that large effects are produced by small changes in binding energy. And it should be remembered that these figures were calculated for an enzyme with only two sites of each kind. If there were four modifier sites, an effect identical with that shown in Figure 5-12 would be produced if each filled modifier site changed the binding energy at each catalytic site by only 1.4 kcal/mole, an amount that is very small in most contexts.

We have recently presented another graphical illustration of the interaction between modifier and substrate that makes the same points in a quite different format (*13*).

GRAPHICAL REPRESENTATION OF ENZYME RESPONSES

Consideration of possible regulatory consequences of the kinetic behavior of an enzyme may be facilitated to an important degree through visualization by means of graphs. The various types of graphical representation are not equally suited to all situations; choice of the most appropriate types of plots is a necessary step in clear presentation of the results of kinetic studies on regulatory enzymes. Because of the importance of graphical treatment in this area, some of the properties of the commonly used plots will be discussed.

Kinetic Orders of Enzymatic Reactions

Assignment of a kinetic order to an enzyme-catalyzed reaction is ambiguous unless the terms are specifically defined. For homogeneous reactions, the concept of reaction order is simple and explicit: a reaction is first order with respect to a reaction component if its velocity is proportional to the concentration (strictly speaking, the activity) of that component, second order if the velocity is proportional to the square of the component concentration, and so on. This dependence of the velocity on reactant concentration is shown in equation 5-16, where n is the order of the reaction.

$$v = k(S)^n \qquad (5\text{-}16)$$

It is evident that the slope of a plot of velocity as a function of reactant concentration will increase with increase in concentration if n is greater than 1, and that the slope at any point will be a simple function of substrate concentration (equation 5-17).

$$m = dv/d(S) = kn(S)^{n-1} \qquad (5\text{-}17)$$

A plot of the logarithm of velocity against the logarithm of substrate concentration is a straight line with slope equal to n, the kinetic order of the reaction, as is seen by taking the logarithm of both sides of equation 5-16.

$$\log v = \log k + n \log(S) \qquad (5\text{-}18)$$

Because of the phenomenon of site saturation, graphical representations of enzyme-catalyzed reactions do not yield such simple plots, and the concept of kinetic order is less simply defined. The order of a reaction catalyzed by an enzyme that exhibits simple Michaelis behavior decreases from one at very low substrate concentration to zero at high concentration as the catalytic sites approach saturation. At any intervening point the order must then have some value between one and zero. Thus, in striking contrast to the homogeneous reaction, the order of an enzyme-catalyzed reaction is a function of substrate concentration. For quantitative assignment of the kinetic order, a definition is required. The convention that seems most obvious because it is the one most consistent with the concept of kinetic order in homogeneous reactions is: the order of a reaction is defined as $d[\ln v]/d[\ln(S)]$; that is, the order at any point is the slope at that point of a plot of the logarithm of velocity against the logarithm of substrate concentration.

For simple Michaelis behavior the order defined in this way is given in equation 5-19. Thus the order is one when the concentration of substrate

$$\text{order} = 1 - \frac{(S)}{(S)_{0.5} + (S)} = 1 - \frac{\phi}{\phi + 1} = 1 - \frac{v}{V_m} \qquad (5\text{-}19)$$

is essentially zero, is 0.5 when the velocity is half of the saturating velocity [when $(S) = (S)_{0.5}$], and approaches zero as the substrate concentration increases and the catalytic sites approach saturation.

The expressions for slope of the various curves as a function of ϕ are tabulated in Table 5-1. As defined previously, ϕ is $(S)/(S)_{0.5}$, the concentration of substrate divided by the concentration at which the reaction velocity is half of the saturation velocity. This function is used in the table for simplicity and generality. It will be recognized that the curves obtained would not be changed if the actual substrate concentration were used rather than ϕ; in plots with (S) rather than ϕ on the abscissa, the scale would merely be multiplied by the constant factor $(S)_{0.5}$ and in plots with a logarithmic scale on the abscissa a constant factor $\ln(S)_{0.5}$ or $\log_{10}(S)_{0.5}$ would be added to the scale.

The derivations of the slopes shown in Table 5-1 are straightforward. The assumptions on which they are based should, however, be stated explicitly. We begin with the basic Michaelis assumption that actual chemical conversions are slow in relation to the binding and dissociation of ligands.

TABLE 5-1

Slopes of Plots of Results of Kinetic Experiments

Type of plot	Infinitely cooperative interactions among n sites		Single site or noninteracting sites	
	Slope	Slope when $\phi = 1$	Slope	Slope when $\phi = 1$
Homogeneous reactions				
v vs (S)	$kn(S)^{n-1}$	—	k	—
$\ln v \ \ln(S)$ $\Big\}$ $\log_{10} v$ vs $\log_{10}(S)$	n	—	1	—
Enzymic reactions				
v/V_m vs ϕ	$\dfrac{n\phi^{n-3}}{(\phi^n + 1)^2}$	$0.25n$	$\dfrac{1}{(\phi + 1)^2}$	0.25
$\ln(v/V_m)$ vs $\ln \phi$ $\Big\}$ $\log_{10}(v/V_m)$ vs $\log_{10} \phi$	$n\left[1 - \dfrac{\phi^n}{\phi^n + 1}\right]$	$0.5n$	$1 - \left[\dfrac{\phi}{\phi + 1}\right]$	0.5
v/V_m vs $\ln \phi$	$n\left[\dfrac{\phi^n}{(\phi^n + 1)^2}\right]$	$0.25n$	$\dfrac{\phi}{(\phi + 1)^2}$	0.25
v/V_m vs $\log_{10} \phi$	$2.3n\left[\dfrac{\phi^n}{(\phi^n + 1)^2}\right]$	$0.575n$	$2.3\left[\dfrac{\phi}{(\phi + 1)^2}\right]$	0.575
$v/(V_m - v)$ vs ϕ	$n\phi^{n-1}$	n	1	1
$\ln[v/(V_m - v)]$ vs $\ln \phi$ $\Big\}$ $\log_{10}[v/(V_m - v)]$ vs $\log_{10} \phi$	n	n	1	1

In addition, it is assumed that binding is infinitely cooperative—that the presence of a molecule of substrate at one site increases the affinities at the other sites so strongly that enzyme molecules already bearing one or more substrate molecules will compete so favorably with unliganded molecules that when one site has been filled the others will be filled almost instantaneously. Then only two types of enzyme molecules will be present, those bearing no substrates and those with all substrate sites filled. The Michaelis equation for partitioning of enzyme between free and liganded forms is then given by equation 5-20, and the overall process can be represented as

$$(E)_T = (E) + (ES_n) \qquad (5\text{-}20)$$

in equation 5-21, where p may be any number from 1 to n. That is, it is of

$$E + nS \rightleftharpoons ES_n \rightleftharpoons ES_{n-p}P_p \rightleftharpoons ES_{n-p} + pP \qquad (5\text{-}21)$$

no consequence in the derivations of the expressions in Table 5-1 whether all of the substrate molecules bound to an enzyme molecule are simultaneously converted to product, in which case $ES_n \rightarrow EP_n$, or not. Since the conversion is assumed to be slow in comparison to dissociation, if the sites act independently the usual occurrence will be $ES_n \rightarrow ES_{n-1}P_1 \rightarrow ES_{n-1} + P$. This seems the most likely situation, but the possibility that enzyme conformational changes accompanying the actual reaction are coupled between catalytic sites so that they act in synchrony cannot be ruled out.

The assumption of infinitely cooperative binding obviously cannot be rigorously true. The consequences of relatively weak cooperativity will be discussed below. But cooperativity is sufficiently strong in many cases to make the entries in Table 5-1 meaningful. Therefore, we will first consider the case on which this table is based, that of infinite cooperativity.

For $E + nS \rightleftharpoons ES_n$, we have equation 5-22, where K is a higher-order

$$K = \frac{(S)^n(E)}{(ES_n)} \qquad (5\text{-}22)$$

dissociation constant with the dimensions of (concentration)^n. Making the Michaelis assumptions, the velocity is taken to be proportional to the concentration of (ES_n). This assumption leads to equation 5-23, which is iden-

$$v(V_m - v) = (S)^n/K \qquad (5\text{-}23)$$

tical with the corresponding relation for ordinary Michaelis behavior (equation 5-7) except for the exponent n. When the reaction velocity is half of the saturating velocity, $v/(V_m - v) = 1$; then $(S)^n = K$. Since $(S)_{0.5}$ is defined as the concentration of substrate at which reaction velocity is half of the saturating velocity, it follows from the preceding sentence that $(S)_{0.5}{}^n = K$. Then, since ϕ is defined as $(S)/(S)_{0.5}$, we obtain equation 5-24.

$$\frac{v}{(V_m - v)} = \left[\frac{(S)}{(S)_{0.5}}\right]^n = \phi^n \qquad (5\text{-}24)$$

Since this equation is identical with the general form of the Michaelis equation except that ϕ^n replaces ϕ, it follows that all derivative forms of the Michaelis equation, including the frequently used logarithmic and reciprocal forms, will apply equally well to enzymes exhibiting higher-order kinetics characterized by essentially infinite cooperativity, if $(S)^n$ replaces the term (S) of the first-order equation.

In Table 5-1 the two right-hand columns give, for "normal" Michaelis enzymes for which $n = 1$, the general expressions for slopes of the various plots as a function of ϕ and also the slope when $\phi = 1$ and $v = V_m/2$. The two left-hand columns give the same information for cooperative enzymes.

In the sense defined above, that the order of a reaction is $d[\ln v]/d[\ln(S)]$, the order of an enzyme-catalyzed reaction is evidently given by the second entry in the listing of enzymic reactions in Table 5-1: the order of an enzyme-catalyzed reaction, when the concentration of product is zero, is $n[1 - \phi^n/(\phi^n + 1)]$. This definition of order is of very little use, however. Some way of expressing the relative order as a property of the reaction (that is, of the enzyme as such), independent of substrate concentration, is needed. The obvious parameter is n, the number of interacting substrate-binding sites and hence the maximal possible kinetic order. This number is equal to the kinetic order of the reaction only for infinitely cooperative enzymes, however.

As we saw earlier, the function $v/(V_m - v)$ may be considered a normalizing parameter, in that equations and plots describing enzyme-catalyzed reactions in terms of this function are similar to corresponding equations and plots in terms of v for homogeneous reactions. Thus in Table 5-1 entries in the last two lines, which relate to plots in terms of $v/(V_m - v)$, are similar to those in the two lines at the top of the table, which relate to homogeneous reactions. In the ideal case of infinite cooperativity, the Hill plot (last line in Table 5-1) is linear with a slope of n. Thus the kinetic order of an enzyme-catalyzed reaction is generally defined as the slope of a Hill plot of the results. This usage, although not strictly correct, seems to be justified. It is unlikely to lead to confusion, since there is no other obvious way in which a fixed order could be assigned to an enzyme reaction. However, since the actual order of an enzyme-catalyzed reaction is variable, depending on the concentration of substrate, it is desirable that any reference to the order of an enzymic reaction should be accompanied by a statement as to what is meant: for example, "The order of the reaction (slope of the Hill plot) is 4." And even that statement is not complete, since what is really meant is the slope of the Hill plot at its midpoint. It is generally assumed that the midpoint of the curve is at zero on the vertical coordinate, and this is true if site-site interactions are symmetrical, that is, if each filled site has the same effect on each unfilled site.

Estimation of Kinetic Parameters

Noncooperative Enzymes

The main difficulty in making Hill plots, as with any use of the parameter $v/(V_m - v)$, is the necessity of knowing the value of V_m. Since the velocity of an enzymic reaction approaches a maximal value asymptotically, the limiting maximal rate is not easy to estimate from any of the direct plots (first four listings for enzymic reactions in Table 5-1). Another approach is needed for evaluation of V_m.

The plot of $v/V_m = \phi/(\phi + 1)$ is a hyperbola (the familiar "Michaelis" plot is of course only part of one limb, in the quadrant where both v and ϕ are positive). Plots of various inverse functions must therefore be linear, with obvious advantages in extrapolating to V_m. The most common form, usually termed the Lineweaver-Burk plot, is obtained by merely inverting the Michaelis equation to obtain equation 5-25. When $1/v$ is plotted against $1/(S)$, the y-intercept is $1/V_m$ and the x-intercept is $-1/(S)_{0.5}$. Thus both

$$\frac{1}{v} = \left[\frac{(S)_{0.5}}{V_m}\right]\frac{1}{(S)} + \frac{1}{V_m} \tag{5-25}$$

of the desired parameters are readily estimated. This is the only linearized form of the Michaelis equation in which v and (S) are separated, but linear forms in which the variables are not separated exist. From equation 5-26

$$\frac{v}{(S)} = \left[\frac{1}{(S)_{0.5}}\right]v + \frac{V_m}{(S)_{0.5}} \tag{5-26}$$

it follows that a plot of $v/(S)$ as a function of v (the Eadie plot) will be linear. The same equation and plot, with the number of ligand molecules bound per macromolecule replacing v and the number of binding sites replacing V_m, is generally used for estimation of the number of ligand-binding sites from a determination of the amount of ligand bound at various concentrations of free ligand. In that application it is usually called a Scatchard plot. Another form of the relationship is shown in equation 5-27 from which a plot of $(S)/v$ against (S) must be linear.

$$\frac{(S)}{v} = \left[\frac{1}{V_m}\right](S) + \frac{(S)_{0.5}}{V_m} \tag{5-27}$$

Any of these three linear variants of the Michaelis equation may be used for the estimation of V_m and $(S)_{0.5}$ for noncooperative enzymes. Since they are algebraic variants of a single equation, they would necessarily yield exactly the same values for these parameters if there were no experimental error. Because of widely differing weighting of points at the high and low ends of the range, however, the different graphical methods, when used with real results, may lead to estimates of V_m and $(S)_{0.5}$ that differ by large factors. Dowd and Riggs (45), in an important computer simulation study, showed that all three plots may yield surprisingly poor estimates for V_m and $(S)_{0.5}$, with the simple double-reciprocal plot being generally the poorest of the three. Their paper should be read by anyone who works with enzymes, as a safeguard against too much faith in V_m and $(S)_{0.5}$ or K_m values, whether they are one's own or are obtained from the literature.

All of the permutations of the inverted Michaelis-Menten equation discussed above are similar in principle. Each experimental determination of velocity at a given concentration of substrate is plotted as a point, and a number of such points determine a line from which the value of maximal velocity and the Michaelis constant can be estimated. The first fundamentally different graphical use of an inverted Michaelis plot was proposed by Eisenthal and Cornish-Bowden (46). When the relationship is put into the form shown in equation 5-28, it is possible, for the sake of the analysis, to consider

$$\frac{V_m}{v} - \frac{(S)_{0.5}}{(S)} = 1 \tag{5-28}$$

v and (S) to be fixed parameters and V_m and $(S)_{0.5}$ to be variables. Thus the equation is viewed as expressing, for any given values of v and (S), the dependence of V_m on $(S)_{0.5}$ (or the inverse). This dependence is obviously linear and can be expressed graphically as a straight line. Thus the Eisenthal–Cornish-Bowden plot differs from other treatments based on the Michaelis equation in that each determination of velocity leads to a line rather than to a point.

The method is illustrated in Figures 5-13 and 5-14. V_m is plotted in the vertical dimension and $(S)_{0.5}$ in the horizontal. This plot seems to fly in the face of reality by taking the fixed parameters that are to be determined and treating them as variables. But of course mathematical relationships are independent of applications; the validity of equation 5-28 will not be

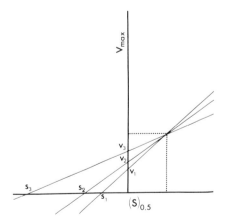

Figure 5-13. Cornish-Bowden plot as it would appear in the absence of experimental error. Each line shows all V_{max}-K_m pairs that are compatible with an observed velocity at a known substrate concentration. The intersection, being the only such pair compatible with all of the measurements, should indicate the values of V_{max} and K_m for the enzyme.

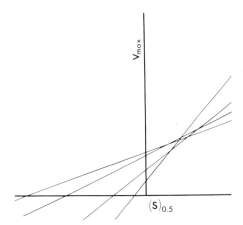

Figure 5-14. Cornish-Bowden plot as it might appear based on experimental results. Because of error, the lines will not intersect at a common point. The median of the values of V_{max} and K_m suggested by all of the two-line intersections supplies the best estimate of these parameters.

affected by the way that we choose to graph it. Each experimental value of v, with the corresponding value of (S), is then used to generate a line on the V_m-$(S)_{0.5}$ graph. When $(S)_{0.5} = 0$, $V_m = v$. Thus the curve crosses the vertical axis at the numerical value of v. When $V_m = 0$, $(S)_{0.5} = -(S)$, so the curve intersects the horizontal axis at the numerical value of $-(S)$. Since, for the purposes of establishing a line, v and (S) are taken as fixed numbers, the line drawn between the two intercepts expresses V_m as a function of $(S)_{0.5}$ for the given values of v and (S). [Since the Michaelis equation relates four properties—v, (S), V_m, and $(S)_{0.5}$—the system is fully defined if any three are specified. So if either V_m or $(S)_{0.5}$ is known, the value of the other could be determined by a single errorless determination of velocity at a known concentration of substrate.] More concisely, the line shows all $(S)_{0.5}$-V_m pairs that are compatible with the experimental values of (S) and v. When a similar line is generated from another v-(S) pair, the intersection of the lines gives the unique values of V_m and $(S)_{0.5}$ that are compatible with both of the v-(S) sets. If there were no experimental error, these would be the true values of V_m and $(S)_{0.5}$, so that all determinations of v would lead to lines intersecting at a single point (Figure 5-13). Since all determinations of v are subject to error, the lines obtained from a real experiment will intersect at different points, with the scatter of points depending on the extent of error (Figure 5-14). The medians of the values of V_m and $(S)_{0.5}$ specified by the intersections are then taken as the best estimates of these parameters. The original paper (*42*) should be consulted for discussion of the statistical basis of the approach, including methods for the estimation of the joint error of the estimates of V_m and $(S)_{0.5}$. These papers also discuss briefly the questionable basis of the least-squares approach to curve fitting and estimation of error in kinetic studies on enzymes, and of the large number of assumptions (few of which are likely to be valid in practice) that are involved in its use. As the authors point out, when this statistical approach of doubtful validity is used in conjunction with the double reciprocal plot, which as noted above has been shown to be the least reliable of all linear permutations of the Michaelis equation, there is little basis for confidence in the parameters that are estimated or in the reaction details that are sometimes deduced from such plots (35–37). These papers will not lead to the rapid abandonment of simple least-squares statistics in enzyme kinetics, but they may contribute to the eventual attainment of that desirable objective.

A statistical criterion for rejection of any observation whose error exceeds some arbitrary value is sometimes added to the least-squares approach. Such automatic rejection is incorporated in some programs supplied for use with computers or programmable calculators. The inherent absurdity of this treatment is seen in a thought experiment in which the error of a single point is progressively increased while all others remain constant. The estimates of V_m and $(S)_{0.5}$ are affected disproportionately by this single point as its error increases, until the arbitrary rejection boundary is reached, when the estimate of the parameters changes discontinuously to that determined by the other points. Thus a very small change in the value of an outlying point, by moving it over the rejection boundary, may have an absurdly large effect on the estimation of parameters. In effect, at the rejection boundary the slope of estimated values of $(S)_{0.5}$ and V_m as a function of the value of one experimental point is infinite. In addition, the degree of error that is required for rejection will depend on the value of v. The double reciprocal equation is probably worst in this regard. It is evident from the equation, and is illustrated graphically by Cornish-Bowden and Eisenthal (42), that a degree of error that will be very large to the eye or to a simple least-squares rejection criterion at one end of the scale will hardly be noticed at the other. A computerized version of the thought experiment described above is used by Cornish-Bowden and Eisenthal to illustrate the superiority of the median, rather than the average, in the estimation of enzyme parameters. This superiority results from the high sensitivity of the average to aberrant values. Packaged computerized treatments of the results of experiments with enzymes are ideally suited to the generation of numbers in minimal time with minimal involvement of the experimenter. But the investigator whose interest is in the properties of the enzyme rather than in numbers, and who is therefore more concerned with the validity of his estimates than with the ease with which they were obtained, should avoid such quick and easy but inherently unreliable expedients as programmed least-squares data processing with automatic rejection of aberrant points.

The Eisenthal–Cornish-Bowden plot, in spite of its unfamiliarity, seems at present to be the method of choice for estimation of $(S)_{0.5}$ and V_m values for noncooperative enzymes. This approach is not directly applicable to results obtained with cooperative enzymes, since here at least two other parameters—the number of interacting sites and the strength of interaction—are involved. In cases of very strong cooperativity, Eisenthal–Cornish-Bowden plots would be valid if $(S)^m$ were plotted on the $(S)_{0.5}$ axis, where m is the slope of a Hill plot. This is not useful in a practical case, since estimation of m requires a Hill plot or its equivalent, for which an estimate of V_m is a prerequisite. And the Hill plot will provide an estimate of $(S)_{0.5}$ [or K_m] that is probably as valid as that obtained from an Eisenthal–Cornish-Bowden plot.

Cooperative Enzymes

When an enzyme-catalyzed reaction is of higher order than first, reciprocal forms of the Michaelis equation such as equations 5-25, 5-26, and 5-27 will give nonlinear curves; thus in such cases they are less useful for extrapolation. Since they are all forms of the same equation, a value of m estimated, for example, from the slope of a Hill plot must apply to all. Thus, the plots will be linearized if $(S)^m$ is used wherever (S) appears in equations 5-25, 5-26, and 5-27 (*71*).

We thus see that in order to obtain a good estimate of V_m from the Eadie or either of the other reciprocal plots, we need m, which is derived from a Hill plot, for which V_m is needed. Evidently recycling from one type of plot to another is necessary in order to obtain the best estimates of these parameters. One approach is to make an Eadie plot, which though nonlinear will allow a rough estimation of V_m, and then to use this value in constructing a Hill plot. The slope of the Hill plot is in turn used as the linearizing exponent in a second Eadie plot, which should give as good an estimate of V_m as is obtainable from the experimental results. If this value differs significantly from the first estimate, it should be used in making a final Hill plot from which to estimate m and $(S)_{0.5}$. Alternatively, in a simple plot of log v as a function of log(S) the slope in the region below half-maximal velocity will usually approximate m closely enough to linearize the Eadie plot satisfactorily and permit a good estimate of V_m, on the basis of which a Hill plot may be made.

Of course these estimations may all be made by computer, eliminating the need for any plots. Most people who work with enzymes will probably prefer, however, to see the graphs. Patterns of variation from smooth or linear curves may suggest unexpected interactions, perhaps of metabolic significance, that would not be suspected if the results were merely processed nongraphically to yield estimates of the desired parameters as digital computer outputs. Further, it should be kept in mind that, as noted above, error is very inhomogeneously distributed in reciprocal plots, and that the common practice of fitting straight lines to points in such plots by least-squares statistical methods is in principle not valid. It is questionable whether such treatment of the results is preferable to drawing a visual best fit with a pencil and ruler, taking into account the relative confidence to be placed in points at the two ends of the curve in whichever type of plot is used. Of course a computer can also be programmed to take this inhomogeneity of error into account.

Our description of enzymes that catalyze reactions of kinetic order greater than 1 has so far been based on the concept of infinitely cooperative binding. That concept is, of course, an abstraction. As we noted above, an infinitely cooperative enzyme in the presence of a ligand would exist either as free enzyme E or with all binding sites filled, ES_n. A real enzyme cannot behave in this way; it will not collide simultaneously with n molecules of substrate, and must necessarily pass through the intermediate stages ES, ES_2, ..., on the way to the fully liganded form ES_n. In some, and probably many, cases cooperativity is so strong that the concentrations of enzyme species with some but not all binding sites filled are negligible, so that binding, and hence kinetic behavior, closely approximates infinitely cooperative behavior. But we must also deal with cases in which the binding interactions are weaker. We will consider first the effects of varying degrees of cooperativity on the graphical representations that are generally used for presentation and analysis of the results obtained with enzymes catalyzing reactions of higher order.

If an enzyme contained n catalytic sites that did not interact in any way, the kinetic consequences would be the same as if the solution contained n times as many enzyme molecules, each bearing one site. The reciprocal plots of Table 5-1 would be linear and the Hill plot would have a slope of 1. If the sites interacted infinitely strongly the Hill plot, as we have seen, would have a slope of n. Hence it is obvious that intermediate degrees of cooperativity must lead to slopes at the midpoint of a Hill plot that fall between 1 and n, depending on the strength of interaction. It is less obvious how the curves would differ at points other than the midpoint. To approach this question, we must consider how the Hill plots representing results obtained with real enzymes differ from the ideal plots considered above.

Whatever the mechanisms by which cooperative binding is produced, it may be described algebraically by the assignment of effective association or dissociation constants to the binding of successive molecules of ligands. This straightforward common-sense approach was applied by Adair (*1*) to the binding of oxygen by hemoglobin, and is sometimes termed the Adair approach. It consists merely in assigning values to the first dissociation constant, K_1, the second dissociation constant, K_2, and to other up to K_n to give the best fit to the empirical binding curve, or to the kinetic response curve in the case of an enzyme.

Even in the absence of cooperativity, the Adair constants for a multisite enzyme are not identical. The differences are small, and stem from very simple statistical considerations. If an enzyme contains a single site at which a ligand may bind, with an intrinsic dissociation constant K, binding may be represented by equation 5-29, where k_a and k_d are velocity constants for association and dissociation of the ligand. The dissociation constant K has

$$\text{E} + \text{S} \underset{k_d}{\overset{k_a}{\rightleftharpoons}} \text{ES} \qquad (5\text{-}29)$$

the value k_d/k_a. If an enzyme molecule contains two such sites that do not interact, equation 5-29 applies to each independently, and the curve of velocity as a function of substrate concentration will be identical to that corresponding to twice as many enzyme molecules, each bearing one site. This conclusion is intuitively obvious; if sites do not interact, it makes no difference whether there are one or many sites per enzyme molecule. The number of enzyme molecules bearing 0, 1, and each number up to n molecules of ligand can be easily calculated. If an enzyme has two identical and noninteracting sites at which a ligand may bind, the molecule as a whole is twice as likely to encounter and bind a ligand molecule as is a single site. Thus the rate of binding is twice as fast for the enzyme molecule as for a single site. But the ES complex has only one bound molecule of ligand; thus the rate of dissociation is the same as for a single site. This situation is schematically illustrated in equation 5-30. Here the dissociation constant

$$-\text{E} - + \text{S} \underset{2k_d}{\overset{2k_a}{\rightleftharpoons}} \text{S}-\text{E} - \qquad (5\text{-}30)$$

for the first molecule of ligand bound, K_1, is equal to $k_d/2k_a$, or $K/2$. Binding of the second molecule of ligand is represented by equation 5-31. Now only

$$\text{S}-\text{E} - + \text{S} \underset{2k_d}{\overset{k_a}{\rightleftharpoons}} \text{S}-\text{E} -\text{S} \qquad (5\text{-}31)$$

one site is available to bind substrate, so the effective binding rate constant is the same as for the single site. But the ligand may dissociate from either site, so the effective dissociation rate constant is twice that for one site. The second Adair dissociation constant, K_a, is then $2k_d/k_a$, or $2K$. The two Adair constants thus differ by a factor of 4. In the absence of cooperativity, the first and last Adair constants will always differ by a factor of n^2. It is easy to show, by an extension of the reasoning applied above to the two-site case, that the successive Adair constants for an enzyme molecule with n noninteracting sites are K/n, $2K/(n-1)$, $3K/(n-2)$, ..., nK. For the important case of four sites, the Adair constants are thus $K/4$, $2K/3$, $3K/2$ and $4K$.

The geometric mean of the Adair constants for noninteracting sites is the intrinsic dissociation constant for a single site. Whether the sites interact or not, the geometric mean of the Adair constants is equal to $(S)_{0.5}$, the ligand concentration at which half of the sites are filled (equation 5-32).

$$(S)_{0.5} = (K_1 K_2 K_3 \ldots K_n)^{1/n} \qquad (5\text{-}32)$$

It is easy to demonstrate, either algebraically or by counting filled and empty sites in a schematic representation, that when half of the sites are filled, the distribution of ligands among enzyme molecules is given by the coefficients of the expansion of $(a + b)^n$ if there is no interaction between sites. Thus for an enzyme with two noninteracting sites, when half of the sites are filled the relative concentrations of E, ES, and ES_2 are 1, 2, and 1. For a four-site case, the relative concentrations of E, ES, ES_2, ES_3, and ES_4 are 1, 4, 6, 4, and 1. These numbers of course are the same as the relative frequencies of $4:0$, $3:1$, $2:2$, $1:3$, and $0:4$ ratios if one were to take random 4-ball samples from a bag containing equal numbers of red and white balls. Thus the Adair constants are of no concern in the absence of interaction. They reflect the distribution of ligand molecules among enzyme molecules, but this distribution has no kinetic consequences if there is no interaction among sites. The case of no interaction had to be considered only for purposes of comparison. Cooperativity of binding is measured by the extent to which the relative values of the Adair constants differ from the statistical pattern described.

We have assumed that cooperative kinetic behavior results from cooperativity in ligand binding. There is another possibility—kinetic cooperativity might instead be a consequence of site-site interaction involving the actual catalytic step. That is, an enzyme might not catalyze any reaction unless all binding sites were occupied. For an enzyme with four catalytic sites, this would mean that no reaction could be catalyzed at any site unless the other three were also filled. Then

$$E + 4S \rightleftharpoons ES_4 \rightleftharpoons ES_3P \rightarrow \cdots$$

or

$$E + 4S \rightleftharpoons ES_4 \rightleftharpoons EP_4 \rightarrow \cdots$$

It would not matter, in terms of our present analysis, whether reaction occurred randomly at individual sites or was obligately simultaneous at all of them. In either case, the reaction would necessarily be kinetically of fourth order, even in the absence of any cooperativity in binding, because the concentration of ES_4 must be proportional to the fourth power of substrate concentration. For a multisite enzyme catalyzing a reaction that involved only one substrate, it would be difficult to distinguish by kinetic measurements between cooperativity in ligand binding and cooperativity in catalyzing a reaction. However, this difficulty is of no concern, since no such enzymes are known. When two or more substrates are involved in the reaction, the kinetic pattern observed when substrate concentrations are individually varied allows for simple distinction between cooperative binding and cooperative reaction. Most regulatory enzymes exhibit cross-cooperativity between substrates and between substrates and modifiers. That is, an increase in the concentration of one ligand changes the affinity of the enzyme for others. In such cases it is clear that the effect of site-site interactions is on binding.

The distinction between cooperative binding and cooperativity in the actual catalytic step can also be made by nonkinetic means. By use of isotopically labeled substrates and equilibrium-dialysis techniques, for example, the amount of substrate actually bound to the enzyme at different concentrations of substrate may be determined. If the kinetic cooperativity is a result of cooperativity in binding, the curves and parameters obtained from the binding study should be similar to those from kinetic analysis.

It is intuitively obvious, and will not be proved here, that the slope of a Hill plot at any point is equal to the average number of ligand molecules that are being added to the enzyme in the equation that is applicable at that point. If the appropriate equation is $E + S \rightleftharpoons ES$, the slope of a Hill plot will be 1; for a nearly infinitely cooperative enzyme, over most of the range the applicable equation is very nearly $E + nS \rightleftharpoons ES_n$, with negligible participation of other forms; in that case the slope will be n. If the cooperativity is weaker, a mixture of E, ES, ES_2, and ES_3 may be converted to a mixture of ES, ES_2, ES_3, and ES_4, and the slope would depend on the relative amounts of the various forms. It must, of course, have a value between 1 and n.

Although it is approached very closely, truly infinite cooperativity in binding ligands is of course not possible for a real enzyme. However strong the cooperativity, there must be a substrate concentration so low that the predominant forms of enzyme are E and ES. For a strongly cooperative enzyme, this condition could only arise at concentrations of substrate very low relative to $(S)_{0.5}$. Consider, for example, a four-site enzyme for which the successive Adair constants differ by a constant ratio of 30, with $K_1 = 2.7\,mM$, $K_2 = 90\,\mu M$, $K_3 = 3\,\mu M$, and $K_4 = 0.1\,\mu M$. The $(S)_{0.5}$ value, the geometric mean of these constants, would be $16\,\mu M$. This would be an exceedingly cooperative enzyme; in fact this degree of cooperativity would appear to be infinite by kinetic criteria. But, in principle, at a very low concentration of substrate, far below that at which it is likely that the rate of reaction could be observed, what little reaction occurred would be due almost entirely to the ES complex. For example, if the concentration of substrate were 1 μM, equilibrium calculations show that the concentration of ES would be 1/2700 that of free enzyme, and that of ES_2 would be 1/2,430,000 that of free enzyme or only 1/900 that of ES. Each molecule of the ES_2 complex would generate product at twice the rate of the ES complex, but even so ES_2 would contribute only 1/450 of the total reaction. The concentrations of ES_3 and ES_4 would be much lower still. Under such circumstances the reaction, if it could be followed, would be found to be kinetically of first order with regard to S, and the slope of the Hill plot in this region would be 1. (Because the velocity of the reaction would be only about 0.03% of V_m, it would in most cases be difficult to estimate the rate with much accuracy.) The situation is exactly analogous at the high end of the curve; concentration of ES_3 will be very low, but still so much higher than the concentrations of forms bearing one or two molecules of ligand that the contribution of those other forms will be negligible and the slope of the plot will again be 1. This region is less experimentally accessible than the extreme lower end because as v approaches V_m the denominator of the Hill function becomes a very small difference between large numbers, with a resulting increase in relative experimental error. If cooperativity is strong, the central region of the Hill plot will be essentially linear with a slope of n. The greater the cooperativity, the longer will be the essentially linear region, as is illustrated in Figure 5-15. Evidently the slope of the Hill plot at its midpoint can be taken to be a good estimate of the number of interacting sites only if the plot has been shown to be essentially linear over a wide range of velocities.

Since the Hill plot for a cooperative reaction has a slope of 1 at each end with higher slope in the middle region, it follows that the displacement of the two linear terminal regions bears a direct relationship to the degree of cooperativity. This is also shown in Figure 5-15. As cooperativity increases, the slope at the midpoint, the velocity range over which the midpoint slope is essentially constant, and the distance between the linear parts of the curve all increase. The perpendicular distance between the asymptotes of the curve is directly proportional to the difference between the free energy of binding of the first and the last ligand molecules (*103, 127*). Differences in the pattern of interaction energy cause displacement of the Hill plot or changes in its shape. If the interaction were expressed entirely as difference between the first two Adair constants K_1 and K_2, while K_3 and K_4 remained in the normal statistical pattern characteristic of noninteracting sites, the whole pattern would move downward, and if the interaction were expressed only in change of relative values of K_3 and K_4 the pattern would move upward.

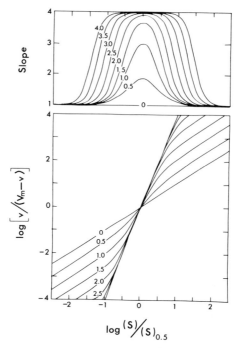

Figure 5-15. Shapes of Hill plots as a function of the degree of interaction between substrate-binding sites. The curves in the lower panel were calculated for an enzyme with four binding sites. Each substrate molecule bound makes the free energy of binding at each other site more negative by the number of kilocalories per mole indicated by the number identifying each curve. The curves in the upper panel show the slopes of the Hill plots in the lower panel. They extend beyond the portions of the Hill plots that are shown in the lower panel.

In neither of these cases would the maximal slope occur at half saturation. More unsymmetrical patterns of interaction would lead to changes in the shapes of Hill plots. Curve b in Figure 5-16 is the response curve that would be observed if the first molecule of substrate bound enhanced binding at other sites very strongly, the second molecule decreased affinity at other sites very strongly, the second molecule decreased affinity at other sites very strongly, and the third molecule again increased affinity at the remaining site. No such extreme situation will be encountered in nature, but this exaggerated case illustrates the fact that Hill plots may vary considerably from the "normal" shape. They will have a maximal slope at the midpoint (when $\phi = 1$) and be symmetrical around that point only if the interaction energy is evenly distributed among the binding steps, as in curve a of Figure 5-16 and the curves of Figure 5-15. Hence all of our previous statements concerning Hill plots refer, strictly speaking, only to cases where the free

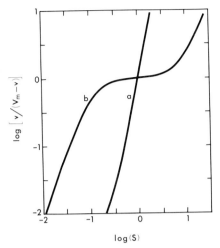

Figure 5-16. Effect of pattern of interaction between binding sites on the shape of the Hill plot in the vicinity of half saturation. Both curves were calculated for an enzyme with four binding sites and a difference between free energy of binding of the first and last ligands of −4.1 kcal/mole. Thus for both curves the distance between the terminal linear portions of the curves would be equal. Curve a was calculated on the assumption that each molecule of substrate bound has the same effect on binding at each other site. Thus this curve corresponds approximately to the 1.5 kcal/mole curve of Figure 5-15. Curve b was calculated on the basis of changes in free energies of binding of −8.5, +8.0, and −3.6 kcal/mole as the first 3 substrate molecules are bound, respectively. Midpoint slopes: curve a, 3.6; curve b, 0.05.

energy of binding changes by approximately equal increments as each molecule of ligand is bound.

An interesting modification of the Hill plot was suggested by Watari and Isogai (*120*). If log(S) is subtracted from each side of the Hill equation, the result is equation 5-33. Thus when the left-hand term of equation 5-33 is

$$\log\left[\frac{v}{V_m - v} \cdot \frac{1}{(S)}\right] = (n - 1) \log S - \log K \qquad (5\text{-}33)$$

plotted against log(S), the slope of the resulting curve at every point will be smaller by one than the slope of a standard Hill plot at the same point (Figure 5-17). The consequence of interest is that at each extreme the curve asymptotically approaches a slope of 0 rather than 1. Since the distance between these terminal linear regions is proportional to the difference between the free energies of binding of the first and last substrate molecules, a scale of change in binding free energy ($\Delta\Delta G_b^0$) may be fitted to the vertical coordinate. Since the scale is to be used only to measure the distance between two lines, the position of zero is undefined, and the scale may be moved vertically to any desired position.

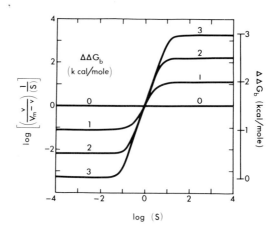

Figure 5-17.   Plot of the usual Hill function minus log(S) against log(S), as suggested by Watari and Isogai (*119*). The curves were calculated on the basis of symmetrical distribution of interaction energy, and thus correspond to the plots for the same $\Delta\Delta G_b$ values in Figure 5-15.

The Watari-Isogai plot is ingenious, and may be of illustrative value in teaching. It does not seem likely to be of much help to experimentalists because of the experimental inaccessibility of very low and especially of very high parts of the velocity range. It might be possible, however, to obtain a rough estimate of $\Delta\Delta G_b{}^0$ by superposing a plot of experimental points onto a graph showing curves for different degrees of interaction (such as Figure 5-17), and seeing which calculated curve is most closely approximated by the experimental points.

Overall Order of Reaction

Our discussion of kinetic orders of reaction has been in terms of order with respect to one substrate. This is probably the only kind of kinetic order that is relevant to enzyme action and regulation *in vivo*, since no significant change in total cell water can be expected. But it is of chemical interest that enzyme-catalyzed reactions may give much higher overall orders than are obtainable with homogeneous reactions.

The overall order of a reaction is measured by diluting the reaction mixture and thus decreasing the concentrations of all reaction components—substrates, activators, inhibitors, modifiers, and catalysts—by the same factor. On first thought, it might appear that the overall order should be the sum of all of the orders with respect to individual components, since all concentrations are changed. In fact, overall orders are generally much lower than this sum, for rather obvious reasons. Even though a complicated homogeneous reaction might involve several components and under appropriate conditions might be shown to be of first or second order with respect to each, under any given set of conditions one step will usually be sufficiently slower than the others so as to be rate determining. Thus the only effects seen on dilution of the reaction mixture will be those on this slow step, and the observed dilution kinetic order will be that corresponding to the slow step. Dilution orders higher than 2 are rare for homogeneous reactions.

With enzyme-catalyzed reactions, the situation is markedly different. Even a simple two-substrate reaction following normal Michaelis kinetics should be expected to exhibit third-order dilution kinetics under appropriate circumstances. For simplicity, we will assume that the two substrates, A and B, bind randomly (not in fixed sequence) to the catalytic site. Then, from equation 5-34, the concentration of the reactive complex is a linear function

$$K_A K_B' = \frac{(E)(A)(B)}{(EAB)}$$

$$(EAB) = \frac{(E)(A)(B)}{K_A K_B'}$$

$$v = k(EAB) = \frac{k(E)(A)(B)}{K_A K_B'} \tag{5-34}$$

of the concentrations of E, A, and B. Third-order dilution kinetics will not be seen, however, in the vicinity of enzyme saturation, where most enzyme reactions are run *in vitro*. On dilution, the concentrations of A and B will decrease by the dilution factor, but the tendency for the concentration of free enzyme to decrease will be countered by dissociation of the EA, EB, and EAB complexes as a consequence of the lower ligand concentrations. When the enzyme is nearly saturated, this dissociation will hold the concentration of E nearly constant so the dilution order will be about 2. As dilution and the resultant dissociation continue, however, (E) approaches $(E)_T$. When $(E) = 0.99(E)_T$, for example, its relative concentration cannot be increased significantly by further dissociation; consequently, on further dilution, the concentrations of E, A, and B will all change by the dilution factor and the dilution kinetic order of the reaction will be three. Since the necessary condition is that nearly all of the enzyme be free, third-order kinetics will be seen only when v/V_m is very small.

With enzyme that bind substrates and modifiers cooperatively, however, much higher orders are obtainable. Indeed, it is clear from the discussion above that the dilution order could theoretically equal the number of components in the reaction complex, including the enzyme. As an illustration, we may consider a hypothetical enzyme that binds six molecules of ligands in the reactive complex [for example, two molecules each of two substrates and two molecules of a positive modifier (equation 5-35)]. The equilibrium constant for this enzyme is shown in equation 5-36. In our illustration we will consider ligand binding to be infinitely cooperative between all sites. Since the relative values of $(S)_{0.5}$ do not matter, we will for simplicity consider all ligands to bind with the same effective $(S)_{0.5}$.

$$E + 2A + 2B + 2M \rightleftharpoons EA_2B_2M_2 \qquad (5\text{-}35)$$

$$K = \frac{(E)(A)^2(B)^2(M)^2}{(EA_2B_2M_2)} \qquad (5\text{-}36)$$

Since binding is assumed to be infinitely cooperative, the enzyme exists only as E and the fully liganded complex. In this case the order of the reaction must approach 7, the number of components in the reactive complex.

It should be emphasized that seventh-order dilution kinetics does not imply a seventh-order velocity constant or the occurrence of a heptamolecular step. The difference between a homogeneous reaction and one catalyzed by an enzyme is strikingly evident here. We assume that the actual chemical reaction is slow relative to binding and dissociation, so that $EA_2B_2M_2$ remains at all times essentially in equilibrium with free ligands and the free enzyme. This assumption leads to equation 5-37, where K is a sixth-order

$$v = k(EA_2B_2M_2) = \frac{k(E)(A)^2(B)^2(M)^2}{K} \qquad (5\text{-}37)$$

dissociation constant (the product of six individual dissociation constants). The predicted seventh-order kinetics thus results from a first-order velocity constant and six first-order dissociation constants. Thus the entropy difficulties that preclude high-order dilution kinetics of homogeneous reactions (the unlikelihood that many molecules will collide simultaneously) are overcome by the specificity, strength, and cooperativity of binding at the evolution-designed binding sites of a cooperative enzyme, which is able to assemble the reaction components into a multimolecular complex.

These theoretical considerations were first tested in 1965 by experiments on yeast DPN isocitrate dehydrogenase (*12a*). The oxidation of isocitrate (equation 5-38) is, on the basis of Hill plots obtained when each component

$$\text{isocitrate} + \text{NAD}^+ \rightleftharpoons \alpha\text{-ketoglutarate} + CO_2 + \text{NADH} + H^+ \qquad (5\text{-}38)$$

is varied individually, fourth-order with respect to isocitrate and second-order with respect to the other substrate, NAD^+, to the cationic cofactor, Mg^{2+}, and to the positive modifier, AMP. All Hill plots were linear over the velocity range observed, about 100-fold. Since binding was thus seen to be highly cooperative, it was suggested that the kinetic orders reflected the actual numbers of interacting binding sites; that is, that each of these slopes was equal to the corresponding n.

When a dilution experiment of the type discussed above was done with this enzyme, in the velocity range between about $10^{-2} V_m$ and $10^{-4} V_m$, the order was found to approximate the theoretical maximal value of 11. This result emphasizes the exceedingly strong cooperativity of ligand binding by this enzyme, since it appears that even when only about 0.01% of the enzyme is in the fully liganded form, the enzyme is still partitioned nearly exclusively between this form and the free enzyme. That is, even at this point, we do not see significant deviations from linearity of the Hill plot.

Dilution experiments of the type described are facilitated by the fact that the ratio of concern is that of free enzyme to total enzyme. Thus when the reaction becomes too slow (as a result of dilution) for accurate determination, the concentration of enzyme may be increased. So long as appropriate control experiments—overlapping each enzyme concentration with the higher and lower concentrations—establish that the reaction is strictly first-order with regard to enzyme concentration, this increase in enzyme concentration will not affect the results.

As discussed earlier for the general case, it is theoretically possible that cooperative kinetics might result from cooperativity in catalyzing the actual reaction rather than from cooperative binding. This possibility is excluded in the case of isocitrate dehydrogenase by the strong mutual cooperativity observed—an increase in the concentration of either substrate, of Mg^{2+}, or of AMP increases the affinity of the enzyme for each of the others, as estimated from kinetic results. The conclusion that the cooperative kinetic behavior of this enzyme depends on cooperative binding was also tested by direct equilibrium binding studies (71). The stoichiometries of binding that had been earlier suggested by the slope of kinetic Hill plots—4 molecules of isocitrate, 2 of NAD^+, 2 of divalent cation and 2 of AMP per molecule of enzyme—were confirmed by the binding studies, as was the strong mutual cooperativity. Indeed, cooperativity of binding is so strong that, with specific activities of the isotopically labeled compounds that were available and concentrations of enzyme that were feasible, it was not possible to measure binding of any ligand unless at least one other (unlabeled) was simultaneously present.

The kinetic patterns of enzyme-catalyzed reactions, and especially of reactions catalyzed by cooperative enzymes, differ from those for homogeneous reactions in many ways, as we have seen. Another example of strikingly different enzymatic behavior is seen in Figure 5-18. Because of

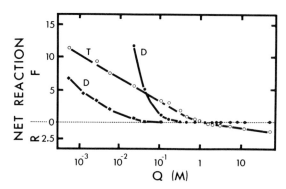

Figure 5-18. Dependence on the reaction parameter Q of the reaction catalyzed by isocitrate dehydrogenases. Reaction mixtures contained 100 mM Hepes-KOH (pH 7.6). 4 mM MgSO$_4$, 3 mM dithiothreitol, 0.2 mM pyridine nucleotide pool (NAD$^+$ + NADH or NADP$^+$ + NADPH), 2 mM substrate-product pool (isocitrate + α-ketoglutarate), NaHCO$_3$ at 20 mM plus the α-ketoglutarate concentration, and enzyme. T: pig heart NADP isocitrate dehydrogenase; D: yeast NAD isocitrate dehydrogenase; ■, enzyme activity under standard assay conditions (initial rate in absence of products) 3.5 times that of the NADP enzyme; ●, activity 70 times that of the NADP enzyme. Note that even at the higher concentration the NAD enzyme becomes nearly inactive before the equilibrium point is reached, and that its catalysis of the reverse reaction is too weak to show on this scale. From Barnes *et al.* (*20*). Reprinted with permission from *Biochemistry* **11**, 4322 (1972). Copyright by the American Chemical Society.

the highly cooperative binding of the substrate and the inhibitory effect of the products, α-ketoglutarate and NADH, the rate of the reaction catalyzed by yeast NAD-specific isocitrate dehydrogenase becomes essentially zero well before equilibrium is reached and the reverse reaction is not catalyzed at a measurable rate at the pH of the experiment (*20*). Thus, this enzyme may be said to be a one-way catalyst. In fact the first indication of the unusual kinetic properties of NAD isocitrate dehydrogenase was the observation by Kornberg and Pricer in 1951 (*63*) that this enzyme would not catalyze the reverse reaction under the conditions employed. In contrast, the NADP-specific enzyme catalyzes the reaction well in either direction.

The phenomenon of unidirectionality shown in Figure 5-18 is strictly kinetic; it does not violate any thermodynamic principle or the concept of microscopic reversibility. The situation is merely that as the concentrations of α-ketoglutarate and NADPH rise relative to those of isocitrate and NAD$^+$ the enzyme becomes progressively less active catalytically, so that before the equilibrium point is reached the enzyme becomes essentially inert.

It does not seem likely that inactivity of the enzyme under conditions near or to the right of equilibrium confers any selective advantage on the cell. Rather this behavior is probably an unimportant consequence of the enzymic properties that have evolved to produce a high degree of cooperativity under physiological conditions (near or beyond the left-hand edge of Figure 5-18). It may be expected that many equally strange patterns will be seen as the behaviors of more regulatory enzymes are studied over reasonably wide ranges of concentrations of substrates and modifiers. The steepness of the curve for the NAD enzyme in the physiological region compared with that for the NADP enzyme illustrates the sharp dependence of a cooperative enzyme on substrate concentration.

BASIS OF COOPERATIVITY

An effect of a bound ligand molecule on the affinity of an enzyme for a second molecule might be exerted in various ways. The simplest is direct competitive exclusion, where the two ligands bind at the same or overlapping sites so that the presence of one prevents binding of the other. Many cases of such competitive inhibition are known in enzyme kinetics and, as we have seen, some of them appear to be of great importance in metabolic regulation. Direct interaction between ligand molecules seems insufficient, however, to account for the broad range of kinetic interactions and modulations that has been observed. Cooperative binding, for example, could in principle result if the first molecule of ligand that binds forms part of the binding site for the second molecule, and so on. But it is hard to imagine how molecules of the same substrate so clustered together could all be able to participate in a reaction. Furthermore, the evidence that multiple sites for binding of the same ligands are normally located on different subunits is compelling. Where many subunits are involved, it becomes geometrically impossible for them to assemble in such a way as to bring all of the binding sites together. Thus it is accepted generally that cooperative substrate binding and modulation of enzyme behavior by metabolites must result from interaction between sites located some distance apart on the enzyme molecule, and frequently on different subunits.

It seems self-evident that the binding of a ligand molecule at one point on an enzyme surface can affect the affinity with which ligands of the same or a different species are bound at a remote site only by changing the conformation and electron distribution of the enzyme molecule. Since the primary structure of the protein—the amino acid sequence—is unchanged, no alternative explanation seems possible. Because the interacting sites are frequently located on different subunits, it is clear that the conformational alterations must be propagated across subunit boundaries. In the process, it is quite possible that what is sometimes referred to as the quaternary structure of the enzyme—the relative positions of the subunits—may change. But because the assembly of subunits depends on the three-dimensional arrangement of functional groups and hydrophobic regions on the subunits, a change in quaternary structure must reflect an underlying change in subunit conformation. In some cases the quaternary structure may change to the maximal extent—involving actual dissociation or association of subunits—as a consequence of modifier action. Even if cases of this kind exist, the primary effect must be on subunit conformation, with a resultant increase or decrease in the free energy of subunit-subunit association.

The means by which the binding of a ligand is associated with change in enzyme conformation are in a sense outside the scope of this book, which is concerned with metabolic correlation and regulatory interactions and the patterns of enzymic behavior by which they are produced. These operational effects are, to a degree, independent of the molecular bases of the responses, just as the function and even design of electronic devices can be discussed with no mention of the underlying physics of semiconductors or of electron emission from a hot metal. A more important reason for not considering at any length the mechanisms responsible for regulatory enzyme behavior is that these mechanisms are as yet not at all well understood.

Induced Fit

Explicit realization that an enzyme is a dynamic mechanism, with conformational changes being involved in the catalytic act, dates from the induced fit concept proposed by Koshland in 1958 (*64*). An early argument for this concept may be cited to illustrate the cogency of purely kinetic evidence for it. A kinase typically catalyzes the transfer of a phosphoryl group from ATP to a specific location (usually an oxygen atom) on a specific substrate molecule. Hexokinase, for example, transfers only to the oxygen on C-6 of glucose or closely related hexoses. In more chemical terms, one specific oxygen atom of hexose attacks the phosphorus atom of the terminal phosphate group, displacing ADP. This specificity would be extremely difficult to reconcile with the classical picture of an enzyme as a rigid jig that binds the substrate and, in the process of binding, distorts it, altering bond angles or lengths and electronic distribution and so activating it for reaction. If this were how a kinase worked, the binding of ATP should be followed by rapid hydrolysis. Bound ATP must be surrounded by water molecules, which are roughly equivalent to alcoholic OH groups in nucleophilic displacement reactions. But hexokinase catalyzes the transfer of phosphoryl to hexose millions of times faster than transfer to water (hydrolysis). Evidently ATP is not activated for reaction except when the specific receptor substrate is bound.

The concept of substrate-induced change in enzyme conformation as an integral part of the catalytic process was not generally popular when it was first proposed, but it now seems to be accepted nearly unanimously. Ligand-induced changes have recently been illustrated by x-ray diffraction studies showing that marked conformational differences at the catalytic sites may result from binding of substrate. It is not possible, of course, to watch the approach and binding of the substrate by means of x-ray diffraction techniques. Thus it might be argued that the enzyme exists in an equilibrium mixture containing a small fraction of molecules in the same conformation as is seen in the enzyme-substrate complex; that only these molecules can bind substrate; and that binding of substrate displaces the equilibrium between the two forms, causing a net conversion of the inactive form to the active form capable of binding substrate. This explanation seems implausible on several grounds. It supplies no explanation for the types of behavior on which the concept of induced fit was originally based, such as the specificity of enzyme reactions. The x-ray studies also supply evidence against the preexistence of the catalytically active form of the catalytic site. In the carboxypeptidase-substrate complex, for example, it seems possible to identify the interaction between the terminal carboxylate group and a positively charged group on the enzyme that leads to a primary change of position, which in turn frees an arm of the enzyme to swing over the substrate, bringing a residue within catalytic range (75, 95). Not only can the train of events be deduced, but the conformation of the enzyme in the enzyme-substrate complex is such that a substrate molecule could not bind to a free enzyme molecule with this same conformation. In effect, the enzyme binds substrate at an open site and then closes over it to catalyze the reaction; a substrate molecule could not enter the closed conformation.

Modifier-Induced Conformational Change

Soon after the discovery that metabolites chemically unrelated to the substrate could alter the affinity of an enzyme for that substrate, Gerhart and Pardee (49) proposed, by a reasonable extension of the induced-fit concept, that binding of the modifier induces a change in conformation of the enzyme that extends to the catalytic site and alters its affinity for substrate. This suggestion fits the observed behavior of cooperative enzymes into the framework of general properties of proteins. It seems as reasonable today, when more is known about both cooperative enzymes and proteins in general, as when it was proposed. The details of interaction must be different for each enzyme, but the basic pattern—change in conformation on binding of a specific ligand, with specific effects on the affinity of the enzyme for one or more specific ligands—is probably general.

The Koshland or "Sequential" Model

Koshland and colleagues (65, 66) have developed a treatment of the kinetics of metabolite-modulated enzymes that is based on ligand-induced conformation changes. Site-site interactions are dealt with in terms of subunit interaction energies. In the simplest form of this treatment, binding of a ligand molecule by one subunit of a multisubunit enzyme causes conversion of that subunit from form A to form B. The pattern of subunit interactions is now changed. Before there had been only A-A interactions, but some of these are now changed to A-B interactions. (The number of interactions, and the number that are changed because of a change in conformation of a single subunit, depends on assumptions as to whether each subunit interacts with all others or only with certain ones. Such details need not concern us here.) If A-B interactions are stronger than A-A interactions, the attachment of ligand to enzyme will be stabilized. More importantly, the presence of one subunit in the B conformation raises the possibility of producing B-B interactions as a consequence of binding a second molecule of ligand. If B-B interactions are stronger than A-B and A-A interactions, it is immediately clear that binding of each molecule of ligand after the first will be facilitated; that is, ligand binding will be cooperative. Although the treatment has been developed mainly in terms of cooperative binding of a single type of ligand, it is evidently equally applicable to cooperative binding involving two or several types of ligand molecules.

This treatment supplies a plausible framework for consideration of the behavior of cooperative enzymes. It should be recognized that we deal here with a formalized abstraction, not with a description of any real case. The all-or-none change implied in the change from conformation A to conformation B in the simplest form of the treatment is, for example, a simplifying formalism. As Koshland (65) has pointed out, the conversion probably goes by way of intermediate steps. Thus when only the first ligand molecule has been bound, the subunit to which it is bound may not, because of constraints imposed by other subunits, have changed fully to the conformation it will finally assume in the fully liganded enzyme, whereas some or all of the other subunits, although unliganded, may have been influenced by the liganded subunit to change their conformation to some intermediate form.

Attribution of intersite interactions to subunit-subunit interactions is also a formalism. If two sites located on different subunits interact, the interaction in a sense is necessarily between subunits. But an assumption that a change in conformation within a single subunit and a change in conformation of one subunit induced by a neighboring subunit are in principle different need not be valid. An amino acid residue in a multisubunit enzyme may not "know" whether a neighboring chain, which bears an attractive or repulsive residue, is a remote (in terms of primary sequence) part of its own polypeptide or is part of a different subunit. Functional groups, hydrophobic regions, and open spaces are arranged to functional advantage. This arrangement depends in part on the three-dimensional structure assumed by each subunit and in part on the specific aggregation of subunits; once the enzyme is assembled the distinction between subunit conformation and subunit interaction may not always be meaningful in a functional sense.

The Monod or "Concerted" Model

Treatments of the Pardee-Koshland type resemble the induced-fit concept of the catalytic site, in that they are based on ligand-induced changes of conformation. An alternative treatment, suggested by Monod, Wyman, and Changeux (86), resembles the concept of preexisting equilibrium between active and inactive catalytic sites, in that it is based on a ligand-independent equilibration of unliganded enzyme between two states. This model envisages equilibration between states with different affinities for ligands, but does not necessarily make the unlikely assumption of a catalytic site that preexists, in the absence of ligand, in the same conformation as in the fully liganded enzyme. In fact, the concept of substrate-induced conformational changes at the catalytic sites, which seems now well-established, could be incorporated into the Monod-Wyman-Changeux model, while retaining the concept of preexisting equilibration between states characterized by different affinities for substrate and other ligands. This suggestion was not made by Monod, Wyman, and Changeux, and it seems probably inconsistent with the views on which the model was initially constructed, but it is a logical permutation of that model.

Briefly, the Monod-Wyman-Changeux model is that of a multisubunit enzyme that exists in the absence of ligands in two forms. T, the predominant form, does not bind ligand, or has a low affinity for it; R, a form existing at very low relative concentrations, has a higher affinity for ligand. It is a fundamental postulate of the model that, because of "conservation of symmetry" (a formalism that could be translated to the formalism "very weak A-B interactions as compared to A-A and B-B interactions" in the Koshland treatment) all subunits in an enzyme molecule must be in the same conformation; thus a 4-subunit enzyme will exist either as R_4 or as T_4. Because of this requirement that all subunits must change conformation simultaneously, the model is often spoken of as the concerted model. When a ligand is present, some molecules of R will bind one or more ligand molecules. Because the model rules out ligand-induced changes in affinity, the intrinsic binding constants for all sites in the R_4 model will be equal, regardless of the number of ligand molecules bound; that is, binding to an R_4 molecule will follow the noncooperative statistical pattern discussed earlier. But because binding of one or more ligand molecules reduces the concentration of free R_4, equilibrium is disturbed and a net conversion of T_4 to R_4 must follow.

The necessary and sufficient condition for cooperative binding is that the free energy of binding for the last ligand be more negative than that for the first. In other words, later ligand-binding steps (or at least the last one) must be characterized by higher affinity, or a lower dissociation constant (after the statistical factor is taken into account) than that characteristic of the first molecule bound. This situation tends to be obscured in the Monod-Wyman-Changeux model by the emphasis that is placed on the "allosteric transition" from T_4 to R_4. Binding of ligand is postulated to affect this conformational change only by removing R_4 and thus disturbing the R_4/T_4 equilibrium. It is clear, however, that in terms of thermodynamics, which is independent of pathway, the effective dissociation constant for the binding of the first ligand, K_1, is larger than that for binding of the second and later ligand molecules because it must be the product of the constants for two steps (equations 5-39 and 5-40). The equilibrium constant for the R to T interconversion is given the symbol L in the Monod-Wyman-Changeux

$$T_4 \rightleftharpoons R_4 \qquad K = 1/L \tag{5-39}$$

$$R_4 + S \rightleftharpoons R_4S \qquad K = 4/K_i \tag{5-40}$$

$$\overline{T_4 + S \rightleftharpoons R_4S \qquad K = 4/K_iL = 1/K_1} \tag{5-41}$$

model. We are here using K_i for the intrinsic dissociation constant of sites in the R_4 molecule. For the statistical reasons discussed earlier, the effective dissociation constant for the first molecule is $K_i/4$ (thus the equilibrium constant for the binding reaction shown above is $4/K_i$). Then K_1 (the dissociation constant for binding of the first molecule of substrate) equals $K_iL/4$. For binding of the second molecule of ligand (equation 5-42), the dissociation constant, K_2, is $2K_i/3$. Thus the ratio K_1/K_2 for this model

$$R_4S + S \rightleftharpoons R_4S_2 \tag{5-42}$$

will be $(K_iL/4)/(2K_i/3) = 0.375L$. Values of L of the order of 1000 were suggested for cases of marked cooperativity (86). This value is seen to correspond to a K_1/K_2 ratio of 375.

The ratios between K_2, K_3, and K_4 will be those characteristic of noncooperative binding, since a fundamental postulate of the model is that binding of ligand molecules does not affect affinities at other sites. Thus the equations that are derived from this model are merely those that specify cooperative interactions in which the whole interaction is between the first and second binding steps.

Differences between the Models

A rather large amount of time and effort has been devoted to comparison of these two models. Since both are formalisms rather than descriptions of mechanisms, and since neither deals with the mechanisms by which cooperative behavior arises, this extended discussion has been generally unproductive, and I do not wish to add to it beyond a brief comment on the nature of the difference between the two approaches.

The two models overlap in some ways and are markedly different in others. The terms "sequential" and "concerted" may be useful names for the two models, but they do not clearly identify the fundamental difference in approach. The Koshland treatment allows for essentially concerted change of conformation, which will occur whenever A–A and B–B interactions are very much stronger than A–B interactions. Although both may be termed thermodynamic models, since both make the Michaelis assumption that enzyme, ligands, and enzyme-ligand complexes are in virtual equilibrium and attribute cooperative kinetic behavior to cooperativity of binding, ironically they differ mainly in terms of assumed pathway (which is a kinetic matter). The fundamental distinction hinges on the question of the sequence of ligand binding and conformational change. In the Koshland model, the conformational change is seen as a consequence of the binding of ligand, which it must therefore accompany or follow. The Monod-Wyman-Changeux model sees the conformational change as independent of binding, and indeed as an obligate prerequisite to binding (or at least as an obligate prerequisite to high-affinity binding). Thus the distinction is a matter of relative rates of different possible pathways, which is kinetics. Are all or most enzyme molecules capable of binding substrates, or is only a very small fraction of them capable of binding? Does the path obligately include a thermodynamically unstable rare form of the unliganded enzyme molecule (form R in the Monod-Wyman-Changeux model) or not? These are the diagnostic questions if the two models are to be compared. In a molecule as large as that of a typical enzyme, there must be many conformations with free energies sufficiently close to that of the predominant form that they will exist at low concentrations. The point at issue here is not whether rare conformations exist (they must), but whether one of them participates obligately in ligand binding, as is required by the Monod-Wyman-Changeux model.

No definite statement on the relation of any models to the behavior of real regulatory enzymes can be made as yet. There is no reason why the mechanistic details underlying the behavior of all enzymes that catalyze reactions of order higher than one, or that are modulated by metabolites, need be similar. The properties of each enzyme have evolved to a considerable extent individually. Just as enzymes catalyze reactions in very different ways—for example, some form covalent bonds with a substrate or an intermediate, but most do not—kinetic behavior patterns with selective advantage must be based on various types of interactions.

As a personal guess I would expect that, as more comes to be known about the properties of proteins and the behavior of enzymes, the concept of obligate participation of rare conformations of enzymes in the initial binding step (the "concerted" model) will fade away.

The Koshland approach is not really a model. Rather it is something that is perhaps more useful: a conceptual framework into which results can be fitted, and a formalized description. In this respect it resembles the Adair approach. Adair pointed out that, whatever the molecular basis for cooperative binding of n molecules of ligand to a protein molecule, the process can be described by n formal equilibrium association equations, in which the n equilibrium constants are treated as assignable parameters; that is, their values are chosen to best fit the data. This approach does not provide any explanation of molecular events, but it supplies a basis for thinking about the changes and for construction of computational models to illustrate various formal aspects of binding. The calculated model response curves presented in this chapter, as well as most such curves published by other workers, were calculated on the basis of systematic variation of the values to be assigned to Adair constants. The Koshland treatment builds on the Adair approach, pointing out that subunit-subunit interactions will be among the factors responsible for changes in Adair constants that are caused by binding of ligand molecules. If all of the conformational and interactive changes that affect the strength of ligand binding are formally attributed to subunit-subunit interactions, we have the Koshland approach.

It would be meaningless to debate whether the Adair treatment is valid or not. It makes no assumptions; it is merely a way of describing or predicting binding response curves. It cannot be invalid; the question in any given context is how useful it will be and, in general, it has been very useful. To a considerable extent similar comments apply to the Koshland approach, which is also a treatment that allows for formal description or prediction of response curves. There is no sense in which it can be proved or disproved, since it is not a suggested mechanism. It is a way of considering experimental results and especially a basis for construction of computational models aimed at illustrating aspects of enzyme-ligand interaction. As a matter of convenience, it assigns all changes to subunit-subunit interactions. It should be evident that this assignment is merely for the sake of convenience. Koshland has pointed out that changes in interaction between subunits must of course result from ligand-induced changes in subunit conformation (65).

BINDING ENERGIES AND ENZYME ACTION

Whatever the molecular mechanisms involved, one aspect of enzyme-ligand interaction seems clear: the large and negative free energy of binding provides the driving force for the conformational changes in the enzyme that are necessary for cooperative binding, for response to changes in modifier concentration, and for catalysis of the reaction. This generalization is obscured in the Monod treatment. Although implicit in the Koshland approach, it is not explicitly emphasized.

The following discussion is compatible with the Koshland treatment, but not with the basic Monod model. It is based on the concept of induced fit, the proposal by Gerhart and Pardee (49) of modifier-induced conformational changes, and suggestions by Low and Somero (77) regarding contributions of protein-ion interactions in attainment of the transition state.

Cooperative Binding

If we consider first the noncooperative binding of a ligand by a protein with only one binding site, we may write formal equations 5-43 and 5-44. The numbers in those equations are assigned for the sake of illustration. The free

$$E \rightleftharpoons E^* \qquad K_{(E \to E^*)} = 10^{-5} \qquad \Delta G_{(E \to E^*)} = 7.0 \qquad (5\text{-}43)$$

$$E^* + S \rightleftharpoons E^*S \qquad K^* = 10^8 \ M^{-1} \qquad \Delta G^* = -11.2 \qquad (5\text{-}44)$$

$$\overline{E + S \rightleftharpoons E^*S \qquad K = 10^3 \ M^{-1} \qquad \Delta G = -4.2} \qquad (5\text{-}45)$$

energy change of the overall conversion of free enzyme and free substrate to the E*S complex, in which the conformation of the enzyme is different than that of the free enzyme (equation 5-45) may be considered for purposes of analysis to be the sum of the free energy change that would be associated with the binding of substrate to an enzyme molecule already in the final conformation (equation 5-44; this free energy change will always be negative) and the free energy change that would be associated with the change in conformation (equation 5-43; this change will always be positive). Imaginary dissection of the overall free energy change into those two components does not suggest that the two steps actually occur separately (as in the Monod model); it is merely a standard thermodynamic approach. The free energy changes accompanying any physical or chemical process must be independent of pathway, so any steps, however unlikely, may be added if their sum is the actual overall process. Our assumption that the conformation change accompanies or follows binding thus has no bearing on the illustrative use of equations 5-43 to 5-45.

In that illustration, the Michaelis constant or $(S)_{0.5}$ value of 10^{-3} M (the reciprocal of the association constant) is considered to be the resultant of the large free energy decrease that would accompany binding if the enzyme were initially in the most favorable conformation and the free energy increase that would accompany the conversion of the enzyme from the conformation most stable in solution to that found in the enzyme-ligand complex. The free energy change may be symbolized by equation 5-46.

$$\Delta G = \Delta G^* + \Delta G_{(E \to E^*)} \tag{5-46}$$

When two or more ligand-binding sites interact, the real situation is far more complicated, but the formal thermodynamic treatment is not different in principle. When a molecule of substrate or other ligand binds in such a case, there is a concomitant change in conformation not only at the site at which that molecule binds but also of other ligand-binding sites. All of these changes are necessarily away from the most stable states in the unliganded molecule; so, when dissected out for analysis, all of the corresponding changes in free energy must be positive. The formal free-energy equations for an enzyme with four interacting sites are similar to equation 5-46 except for having more terms. For the first ligand molecule bound, we have equation 5-47, where ΔG^*, as before, is the free energy change that would accompany binding if all conformations were initially optimal. $\Delta G_{(A \to A^*)}$ is equivalent to the last term in equation 5-46; it is the free energy change involved in changing the site at which the ligand binds from the unliganded to the liganded conformation. The other terms are the free energy changes accompanying the changes in conformation of the other subunits that result from site-site interactions that follow or accompany the conformational change at site A. These terms may all be equal, though they need not be. In most or all cases the sites are on separate subunits, so the general term site-site interaction could be replaced by subunit-subunit interaction. The site at which the first molecule of ligand binds is designated A only for convenience. It is assumed that the sites were identical before binding, and that it is a matter of chance which one first acquires a molecule of ligand.

Since site (or subunit) A must be changed all the way to the liganded conformation, it may be assumed that the term $\Delta G_{(A \to A^*)}$ will be larger than the other conformational terms in equation 5-47, which correspond to the less extensive conformational changes in the other subunits. The free energy changes accompanying binding of the second, third, and fourth molecules of ligand are given by equations 5-48, 5-49, and 5-50. It is assumed that ΔG^*

$$\Delta G_1 = \Delta G^* + \Delta G_{(A \to A*)} + \Delta G_{(B \to B')} + \Delta G_{(C \to C')} + \Delta G_{(D \to D')} \quad (5\text{-}47)$$

$$\Delta G_2 = \Delta G^* + \Delta G_{B' \to B*} + \Delta G_{(C' \to C'')} + \Delta G_{(D' \to D'')} \quad (5\text{-}48)$$

$$\Delta G_3 = \Delta G^* + \Delta G_{(C'' \to C*)} + \Delta G_{(D'' \to D''')} \quad (5\text{-}49)$$

$$\Delta G_4 = \Delta G^* + \Delta G_{(D''' \to D*)} \quad (5\text{-}50)$$

is constant. Each equation has one less positive term than the preceding equation. In addition, the first conformational term in each equation should be smaller than the corresponding term in the preceding equation. When the first molecule of ligand binds, site (or subunit) A must undergo the full change from the unliganded to the liganded conformation. In contrast, before a molecule of ligand binds at site B, the local conformation has already been changed toward the liganded conformation as a consequence of binding at site A. Thus the free energy increase corresponding to the remaining necessary change (B' → B*) should be less than that at site A. Binding of the second ligand causes further changes at sites C and D, so that the third molecule of ligand to bind should encounter less conformational resistance than the second. Similarly, the last site is affected by three liganded sites, and the positive free energy associated with the change D''' to D* should be still smaller than that at the third site. Thus, because each binding equation contains one less positive term than the preceding one and because the largest of these terms should progressively decrease as sites become occupied, the overall free energy of binding for each ligand molecule will be more negative than that for those previously bound. This is the necessary condition for cooperative binding.

It is customary to say that the binding of a molecule of ligand by a cooperative enzyme enhances binding at other sites. This is a valid statement, but the same relationship might be stated in an apparently reverse manner. Coupling to conformational changes at other sites hinders binding of the first ligand, as illustrated by the last three terms in equation 5-47. Thus instead of saying that filled sites enhance binding at other sites, it might be equally valid, and more helpful to understanding the interactions involved, to say that empty sites impede binding at other sites. Part of the free energy decrease that inherently accompanies the interaction between the first binding site and the ligand molecule is invested for future benefit, as it were, in forcing other sites part way toward the conformation most favorable for binding.

Hemoglobin and aspartate transcarbamylase retain the ability to bind ligand when the subunits are partially dissociated. In both cases, the relative affinities of the native protein and of the dissected moieties are consistent with the viewpoint expressed in the last paragraph. When hemoglobin is dissociated into $\alpha\beta$ units, cooperativity of binding is lost but the affinity for oxygen is strongly enhanced. When aspartate transcarbamylase, which contains six catalytic and six regulatory subunits, is partially dissociated one of the products is a trimer of catalytic subunits that retains catalytic activity. Again, cooperativity of reaction and of substrate binding is lost, but the affinity for aspartate is increased [the value of $(S)_{0.5}$ is decreased].

It is only the free energy of specific interactions that can supply the driving force for construction of the functional machinery of a cell from linear chains of amino acids. (Kinetic factors, of course, play a key role in determining which thermodynamically favorable interactions actually occur.) A simple formalized verbalization of the last stages in the construction and of the functioning of a protein that binds a ligand cooperatively may be useful as a basis for thinking about cooperativity. First, as with any protein, the polypeptide chain must fold into a specific three-dimensional conformation, or a family of closely similar conformations. In some cases, and perhaps in most, these subunits, if sufficiently stable for this property to be evident, have relatively high affinity for one or more specific ligands. When the subunits associate to form the native oligomeric enzyme, the attractive forces that stabilize the oligomer distort the individual binding sites in such a way as to reduce their affinity for ligand. Thus for association of subunits we could write an equation similar to equation 5-47. The negative free energy change that accompanies the oligomerization is opposed by the positive changes that accompany changes in subunits from the conformation which is most stable for free subunits to that specified by the subunit-subunit interactions. These interactions are evolutionarily tailored not only to decrease the affinities of all binding sites, but to be overcome by the effects of binding (equations 5-47 to 5-50).

The picture of opposition between the conformational effects of subunit-subunit interactions that accompany association and the subunit-ligand interactions that accompany ligand binding may seem strange or even counterproductive. Why should cooperative enzymes have evolved so that one type of complex and sophisticated enzyme responses would be abolished by another? The answer obviously lies in the fact that positive regulation always implies the prior imposition of limitations to optimal response. Positive cooperativity is possible only if binding sites are initially at a less-than-optimal conformation; subunit-subunit interactions provide one way for distorting binding sites away from the best conformation for binding.

The pattern of interactions suggested in the last two paragraphs need not hold in detail for all cooperative enzymes. It is not necessary that the individual subunits have high affinity for a ligand. What is necessary is that the conformation of subunits that is stabilized by the subunit-subunit interactions in the native oligomer must not allow optimal ligand binding, but that stabilization of this conformation may be overcome by binding of ligand.

Modifier Effects

Some modifiers of enzyme action change the maximal velocity of the reaction, but, as we have seen, most of them affect the affinity of the enzyme for one or more substrates; that is, they change at least one $(S)_{0.5}$ value. The types of interactions between modifier sites and substrate-binding sites are probably very similar to those among substrate-binding sites, and at the formal thermodynamic level the equations are essentially identical. The binding of a molecule of modifier increases or decreases the free energy of binding at catalytic sites. In addition, the modifier-binding sites generally or always interact positively among themselves. By simple considerations of reciprocity, it follows that if binding of a modifier affects the affinity of the enzyme for a substrate, binding of the substrate must affect the affinity of the enzyme for the modifier. Thus equations like 5-47 through 5-50 could be written in which each molecule of ligand bound, whether substrate or modifier, affected the conformation of each empty site and enhanced its affinity for the appropriate ligand. The form of such equations is obvious, and since they are long, there seems no reason to include them here. The conformational changes that occur on binding a positive modifier are in the appropriate direction to oppose the constraints of the oligomeric regulatory enzyme that decrease the affinity of catalytic sites for substrate. Thus as modifier sites are filled, the substrate-binding sites are caused to change to higher-affinity conformations.

The same treatment applies to the action of a negative modifier, except that in this case the binding of modifier leads to a conformation change that decreases the affinity of the catalytic sites for substrate. In such cases, the binding of modifier is usually cooperative, and so is binding of substrate. Thus the pattern of interactions is complex. The effective affinity of unliganded catalytic sites for substrate will be a resultant of the number of modifier and catalytic sites that are filled, and may be either greater or smaller than the affinity for the first substrate molecule in the absence of modifier.

Catalysis

Since catalysis, as well as binding, must involve conformational changes, and since free energies of interaction of the protein with ligands, other solutes, and solvent are the only sources available to drive conformation changes, it seems that the formal thermodynamic treatment applied above to cooperative binding and modifier action should be applicable also to the catalytic action of enzymes. This application is illustrated in equations 5-51 through 5-56. In these equations the asterisks are shown to the left of the letter E to

$$E + S_1 \rightleftharpoons {}^*ES_1 \tag{5-51}$$

$$^*ES_1 + S_2 \rightleftharpoons {}^*_*E {\Large\diagdown_{S_2}^{S_1}} \tag{5-52}$$

$$^*_*E {\Large\diagdown_{S_2}^{S_1}} \rightleftharpoons {}^\ddagger_*E {\left({\overset{S_1}{\underset{S_2}{|}}} \right)}^{\ddagger} \tag{5-53}$$

$$^\ddagger_*E {\left({\overset{S_1}{\underset{S_2}{|}}} \right)}^{\ddagger} \rightleftharpoons {}^*_*E {\Large\diagdown_{P_2}^{P_1}} \tag{5-54}$$

$$^*_*E {\Large\diagdown_{P_2}^{P_1}} \rightleftharpoons {}^*EP_1 + P_2 \tag{5-55}$$

$$^*EP_1 \rightleftharpoons E + P_1 \tag{5-56}$$

indicate that the conformational changes that we deal with here are different from those considered in equations 5-43 to 5-50 (although they must, of course, occur simultaneously).

Equation 5-51, like equation 5-45, can be dissected for thermodynamic analysis into two components: binding of substrate to enzyme and change of the enzyme from its most stable conformation, E, to a conformation that is inherently much less stable, $^*E$. The change in free energy associated with the conformation change is necessarily large and positive. The conversion is made thermodynamically favorable, however, because of the larger negative free energy change associated with substrate binding. The net free energy for equation 5-51 will be negative (but see the discussion of this point later in this section). Similarly, the free energy change for reaction 5-52 will be the sum of a large positive change associated with the further distortion of the enzyme molecule to a still less stable conformation and a larger negative change associated with binding of the second substrate molecule. In the $^*_*ES_1S_2$ complex the substrate molecules are held in proximity on an energetically loaded (conformationally unstable) enzyme molecule. Two points should be noted. First, there is no reason why the binding need be sequentially ordered; presumably the same strained configuration of the enzyme would be reached if S_2 bound first. Thus this treatment is compatible with the fact that many or most enzymes bind their substrates in random order. Second, description of $^*_*E$ as a highly unstable conformation of the enzyme might be ambiguous. That conformation would be highly unstable in the absence of ligands, but it is of course stabilized by enzyme-substrate interactions so that it becomes the most stable conformation in the ES_1S_2 complex.

The transition state is, by definition, the state of highest free energy in the reaction pathway and hence the stage at which the reaction is equally likely to proceed in the forward or in the reverse direction. In the simplest sense, the rate of a reaction depends on the probability of the transition state, and hence catalysis consists of provision of a more likely transition state (one of lower free energy) than would be available in the absence of the catalyst. Equation 5-53 represents the forcing of the reactants into their transition state conformation, by whatever combination of pushing them closer, stretching bonds, distorting bond angles, polarization, proton donation or abstraction, or other effects is necessary (the free energy change associated with these changes will obviously be large and positive), at the expense of relaxation of the enzyme from its highly strained conformation $^*_*E$ to what we represent as $^‡E$. The transition state symbol $‡$ here indicates only that this conformation of the enzyme is associated with the reaction transition state; the conformation $^‡E$ is inherently much more stable than $^*_*E$, and it is the large negative change in free energy associated with the conformational change of the enzyme that causes the overall free energy change for reaction 5-53 to be small. It must, of course, be positive, since in speaking of the transition state we are arbitrarily choosing the state of highest free energy.

The transition-state complex is equally likely to revert to the $^*_*ES_1S_2$ complex (reverse of equation 5-53) or to go to an enzyme-product complex (equation 5-54). In either case the ligands go to a much more thermodynamically stable conformation and the enzyme to a less stable conformation. Asterisks are used as a general indication of conformations of the enzyme that would be unstable in the absence of stabilizing ligands, and do not indicate specific states. The exact conformation of the enzyme indicated by two asterisks in equation 5-54 is presumably not the same as that in equation 5-53, but both are inherently highly unstable.

Dissociation of the product molecules (equations 5-55 and 5-56) may be considered to be facilitated by relaxation of the enzyme from its unstable conformation $^*_*E$ to the stable E. Of course when the enzyme catalyzes the reverse reaction, the free energy of binding of P_1 and P_2 would be associated with the distortion of enzyme to $^*_*E$, and the dissociation of S_1 and S_2 would be facilitated by enzyme relaxation.

The equilibrium constants for substrate-binding steps (reciprocals of the Michaelis constants) are typically around 10^3 to 10^5 M^{-1}, and the corresponding ΔG^0 values are in the range between about -4 and -7 kcal/mole. Thus reactions 5-51 and 5-52 may be said to be thermodynamically highly favorable. It should be remembered, however, that equilibrium constants and standard free energy changes depend on the arbitrarily chosen standard states. If instead of the standard state of 1 M that is routinely used in thermodynamic calculations we were to take a concentration of 10^{-4} M as our standard state, the equilibrium constants for substrate binding would be near 1 and the corresponding ΔG^0 values would be near zero. Thus, unless we remember to do the mental calculations each time, it is ambiguous, if not misleading, to refer to reactions 5-51 and 5-52 as having large equilibrium constants. The binding interactions and conformational energy-loading interactions seem to have been adjusted in the course of evolutionary design so that at physiological concentrations of substrate they are nearly equal, and the ratio between free enzyme, E, and the liganded complex, $_*^{}ES_1S_2$, will not be either very large or very small. That statement is equivalent to our observation in Chapter 4 that Michaelis constants are typically in the range of, and usually a little larger than, the physiological concentrations of the substrates.

In the reaction sequence illustrated by equations 5-51 through 5-56, all of the change of conformation of the substrate molecules is shown as occurring in reaction 5-53 (and 5-54). This representation is for the sake of simplicity only. It may be expected that the first two reactions (5-51 and 5-52) must involve some distortion of substrate molecules in the direction of the transition state, as well as energy loading of the enzyme, and there is experimental evidence that this is true. In several cases, compounds that have been designed to be sterically similar to the presumed transition-state conformation of a substrate have been shown to be very good inhibitors of the reaction, being bound by the enzyme with greater net affinity than the substrate itself (73). This is not a surprising finding. In our earlier discussion of reaction 5-51 we ignored changes in conformation of substrate. We must now note that the overall free energy change associated with that reaction will be the sum of three rather than two components: the free energy of binding (negative) and the free energy changes corresponding to conformational distortion of enzyme and of substrate (both positive). If the investigator provides a substrate analog that is already constrained by its molecular architecture into a form similar to the conformation that the normal substrate will assume in the enzyme-substrate complex, and if the analog has the proper groups to allow it to interact with the enzyme as strongly as the substrate, the free-energy component associated with distortion of the ligand will be decreased and ΔG^0 for reaction 5-51 will become more negative (the analog will be bound more strongly than the substrate).

It might reasonably be asked whether binding free energies are adequate to overcome the large free energy change incurred in going from the individual substrate in solution to the transition state. However, there seems to be no difficulty here. Inherent binding energies may be very large. Avidin, for example, binds biotin with an association equilibrium constant of about 10^{15} M^{-1}, and a corresponding free energy of about -21 kcal/mole. Typical net association constants (reciprocals of Michaelis constants) for substrates are around 10^4 M^{-1}, corresponding to about -6 kcal/mole. The difference between the avidin-biotin binding free energy and a typical residual or effective substrate binding energy is thus about 15 kcal/mole. If the two substrates of a reaction interacted with the enzyme as strongly as biotin with avidin, they could thus provide for a conformational change with a free energy increase of 30 kcal/mole while still having effective binding constants [and thus Michaelis constants or $(S)_{0.5}$ values] in the normal range. Such a change would allow for adequate catalytic effect. In principle, although such calculations should not be taken too seriously, a decrease of 30 kcal/mole in the effective free energy of the transition state would correspond to a rate acceleration of about 10^{21}, which is perhaps around a million or a billion times greater than a typical enzyme effect.

Whatever the mechanism or pathway of enzymic reactions, the considerations of the preceding paragraph apply. The inherent binding energy must exceed the apparent binding energies by enough to make the transition configuration a relatively probable state. If the general pathway implied in equations 5-51 through 5-56 is true, a rather large amount of energy must be stored in the unstable enzyme conformation $^*_*E$. When considered in relation to the size of a typical enzyme molecule and the number of interactions among its parts and between the enzyme and the solvent and solutes, the necessary energies are, however, quite small. It may be that one reason for the large size of an enzyme relative to the active site itself is the need to delocalize conformational energy among a large number of interactions.

Of course the conformational changes discussed earlier that lead to alteration of binding affinities of unfilled sites in response to binding of substrate or modifier molecules and thus give rise to cooperative kinetics or to regulatory effects, and the conformational changes that are involved in actual catalysis must occur in the same molecule and overlap in time. Our appreciation of these changes may be aided by such formal abstractions as the kind of equations used here, but we should remember that the actual conformational events are not abstractions. They are highly specific changes of positions of functional groups and portions of polypeptide chains, mediated by real interactions between real groups. The molecular design that makes these complex responses possible is at present entirely beyond our comprehension.

SUMMARY

The control functions of enzymes are as important as their catalytic properties. The two types of properties have evolved together, and are probably less distinct in terms of interactions between enzymes and ligands, conformational changes, and the actual catalytic event than they may seem to us. The historical pattern of enzyme chemistry and the standard textbook approach to the subject may give the appearance of a greater dichotomy between catalysis and regulation than is warranted. Both must depend mainly on conformational changes and must be driven by enzyme-ligand interaction energy.

The most common regulatory response of enzymes appears to be a change in affinity for the substrate. Thus the classical Michaelis assumption of quasi-equilibrium between substrate and enzyme, with the actual catalytic step (in which bonds are broken and formed) being the slow step, seems the most useful conceptual framework for consideration of metabolic regulation. The $(S)_{0.5}$ values, or apparent Michaelis constants, of most enzymes for substrates that are metabolic intermediates of the usual type appear to be somewhat larger than the usual physiological concentrations. In consequence, the catalytic sites are much less than fully saturated under ordinary conditions, and reaction rates can be caused to vary either upward or downward by modification of the affinity. In contrast, the affinities of catalytic sites for such coupling agents as the adenine and pyridine nucleotides are generally strong enough [the $(S)_{0.5}$ values are sufficiently smaller than the physiological concentrations] to ensure that the binding sites for these coupling agents will be essentially saturated at all times. This allows the rates of the corresponding reactions to depend on such ratios as $(NAD^+)/(NADH)$, $(ATP)/(ADP)$, and $(ATP)/(AMP)$, rather than on the actual concentrations of the individual nucleotides.

Cooperative binding, a common characteristic of regulatory enzyme behavior, leads to much sharper responses to changes in concentrations of both substrates and modifiers than would be possible if metabolic reactions were all catalyzed at separate and kinetically independent sites, and is probably an essential condition for the evolution of sensitive metabolic control and thus of life.

6

Interactions between Regulatory Parameters

Interactions between metabolic sequences are necessarily complex. A metabolite may participate in two or more sequences, and may or may not be physically compartmented; that is, the pool of the compound available to one sequence may or may not be the same as the pool available to another. Sequences compete for limited resources of material and energy. Because of these functional interactions, the systems by which metabolic sequences are regulated must also interact.

A given sequence may serve two or more functions, which may be quite different. It is thus clear that several inputs must contribute to the regulation of a typical metabolic sequence. Even in the simple case of a linear synthetic sequence with the sole function of providing a single end product, there must be at least two inputs, one indicating the cell's momentary need for the synthesis and the other indicating the cell's momentary energy status. Because of this need for interacting controls, metabolic regulation is far more complex than would appear from the discussion in Chapter 4 of control by the adenylate energy charge, or from a discussion of control by biosynthetic end products or by any other single input. Relatively little definitive information on interaction between regulatory parameters is yet available, but some of the most obviously necessary types have been suggested and supporting evidence has been obtained from kinetic studies *in vitro*. This chapter summarizes some of those discussions and experiments.

AMPHIBOLIC SEQUENCES

The central catabolic processes (glycolysis, the citrate cycle, and the pentose phosphate pathway) supply the starting materials for biosynthesis, as illustrated in the metabolic block diagram, Figure 3-1. It is thus somewhat misleading to refer to these sequences simply as catabolic or degradative, since they also serve an essential anabolic function. Such pathways are sometimes termed amphibolic to indicate their dual roles in catabolism and anabolism. Regulation of these pathways must, of course, reflect this dual function. A response of the R type to variation in energy charge is necessary in view of the fact that nearly all of the regeneration of ATP in aerobic heterotrophic cells occurs as a consequence of the degradation of foodstuffs by these pathways. But if glycolysis and the citrate cycle were regulated by the energy charge alone, the flux through these pathways would be severely decreased whenever the cell's energy status was favorable. This would limit not only the rate of regeneration of ATP but also the rate of production of the biosynthetic starting materials that are needed for growth and repair. Therefore the cell's ability to grow would be impaired just when growth is most appropriate—when the supply of energy is plentiful.

Faced with the need to regulate a process that simultaneously serves two functions, an engineer would design a control system responding to two inputs. Such a design is logically necessary; a system cannot respond appropriately to two needs unless it receives an input signal relevant to each. This necessity applies with equal cogency to systems designed by evolution; thus we may take it to be necessarily true that amphibolic sequences must respond, at the least, to two input signals, one indicating the level of biosynthetic intermediates and the other indicating the energy level of the cell. When either is low, glycolysis should proceed; when both are in a normal range, the functions of glycolysis have been adequately served and flux through this pathway should be throttled down. Of course glycolysis will never be totally turned off in a cell that is metabolizing glucose, because ATP is used continuously. Here as elsewhere we deal usually with quantitative adjustments of flux rates, not with simple on-off control. In a cell metabolizing under essentially steady-state conditions, the adjustments of flux rates will presumably be small. The system must also be capable of causing very large changes in metabolic fluxes when necessary—for example, when an animal awakes from peaceful sleep to find a predator approaching, and flees for its life.

Dual or multiple control of amphibolic sequences has received little attention as yet, and our information in this area is inadequate. It is clear that there must be controls that are based, directly or indirectly, on the concentrations of the small number of compounds that serve as precursors for biosynthesis: the sugar phosphates, keto acids, coenzyme A esters, and phosphoenolpyruvate shown in Figure 3-1.

The type of interaction between energy charge and the concentrations of biosynthetic intermediates that is to be expected in regulation of amphibolic sequence is shown in Figure 6-1. A pattern similar to this has been observed

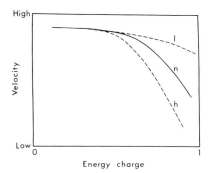

Energy charge

Figure 6-1. Expected interaction between the adenylate energy charge and the concentrations of biosynthetic starting materials in regulation of rates of amphibolic sequences. l = low levels of intermediates; n = normal levels; h = high levels. From Atkinson (5). Reprinted with permission from *Biochemistry* 7, 4030 (1968). Copyright by the American Chemical Society.

with phosphofructokinase, which catalyzes a reaction that appears to be a major metabolic control point in glycolysis. Citrate is a strongly negative modifier for phosphofructokinase. It seems likely that the level of citrate serves as an indirect indication of the availability of α-ketoglutarate, succinyl coenzyme A, and oxaloacetate, all of which can be made from it, as well as of cytoplasmic acetyl coenzyme A in eukaryotic organisms. When the level of citrate is relatively high, all of these biosynthetic precursors can be produced, so metabolic control by the citrate level should assure an adequate supply of them. When the energy charge responses of rabbit muscle phosphofructokinase were determined at different concentrations of citrate, curves like those of Figure 6-1 were obtained (*110*).

The fact that the overall interaction between citrate concentration and adenylate energy charge in regulation of phosphofructokinase closely resembles the pattern predicted on the basis of metabolic function is gratifying. (It could not be predicted, of course, which later intermediate would be a negative modifier for phosphofructokinase but only that at least one must be.) However, the details of the interaction are obscure, especially in eukaryotic cells, and there are obvious and important questions for which answers are needed. It is, of course, cytoplasmic citrate that affects phosphofructokinase and that is a precursor of cytoplasmic acetyl coenzyme A by way of the ATP-utilizing citrate cleavage reaction (equation 6-1). It seems

$$\text{citrate} + \text{ATP} + \text{HSCoA} \rightarrow \text{OAA} + \text{AcSCoA} + \text{ADP} + P_i \qquad (6\text{-}1)$$

clear that cytoplasmic citrate arises from mitochondrial citrate, but the factors that regulate the rate of export of citrate (or of some product and potential precursor of citrate, such as glutamate) from the mitochondrion have not been established. The observed effect of citrate on the kinetic properties of phosphofructokinase allows us to conclude only that the concentration of citrate in the cytoplasm is probably an important factor in the kinetic control of phosphofructokinase *in vivo*.

The sequence of reactions catalyzed by the pyruvate dehydrogenase complex of *E. coli* (the oxidation of pyruvate to AcSCoA and CO_2 at the expense of NAD^+) is inhibited by AcSCoA, and the pattern of interaction between AcSCoA concentration and energy charge is again similar to that shown in Figure 6-1 (*109*). This is an example of feedback rather than direct product inhibition because the effects of both AcSCoA and the adenine nucleotides are exerted on the enzyme catalyzing the first step in the sequence, and AcSCoA is produced in a later step.

Although more experimental work will be required before the interactions between energy charge and feedback signals in the regulation of amphibolic pathways are well understood, some additional insight may be gained by consideration of the number and placement of control points at which the reactions of glycolysis and the citrate cycle are regulated by energy charge. It would appear that one or two controls early in the sequence should suffice to regulate the rate at which free glucose or storage polysaccharides can be used. However, at least five enzymes have been observed to give an R-type response to variation in energy charge (not including the effect of AMP on phosphorylase) (*6*). The locations of these regulatory points are shown in Figure 6-2. Three of these control enzymes come immediately after major branch points at which intermediates of this pathway may be removed for

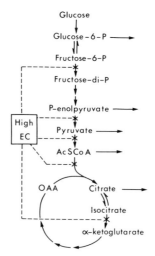

Figure 6-2. Reactions of glycolysis and the citrate cycle that have been shown to be regulated by the adenylate energy charge. Arrows to the right indicate alternate pathways (mainly biosynthetic) that compete for some of the intermediates in these pathways.

use in biosynthesis. Each of the other two control enzymes follows a branch-point by one reaction, and in each case the intervening reaction seems likely to be very near equilibrium *in vivo*. If they are actually at virtual equilibrium, such metabolite pairs as glucose 6-P and fructose 6-P, or citrate and isocitrate, can be considered a single metabolite for control purposes. Each of the points at which energy charge has been found to regulate reactions in glycolysis or the citrate cycle is then seen to occur effectively at a metabolic branch point. Partitioning at branch points will be discussed further in a later section.

It may seem odd that the major control of the rate of glycolysis should occur at the phosphofructokinase step, which appears to be rather well along the sequence, rather than at an earlier step. When the compounds and reactions involved are considered, however, this placement of the control point is easily understood (Figure 6-3). The three hexose monophosphates, glucose 1-P, glucose 6-P, and fructose 6-P, are interrelated by freely reversible reactions with equilibrium constants near 1. As noted above, when two or more intermediates are near equilibrium under physiological conditions they may be considered to constitute, in effect, a single pool. The phosphofructokinase reaction is thus the step by which carbohydrate becomes committed to glycolytic breakdown. Control at this point is in agreement with the generalization that regulatory effects should be exerted on enzymes that catalyze reactions in which the substrate becomes committed to a specific metabolic fate.

According to Figure 6-3, the interconversions of carbohydrates leading toward degradation in typical aerobic heterotrophic cells can be divided into three parts: (a) interconversion between hexose monophosphates and glucose or glycogen, (b) glycolysis, and (c) the pentose phosphate shunt path-

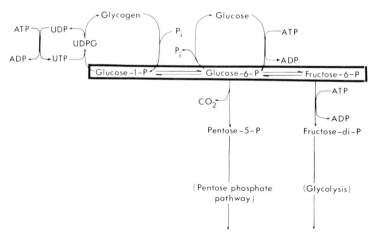

Figure 6-3. Central role of the hexose phosphates in amphibolic metabolism.

way. Because of the central position of these pathways in energy metabolism, they must be especially important quantitatively in the regulatory systems that are responsible for stabilization of the adenylate energy charge.

Interconversions between Hexose Monophosphates and Glycogen or Glucose

The hexose monophosphate pool can be replenished from glucose by the action of hexokinase. Under some circumstances, free glucose is formed by hydrolysis of glucose-6-P. This reaction is especially important in liver, where it contributes to maintenance of the blood glucose level. Glycogen, which serves as a storage form of carbon, ATP, and reducing power or NADPH, is made from hexose monophosphate by way of UDP-glucose, and can break down to hexose monophosphate through the action of phosphorylase. In each case (glucose/glucose 6-P and glycogen/glucose 1-P) a pair of oppositely directed reactions or reaction sequences makes up a pseudocycle of the type discussed in Chapter 3. As in all such cases, these pseudocycles allow for kinetic regulation. In spite of their importance for energy metabolism, neither of them has been the object of thorough study in terms of regulation. Many observations that are clearly related to regulation have been reported for each case, but no serious attempt to construct an integrated metabolic picture has been undertaken. This is clearly an area that deserves greater attention than it has yet received.

Inhibition of hexokinase by glucose 6-P must contribute to stabilization of the hexose monophosphate pool. The same reaction is catalyzed by another enzyme, glucokinase, which, because of its lack of response to glucose 6-P and its low affinity for glucose, is believed to function primarily under conditions when glucose is present at high levels and conversion to glycogen would be appropriate. A careful study of the regulatory interactions between these enzymes and glucose-6-phosphate phosphatase should be rewarding.

Although far more work has been done on the glycogen/glucose 1-P pseudocycle, the basic regulatory interactions are still poorly understood. The very interesting and highly complex cascade system by which phosphorylase *b* is converted to phosphorylase *a* in response to epinephrine has tended to divert attention from the regulation of glycogen breakdown under more normal conditions. The action of epinephrine, like many or most hormonal effects, may be seen as an override of local metabolic controls in the interests of the needs or anticipated needs of the organism as a whole. Epinephrine is a signal causing the mammalian body to prepare for fight or flight. One facet of this preparation is the conversion of phosphorylase *b*, which is responsive to the energy charge as an indication of local needs, to phosphorylase *a*, which is active even when the local energy charge is high.

(That statement is based on the reported effects of AMP and ATP on the action of phosphorylase *b*; no direct energy charge experiments appear to have been done with this enzyme.) Thus a need that is anticipated by the central nervous system leads to removal of phosphorylase from control based on the local energy charge, and causes breakdown of glycogen in advance of need.

Because of the dramatic complexity of the cascade system controlling the conversion of phosphorylase *b* to phosphorylase *a*, textbooks tend to give the impression that this system is responsible for primary regulation of phosphorylase action. That implication seems unlikely to be correct. Phosphorylase *b* appears quite capable of responding to local and momentary needs in such a way as to meet even heavy demands for energy. Morgan and Parmaggiani showed that when a perfused heart was made to do heavy work, by causing it to pump against a relatively high pressure, there was little if any conversion of phosphorylase *b* to phosphorylase *a* (*87*). Evidently the range of response of phosphorylase *b* to the adenylate energy charge and other regulatory inputs is great enough to supply glucose 1-P at the high rate needed in such cases. A more general demonstration of the competence of phosphorylase *b* to meet all of the needs of an organism comes from the observation that a strain of mice lacking phosphorylase kinase, and thus unable to produce phosphorylase *a*, is perfectly viable, and indeed the individuals seem normal and healthy (*78*) under laboratory conditions. Phosphorylase *a* and the system responsible for its production seem to be called on primarily in emergencies. If this system allows an organism to escape from an enemy, to defeat an enemy, or to capture prey, it is very important to the organism. It will have great selective advantage and will be perfected by evolutionary design. But it should be recognized that this cascade system may be quite outside the mainstream of normal metabolic regulation. The action of AMP on phosphorylase *b* was the first effect of an adenine nucleotide to be recognized as probably having regulatory significance (*41*). Study of the regulation of this enzyme in terms of current concepts and information is overdue.

Glycolysis

As discussed above and illustrated in Figure 6-3, the reaction catalyzed by phosphofructokinase is the first step in the degradation of hexose phosphate. It is by virtue of this reaction that the substrate becomes committed to glycolysis. This is therefore the appropriate place for primary control of the flux through the glycolytic sequence. Phosphofructokinase is a particularly interesting regulatory enzyme because it catalyzes an ATP-utilizing reaction in an ATP-regenerating sequence. The regulatory properties of the enzyme must of course be consistent with the function of the sequence rather than with the chemistry of the reaction. Accordingly, phosphofructokinase gives a sharp R-type energy charge response curve (110). Some of the regulatory properties of this enzyme were discussed in Chapter 5, and they need not be repeated here.

Other enzymes of glycolysis for which R-type responses have been observed *in vitro* were identified in Figure 6-2. Because it is, in typical aerobic heterotrophic metabolism, the major supplier of acetyl coenzyme A for oxidation in the citrate cycle with concomitant regeneration of ATP, and is also the source of several biosynthetic starting materials, glycolysis contains several major metabolic branchpoints. As illustrated in Figure 6-2, the location of enzymes that respond to variation in the value of the energy charge reflect the positions of these branchpoints.

Positive Feed-Forward Effects

In addition to the negative feedback effects that have been the main subject of study in research on regulatory enzyme modulation, several examples of positive feed-forward interactions have also been observed. That is, some metabolic intermediates are positive modifiers for enzymes that catalyze reactions occurring later in the sequence. Thus a high concentration of early intermediates will facilitate flow of material through the sequence by which these intermediates are used. Conversely, when the concentrations of early intermediates are low the flux through the sequence will be reduced below the value that would otherwise result from interactions between the other regulatory inputs and the concentrations of the immediate substrates of the regulated enzymes, so that the rate of use of the depleted intermediates will be decreased. Such effects can obviously contribute to homeostasis and to effective use of resources.

Pyruvate kinase is a striking example of positive feed-forward modulation. The velocity of the reaction catalyzed by this enzyme under assay conditions *in vitro* is increased by as much as twentyfold by fructose diphosphate and the hexose phosphates in their physiological concentration ranges (72). Relatively little work on feed-forward controls has been reported, and their frequency and general importance in metabolic control cannot be evaluated at present.

Pentose Phosphate Pathway

Transaldolase and transketolase catalyze interconversions between sugar phosphates containing 3, 4, 5, 6, and 7 carbon atoms. Williams (121) has suggested a more complex reaction sequence that involves an 8-carbon intermediate. The metabolic roles of these interconversions, and even their directions, may change under different conditions, and neither the relation of these reactions to other metabolic sequences nor their regulation is at all clear at present. Glucose-6-phosphate dehydrogenase, a lactone-hydrolyzing enzyme, and 6-P-gluconate dehydrogenase convert hexose monophosphate to pentose monophosphate, reducing two moles of $NADP^+$ for each mole of hexose utilized. It is assumed that production of NADPH for use in biosynthetic reductions is the function of these reactions. The fate of the pentose phosphate (a pool made up of ribose 5-P, ribulose 5-P, and xylulose 5-P) is less well defined. Ribose 5-P is of course needed for the synthesis of nucleotides and of histidine and tryptophan, and oxidation of glucose 6-P is one route for its production. However, ribose 5-P can also be made by carbon shuffling, using the transaldolase and transketolase reactions, starting from triose phosphate and hexose phosphate without the oxidative steps.

Because of the uncertainty as to the metabolic role of the pentose phosphate pathway, determination of the response of the first enzyme to variation in the energy charge seemed especially interesting. In all other cases where energy charge responses have been looked for, the sequence was clearly classified as to function, either ATP-regenerating or ATP-utilizing. If a response curve of the inappropriate type had ever been observed (an R-type curve for an enzyme in an ATP-utilizing sequence or vice versa), the observation would have posed a serious paradox. But for the first enzyme in the pentose phosphate pathway, glucose-6-P dehydrogenase, a response of either type could have been rationalized. Either rationalization would have had implications as to metabolic interrelations of the sequence. Thus this is the only case to date in which determination of the response to variation in energy charge supplied information relevant to assignment of function of the metabolic sequence. The response of glucose-6-phosphate dehydrogenase is of the R type (15). This observation is consistent with the view, which has gained general acceptance on the basis of various types of indirect evidence as well as of apparent plausibility, that the pentose-P pathway is an alternate route from hexose phosphate to triose phosphate, paralleling glycolysis, rather than a self-contained cyclic oxidation of hexose phosphate, as has sometimes been suggested.

A possible relationship between the pentose phosphate shunt pathway and the normal glycolytic pathway is illustrated in Figure 6-4. The two sequences are assumed to join at triose phosphate, and further metabolism through pyruvate and into the citrate cycle is identical in both cases. This description is based on the assumption that fructose 6-phosphate and triose phosphate produced by the action of transaldolase and transketolase are freely available to the enzymes of the normal glycolytic sequence. It is of course possible that there may be some degree of compartmentation between the two sequences, in which case their interrelationships would be less simple

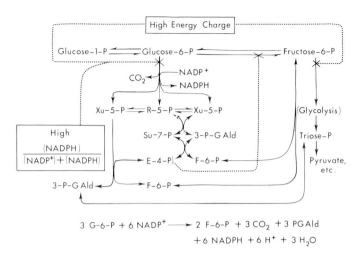

$$3 \text{ G-6-P} + 6 \text{ NADP}^+ \longrightarrow 2 \text{ F-6-P} + 3 \text{ CO}_2 + 3 \text{ PGAld}$$
$$+ 6 \text{ NADPH} + 6 \text{ H}^+ + 3 \text{ H}_2\text{O}$$

Figure 6-4. Relation between the pentose phosphate shunt pathway and glycolysis. Broken lines indicate regulatory interactions, and a negative effect is indicated by an × across the reaction arrow.

than is suggested by Figure 6-4. Since little is known with certainty regarding the relationships between the pentose pathway and other metabolic sequences, our discussion must be speculative, and we will therefore make use of the simplest assumptions.

As shown in Figure 6-4, the difference between glycolysis and the pentose phosphate pathway, in this view, is that one-sixth of the carbon atoms of hexose phosphate are oxidized to CO_2 in the pentose phosphate pathway, with transfer of electrons to $NADP^+$, whereas conversion of hexose phosphate to triose phosphate in the glycolytic pathway involves no oxidative steps. Both pathways thus lead hexose phosphate toward pyruvate and the citrate cycle, and R-type regulation of the first reaction of each step by the adenylate energy charge is appropriate. If the pentose phosphate pathway was really a closed cycle serving only to regenerate NADPH, either no response to energy charge or, more likely, a U-type response would be expected. Since NADPH is used almost exclusively in biosynthetic sequences, it would not make metabolic sense for a cycle with the sole function of producing NADPH to be inhibited by high values of energy charge (an R-type response), because biosynthesis is appropriate and is favored when the energy charge is high. But if this pathway serves the dual functions of regenerating NADPH and of leading to the regeneration of ATP (by providing triose phosphate), it must be regulated by an R-type response to energy charge as well as by response to the $NADPH/NADP^+$ ratio or the mole fraction of NADPH. This latter control has also been observed (15), and the interactions between the responses to energy charge and to NADPH mole fraction are being investigated.

The regulatory interactions shown in Figure 6-4 allow for only the most tentative and preliminary discussion of correlation of these sequences. Since both pathways lead to oxidation of hexose phosphate and regeneration of ATP, it is appropriate that the first step of each is under R-type control by the adenylate energy charge. Regulation of the pentose phosphate pathway by the mole fraction of NADPH is also clearly appropriate. These effects suggest a simple type of basic control: both sequences, and hence the total rate of consumption of hexose phosphate, are regulated by the energy charge, whereas the fraction of that total that begins its journey by way of the pentose phosphate pathway is regulated by the momentary need of the cell for NADPH.

The functional advantage of the reported inhibition by erythrose 4-phosphate of hexose phosphate isomerase, which catalyzes the interconversion of glucose 6-phosphate and fructose 6-phosphate, is not clear. In general, metabolic reactions that are near equilibrium in the cell are not likely points for kinetic regulation. However, the position of this particular equilibrium reaction is rather unusual. According to the interpretation of carbohydrate metabolism illustrated by Figure 6-4, two-thirds of the carbon atoms that enter the pentose phosphate join the glycolytic sequence at fructose 6-phosphate, one-sixth join at triose phosphate, and one-sixth are oxidized to CO_2. (This bookkeeping ignores the amount of ribose 5-phosphate that is drained from the pathway for use in the synthesis of nucleotides, tryptophan, and histidine, and the erythrose 4-phosphate used in synthesis of the aromatic amino acids and the folate coenzymes.) If this interpretation is correct, for two-thirds of its total flux the whole pentose phosphate pathway parallels the single reaction catalyzed by hexose phosphate isomerase. In effect, the isomerase reaction might be considered to shortcircuit the pentose phosphate pathway, and thus to deprive it of any thermodynamic driving force. Under conditions when pentose phosphate was produced rapidly because of a high demand for NADPH, the intermediates of the pentose phosphate pathway might tend to accumulate. It seems at least plausible that modulation of the isomerase reaction by erythrose 4-phosphate is the means that has evolved to prevent such accumulation. If, as a result of an increase in the concentration of erythrose 4-phosphate, the activity of hexose isomerase were decreased, the concentration of fructose 6-phosphate would tend to fall. This would drain sugar phosphates from the pentose phosphate pathway, and the concentrations of all of the intermediates, including erythrose 4-phosphate, should decrease. It must be emphasized that this interpretation is speculative. If it is correct, the regulatory effect of erythrose 4-phosphate is of an interesting type. Although the actual effect of the modulator on its target enzyme is negative, the overall consequence would be a positive feed-forward control, since the reaction by which erythrose 4-phosphate is metabolized would be facilitated by the decrease in the concentration of fructose 6-phosphate caused by inhibition of hexose isomerase. Since the equilibrium constant of the reaction catalyzed by phosphofructokinase is high, a slight decrease in the concentration of fructose 6-phosphate should not hinder glycolysis.

ANABOLIC SEQUENCES

Biosynthesis

As noted earlier, biosynthetic sequences, in which energy and other resources of the cell are expended, must be controlled by at least two parameters, one reflecting the momentary need of the cell for the product of the sequence and the other indicating the momentary level of the cell's resources. The most obvious measure of need for an end product is the concentration of that product. Thus the rate of production of a building block compound such as an amino acid can be kept equal to the rate of its utilization by feedback controls that sense and stabilize the concentration of the product. In the type of negative feedback regulation discovered by Umbarger (*118*) and Yates and Pardee (*128*) and now well known and recognized to be a general feature of biosynthetic metabolism, the end product of a sequence is a negative modifier for the enzyme catalyzing the first step specific for synthesis of that product. Thus the concentration of the end product can be held within rather narrow limits even when the rate of its utilization fluctuates widely. The energy status of the cell may be expressed by the value of the adenylate energy charge, and is usually sensed by the regulated enzyme as a ratio of concentrations, either ATP/ADP or ATP/AMP. Thus interaction of these two regulatory inputs may be expected to result in enzyme responses like those illustrated in Figure 6-5. Such interactions have been seen in the few cases where they have been looked for (*23, 34, 61*). They should insure that a product will be made only when it is needed and when the cell can afford the synthesis. Little or no synthesis will occur if the concentration of the product is already high, no matter what the value of the energy charge (curve h) or if the value of energy charge is low, no matter how low the concentration of product (left-hand part of the figure). The property of a regulatory enzyme that usually varies in response to variation in regulatory parameters is its affinity for substrate. Thus the vertical coordinate of Figure 6-5 can properly be labeled "Biosynthetic Flux" only if it is assumed that the concentration of the substrate for the first reaction of the sequence is con-

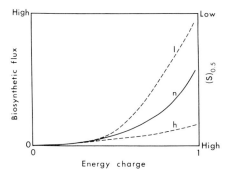

Figure 6-5. Modulation of the energy charge response of a biosynthetic sequence by the concentration of the end product. l = low concentration of the end product; n = normal concentration; h = high concentration. From Atkinson (5). Reprinted with permission from *Biochemistry* **7**, 4030 (1968). Copyright by the American Chemical Society.

stant. In a more general treatment, the vertical scale should be considered to represent affinity for substrate, as indicated on the right-hand vertical coordinate, where affinity increases from the bottom to the top of the scale as the value of $(S)_{0.5}$ falls. As discussed in Chapter 5, the fraction of sites occupied by substrate, and thus the velocity of an enzymic reaction, is a function of $(S)/(S)_{0.5}$, the ratio of substrate concentration to the concentration required for half-maximal velocity. Thus Figure 6-5 is seen to illustrate control by three variables. The first enzyme of the sequence senses the concentration of the end product of the sequence and the value of the adenylate energy charge, and its affinity for substrate [the value of $(S)_{0.5}$] is adjusted accordingly. The concentration of the substrate for this first enzyme enters directly as the term (S) of the controlling ratio $(S)/(S)_{0.5}$. (This is merely to say that the flux through a sequence cannot be high, no matter how favorable the properties of the regulatory enzymes, if the concentration of the starting material is severely limiting.) Thus a low concentration of substrate, as well as a low value of energy charge or a high concentration of the product, will tend to decrease the rate of a biosynthetic reaction. All three of these parameters are clearly appropriate, and their effects are in the appropriate directions, for effective regulation.

Growth and Storage

In addition to the sequences by which intermediates of low to moderate molecular weight are synthesized, there are other metabolic processes that consume ATP and other cell resources. Most of these may be classified either as growth (production of macromolecules, etc.) or as storage of carbon and potential ATP and NADPH in such forms as polysaccharide or lipid. It is a matter of common observation that these processes are regulated in a hierarchical manner: fat is stored when the supply of nutrients is high; a decrease in intake will decrease or abolish storage while allowing growth to continue; further severe limitation of nutrient supply will limit or prevent growth although the organism survives; and total starvation must lead to death. These relationships must have been recognized by prehistoric man, and they obviously are functionally advantageous and hence have survival value. It seems likely that many of the regulatory interactions at the molecular level that underlie this functional hierarchy can be illustrated in a general way by diagrams similar to Figure 6-5. The suggested relationships are shown in Figure 6-6. The curve marked "Synthesis" represents the general response of regulatory enzymes in ordinary biosynthetic sequences to variation in energy charge. It thus resembles curves l or n of Figure 6-5. The curve marked "Growth" illustrates the response to the value of the adenylate energy charge that seems appropriate for regulatory enzymes that control the rate of synthesis of macromolecules or of other steps necessary for growth. These enzymes should be more sensitive to decrease in the value of the energy charge than are enzymes in the central pathways of intermediary metabolism. The curve marked "Storage" shows the response expected for regulatory enzymes in sequences that lead to the production of storage compounds. Such sequences should be active only when the cell has excess energy available beyond momentary requirements, so the corresponding regulatory enzymes should respond very sharply to decreases in the value of the energy charge.

The curves of Figure 6-6, like any real or suggested curves showing responses of regulatory enzymes to a single regulatory parameter, are simplified and incomplete in terms of actual physiological function. Any sequence will

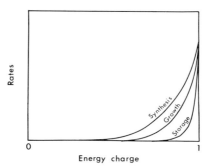

Figure 6-6.   Suggested relationship between energy charge responses of regulatory enzymes in sequences leading to synthesis of small molecules (Synthesis), in sequences leading to macromolecular synthesis, and in other processes required for growth (Growth), and in production of storage compounds (Storage).

be controlled in the intact cell by a variety of regulatory inputs. As discussed in the preceding section, for example, fluxes through biosynthetic sequences will be very low when the end product is present at adequate levels. Thus the response curve for a given synthetic sequence might rise very little at any value of energy charge; such curves would of course cross the growth and storage curves of Figure 6-6. But in trying to understand a complex system it is often useful to consider individual effects of the various factors that are involved, even if it may not be possible to isolate them experimentally. The curves of Figure 6-6 represent such an attempt to visualize the probable relative effects of variation in the value of the energy charge when other factors are relatively favorable for each type of sequence. Results of some experiments with enzymes *in vitro* are consistent with the pattern suggested in the figure.

Growth

The nucleoside triphosphates are strongly specific with regard to metabolic function. Since the adenylates are the general energy transduction system of metabolism, ATP is involved in all sequences of intermediary metabolism, both amphibolic and anabolic. However, it is noteworthy that, as schematically indicated in Figure 3-1, ATP is not used directly in the synthesis of macromolecules (except for the charging of tRNA in preparation for protein synthesis). Each of the other common ribonucleoside triphosphates has a specific role in the synthesis of macromolecules. GTP is required for synthesis of proteins (and of some carbohydrate cell wall precursors); UTP for synthesis of complex carbohydrates; and CTP for synthesis of phospholipids. It seems probable that these specializations of the individual nucleotides have advantageous consequences which we as yet do not understand. However, a possible advantage of the general feature (use of nucleoside triphosphates other than ATP for macromolecular synthesis) is obvious. Since the energy transductions involved in macromolecular synthesis are mediated by GTP, UTP, and CTP, all macromolecular syntheses could be regulated in response to the energy status of the cell by energy charge control of the regeneration of these triphosphates from the corresponding diphosphates. As this speculation might predict, GTP, UTP, and CTP are all regenerated through the action of the same nonspecific enzyme, nucleoside diphosphate kinase (equation 6-2). This enzyme has been found to give a sharper R-type response

$$\text{ATP} + \text{NDP} \rightleftharpoons \text{ADP} + \text{NTP} \qquad (6\text{-}2)$$

curve in energy charge experiments than do typical biosynthetic enzymes (*60, 116*). Further, the rate of the reaction is nearly independent of the concentration of the acceptor nucleotide in the physiological range, which suggests that the properties of the enzyme have evolved to place maximum emphasis on the energy charge response.

Since all macromolecular syntheses require GTP, UTP, or CTP, and since regeneration of these nucleotides depends entirely on nucleoside diphosphate kinase, it seems a possible working hypothesis that nucleoside diphosphate kinase is a key control enzyme in the regulation of growth and macromolecular synthesis, and that the energy charge response of this enzyme (which resembles the growth curve of Figure 6-6) may play a major role in establishing the necessary functional hierarchical relationships between intermediary metabolism and macromolecular synthesis. It is of interest in this connection that the same enzyme also catalyzes the phosphorylation of the deoxynucleoside diphosphates. The energy charge response curves for production of the deoxynucleoside triphosphates that are required in the synthesis of DNA are virtually identical with those for production of ribonucleoside triphosphates (60); thus the synthesis of DNA would also appear to be under indirect but potent energy charge control. It may be that the advantage of reduction of ribonucleotides to deoxyribonucleotides at the diphosphate level instead of the triphosphate level is that it allows for kinetic control, based on the energy status of the cell, at the last step before DNA assembly (phosphorylation of the deoxyribonucleoside diphosphates). However, this suggestion in this simplest form would not predict that DNA synthesis, once initiated, should proceed at about the same rate whatever the nutritional state or growth rate of the cells, as has been observed. Clearly other regulatory factors are involved.

Little is yet known about regulation of the reactions that follow nucleoside diphosphate kinase in metabolism—those in which the nucleoside triphosphates other than ATP are used. Uridine diphosphate glucose synthase seems to respond mainly to the product/substrate ratio UDPG/UTP, without direct response to the adenylate energy charge (99).

To summarize this section: It is a striking fact that GTP, CTP, and UTP (and the four deoxynucleoside triphosphates) are used in macromolecular synthesis, and that all of these compounds are produced through the action of a single enzyme, nucleoside diphosphate kinase. The energy charge response of nucleoside diphosphate kinase is steeper than those of typical biosynthetic enzymes. These three facts are consistent with the hypothesis that nucleoside diphosphate kinase is a master enzyme whose properties regulate growth rates and contribute to a heirarchical relationship with intermediary metabolism like that shown in Figure 6-5. Much further evidence will be needed before the hypothesis can be confirmed, modified, or disproved. It may be noted that mutations leading to altered regulation of nucleoside diphosphate kinase might cause the growth curve of Figure 6-6 to shift to the left. The resulting pathological enhancement of growth as compared to storage or intermediary metabolism might be a factor in hyperplasia or neoplasms.

Storage

As noted above, regulation of energy storage sequences has not been studied in detail. In mammals and other complex organisms the interplay between controls at the cellular level and at the organismal level by way of hormonal override of local control must necessarily complicate the picture.

In green plants and many bacteria, adenosine diphosphoglucose (ADPG) is used for the synthesis of storage polysaccharide. Uridine diphosphoglucose is used, as in other organisms, for hexose epimerizations and for the synthesis of structural carbohydrates. Regulation of storage is thus much more easily studied in bacteria than in mammals, for example, where UDPG is used in glycogen production (storage) as well as in synthesis of structural compounds (growth and repair). Since ADPG is used by *E. coli* only in glycogen production, synthesis of ADPG is the step that commits the glucosyl unit to storage. The reaction catalyzed by ADPG synthase (equation (6-3)

$$\text{ATP} + \text{glucose 1-P} \rightarrow \text{ADPG} + \text{PoP}_i \qquad (6\text{-}3)$$

should therefore be the site of regulation of glycogen synthesis. Preiss has confirmed this expectation and has extensively studied the properties of the enzyme (*94*). The energy charge response of ADPG synthase is the sharpest such curve yet observed (*109*), and compares to typical U-type curves about as the storage curve of Figure 6-6 compares with the synthesis curve. Thus, as in the case of nucleoside diphosphokinase, the properties of ADPG synthase are consistent with, although of course they cannot by themselves prove, the hypothesis illustrated by Figure 6-6.

INTERACTIONS BETWEEN SEQUENCES

Biological homeostasis must depend, at the most fundamental level, on regulatory interaction between metabolic sequences and on the functional properties of membranes. Much of this book, especially Chapters 3 and 4, deals with interactions between sequences, and the basic R-type and U-type energy charge responses illustrated in Figure 4-2 supply probably the most general basis for such interactions. This section deals with some aspects of interactions that are especially relevant at this point.

Overlap of Modulated Energy Charge Responses

Discussions in this chapter and elsewhere (*5, 6, 8, 9, 11*) have emphasized that the simple R-type and U-type response curves must be modulated by other regulatory parameters. Figures 6-1 and 6-5 showed that, as a consequence of such modulation, both R-type and U-type responses should be thought of as fan-shaped families of curves rather than as single curves. If these two figures are combined, we obtain Figure 6-7. Here R-type and U-type responses are seen to overlap over a rather wide area rather than to intersect cleanly as in Figure 4-2. This view of regulatory interaction does not lead to prediction of any lack of precision in stabilization of the energy charge, however. Although the responses of individual biosynthetic sequences may lie anywhere within the U area, there must be a weighted average response—the average of the response curves for all biosynthetic sequences, each weighted in proportion to its rate and to the amount of ATP it consumes—such as that indicated by the broken line labeled U_{ave}. This weighted average response will determine the interaction of biosynthesis, taken as a whole, with amphibolic sequences; curve U in Figure 4-2 represents such a weighted average.

There are far fewer sequences in amphibolic metabolism than in biosynthesis, and the various R-type regulatory enzymes in these sequences probably respond to many of the same modulating regulatory parameters. Thus the weighted average curve R_{ave} represents a much simpler situation than does curve U_{ave}. Nevertheless the situation is in principle the same in both cases, and curve R of Figure 4-2 represents the weighted average response R_{ave}.

It is clear that the argument that steeply intersecting R and U curves must lead to stabilization of the energy charge loses none of its cogency when the curves are recognized to be average responses, rather than representations of the behaviors of individual enzymes. It is the overall fluxes of adenylate interconversions in the two types of pathways that are relevant here, and the weighted average curves reflect those overall fluxes.

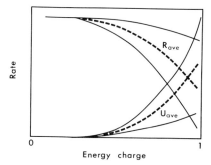

Figure 6-7.   Interaction between R-type and U-type regulatory responses to the value of the adenylate energy charge. Solid lines indicate the approximate limits of the responses of individual enzymes to the energy charge, and the broken lines represent weighted-average responses for R-type and U-type enzymes collectively.

The type of metabolic interactions illustrated by Figure 6-7 is extremely flexible in its ability to regulate overall metabolic fluxes and individual sequences appropriately and simultaneously. With no need to sense total flux—or indeed any need to sense fluxes at all—the system, as a consequence of the individual responses of many enzymes, each sensing concentrations and concentration ratios, balances overall amphibolic and anabolic fluxes with such exquisite precision as to stabilize the energy charge within a very narrow range. At the same time each sequence is independently regulated so as to produce as much of its product as is momentarily required to maintain an essentially constant concentration. If, to illustrate with an extreme example, one amino acid should become available in the environment at an adequate level, the rate of the synthetic pathway leading to that amino acid would fall nearly to zero. This would, however, not affect overall regulation; the weighted average of the remaining sequences would continue to interact with the weighted average of amphibolic sequences just as before. It is striking that both types of controls, the general and the specific, result from the same modulations of enzyme behavior. Although it is complex because of the number of reactions and sequences involved, the system is awesomely simple in principle; it seems impossible to imagine another approach that could attain the same results in as economical a manner. And the solidity of biological homeostasis shows that the system is extremely effective.

Branchpoints

Metabolic regulation is exerted primarily at branchpoints, where a metabolic intermediate is partitioned between two pathways. The branchpoint metabolite is the substrate for two enzymes, and the relative amount of the metabolite that enters each pathway depends on competition between the two enzymes. As discussed in Chapter 5, the outcome of such competition depends largely on the relative affinities of the two enzymes for their common substrate, and changes in these affinities in response to changes in concentrations of other substrates or in concentration ratios of coupling agents is the usual basis for regulation of the relative fluxes through the two pathways. This modulation of the affinities of competing enzymes must lead to a kind of interaction between sequences. As discussed in connection with Figure 5-8, a change in substrate affinity of one of the coupling agents will tend to change the concentration of the common intermediate and thus to affect the rate of the reaction catalyzed by the other enzyme. Thus if enzymes A and B compete for branchpoint metabolite M, an increase in the affinity of enzyme A for the substrate [a decrease in its $(S)_{0.5}$] will not only cause an increase in the rate of the reaction catalyzed by A but, by decreasing the concentration of M, will also cause a decrease in the rate of the reaction catalyzed by B. This type of interaction between sequences is an inevitable feature of this type of regulation, and it sharpens regulatory responses to variations in the values of control parameters.

Metabolism contains a large number of branchpoints, and probably each is subject to regulation. The branchpoints are of several types. When a pathway provides for the synthesis of two amino acids, for example, there must be a point at which the two syntheses diverge. Many branchpoints are of the type shown in Figure 6-2, where a synthetic pathway branches off from a main amphibolic sequence. Although similar in principle, the types of controls that are appropriate at these various types of branchpoints will differ in detail.

The question naturally arises whether there is any key or master branchpoint between catabolic and anabolic metabolism. Because of the complexity of metabolism, the answer is clearly that there can be no such master control point in a strict sense. This is obvious from Figure 6-2, which shows a number of individual branchpoints in glycolysis. However, in aerobic heterotrophic cells metabolizing glucose, one branchpoint comes nearer than any other to providing a clean partition between the major catabolic sequence and the supply of many major biosynthetic starting materials. This branch is at pyruvate in eukaryotic organisms and at phosphoenolpyruvate in many prokaryotes.

In normal operation of the citrate cycle as an oxidative sequence, every intermediate is regenerated at the same rate as it is used; thus none is consumed in a stoichiometric sense. Only acetyl-SCoA can be oxidized by the cycle. By the same token, since each turn of the cycle takes up one acetyl group and produces two molecules of carbon dioxide, acetyl-SCoA cannot contribute to the production of biosynthetic intermediates. Thus although the two functions of the cycle—reduction of NAD^+ leading to regeneration of ATP, and the provision of biosynthetic starting materials—involve the same reactions, they require different inputs. Each molecule of α-ketoglutarate, succinyl-SCoA, or oxaloacetate that is removed for use in biosynthesis must be balanced by addition of a molecule of some intermediate of the cycle; otherwise the level of oxaloacetate would decline and the cycle would stop.

The balance between these two main functions of the citrate cycle thus depends on the relative rates of the two entries into the cycle, one (acetyl-SCoA) supporting oxidation and the other (usually oxaloacetate) supporting the production of biosynthetic intermediates. In typical heterotrophs metabolizing carbohydrate, this branchpoint thus entails partitioning at the 3-carbon stage between decarboxylation to the 2-carbon fuel acetyl-SCoA and carboxylation to the 4-carbon replenishment compound oxaloacetate. These relationships are illustrated in Figure 6-8, where solid arrows indicate

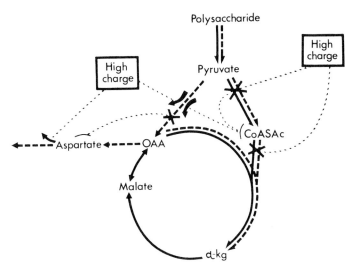

Figure 6-8. Apparent regulatory interaction at the pyruvate branchpoint, based on results obtained with yeast grown on glucose. The broken lines indicate biosynthetic sequences and the solid lines indicate catabolic or energy-yielding pathways. Light broken lines connect modifiers to the reactions that they affect; a curved arrow indicates a positive effect and a cross, a negative effect. "High charge" indicates a high value of the adenylate energy charge. From Miller and Atkinson (*83*).

catabolic reactions leading to the production of carbon dioxide with concomitant reduction of NAD^+, and broken arrows indicate pathways leading to provision of biosynthetic intermediates. The metabolic roles of acetyl-SCoA and oxaloacetate discussed above and shown in the figure refer to stoichiometry rather than to the fates of individual carbon atoms. That is, each molecule of acetyl-SCoA that reacts with oxaloacetate to form citrate is balanced by loss of two molecules of carbon dioxide in the ensuing turn of the cycle, but the two carbon atoms lost are not the same ones that entered at the beginning of that cycle. This mixing of atoms has no metabolic consequences, of course; only stoichiometric relationships matter in such contexts.

As shown in Figure 6-8, the partitioning at pyruvate is not quite clean. All of the oxaloacetate produced by carboxylation of pyruvate is destined, stoichiometrically speaking, for replenishment of cycle intermediates to replace compounds used in biosynthesis. However, not quite all of the carbon atoms that enter as acetyl-SCoA will be oxidized. Of the 5 carbon atoms in each molecule of α-ketoglutarate that is used for synthesis of glutamate and related amino acids, one is derived, stoichiometrically, from acetyl-SCoA. Each molecule of citrate that is exported from the mitochondrion for use in cytoplasmic synthetic or storage processes contains two carbon atoms from acetyl-SCoA. However, regulation of the competition for pyruvate between pyruvate carboxylase and the pyruvate dehydrogenase complex is especially interesting because this competition comes so close to providing a clean separation between major anabolic and catabolic pathways.

The controls shown in Figure 6-8 are based mainly on work with yeast (83), but are probably typical for aerobic heterotrophic eukaryotes. As is to be expected, a high value of the adenylate energy charge facilitates carboxylation of pyruvate, leading to biosynthetic starting materials, and decreases the affinity of the pyruvate dehydrogenase complex for pyruvate, thus decreasing the tendency for pyruvate to be oxidized to acetyl-SCoA. If the charge falls slightly, the resulting decrease in carboxylation and increase in oxidative decarboxylation of pyruvate would obviously tend to counteract the change in charge. Interactions at this branchpoint are probably quantitatively among the most important of the effects that stabilize the energy charge. The other regulatory modulations shown in the figure appear to allow for other inputs while also reinforcing the direct effects of energy charge. The affinity of yeast citrate synthase for acetyl-SCoA is strongly affected by the value of the energy charge (57).

When the energy charge rises, the resulting increase in $(S)_{0.5}$ of citrate synthase for acetyl-SCoA must cause an increase in the concentration of acetyl-SCoA. The resulting effects on pyruvate carboxylase and pyruvate dehydrogenase are in the same direction as the effects of increased energy charge on those enzymes; thus the indirect effects of energy charge, as noted above, reinforce the direct effects. But the responses of the competing enzymes to the concentration of acetyl-SCoA must have additional consequences beyond amplifying the effect of energy charge. If the concentration of oxaloacetate falls to the extent that the rate of the citrate synthase reaction is decreased because of substrate limitation, the decrease in rate of consumption of acetyl-SCoA should cause the concentration of that metabolite to rise. The result will be a shift in the partitioning of pyruvate in the direction of increasing the rate of production of oxaloacetate; thus the concentration of this important metabolite will be stabilized. The feedback control of pyruvate carboxylase by aspartate similarly will be to some extent an indirect effect of energy charge, but is presumably primarily a mechanism for the stabilization of the concentration of aspartate, which not only is required directly in protein synthesis but is also the precursor of four other amino acids.

In prokaryotes that produce oxaloacetate by carboxylation of phosphoenolpyruvate rather than pyruvate, the 3-carbon/4-carbon branchpoint is at phosphoenolpyruvate, and the competing enzymes are pyruvate kinase and phosphoenolpyruvate carboxylase. This relation, for *Azotobacter vinelandii* growing on carbohydrate, is shown in Figure 6-9. The R-type response

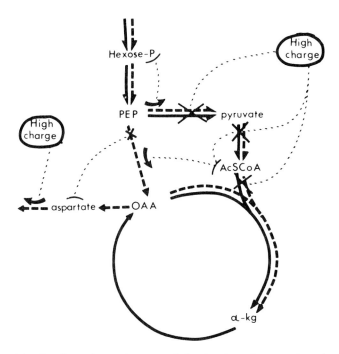

Figure 6-9. Regulatory interactions around the phosphoenolpyruvate branchpoint, based on results obtained with *Azotobacter vinelandii* grown on sucrose. Solid arrows indicate the catabolic sequence leading to regeneration of ATP, and broken arrows indicate anaplerotic or biosynthetic sequences. Light, obliquely broken lines connect modifiers to the reactions that they modulate. A curved arrow indicates stimulation (usually increase in affinity for substrates), and a cross indicates inhibition. "High charge" refers to the energy charge of the adenine nucleotide pool. Abbreviations used are PEP, phosphoenolpyruvate; OAA, oxaloacetate; α-kg, α-ketoglutarate; AcSCoA, acetyl coenzyme A. From Liao and Atkinson (*72*).

of pyruvate kinase to variation in energy charge must be a major determinant of the amount of phosphoenolpyruvate that is converted to acetyl-SCoA. The overall pattern is very similar to that shown in Figure 6-8, except that no direct effect of the adenylate energy charge on phosphoenolpyruvate carboxylase was observed. The effect of acetyl-SCoA on this enzyme must provide, as discussed above in connection with the acetyl-SCoA modulation of pyruvate carboxylase in yeast, both stabilization of the oxaloacetate level and an indirect response to the value of the energy charge.

When an organism grows with a 3-carbon compound such as lactate as the sole source of carbon and energy, regulatory needs are rather different than when carbohydrates are utilized. Since carbohydrates are components of cell walls and perhaps of other structural elements, gluconeogenesis is in effect a biosynthetic path in this case; it may also supply precursors for production of storage polysaccharide. Regulatory interactions in *Escherichia coli* growing on lactate are illustrated in Figure 6-10. Again an important branchpoint occurs at phosphoenolpyruvate, but the partitioning is only between two anabolic pathways, both leading to the production of biosynthetic intermediates. The primary partition between anabolic and catabolic functions is at pyruvate, and the competing enzymes in this case are phosphoenolpyruvate synthase and the pyruvate dehydrogenase complex. Reversal of the pyruvate kinase reaction would be thermodynamically unfavorable. The interconversions of pyruvate and phosphoenolpyruvate make up a pseudocycle of the type discussed in Chapter 3. In prokaryotes the phosphorylation of pyruvate is catalyzed by phosphoenolpyruvate synthase

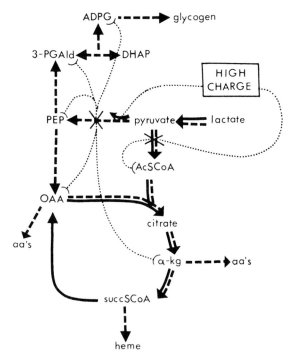

Figure 6-10. Regulatory effects on PEP synthetase and pyruvate dehydrogenase that seem to have evolved to control the partitioning of pyruvate between conversion to PEP for biosynthetic purposes and conversion to acetyl coenzyme A, which is used mainly in the regeneration of ATP, based on results obtained with *Escherichia coli* grown on lactate. Solid arrows are used for the sequence of reactions by which lactate is oxidized to CO_2, with regeneration of ATP, and broken arrows for biosynthetic sequences. Broken lines connect modifiers to the reactions that they affect; a cross indicates inhibition and a curved arrow indicates stimulation. "High charge" refers to a high value of the adenylate energy charge. From Chulavatnatol and Atkinson (*34*).

which, because it converts ATP to AMP, has a coupling coefficient of -2 (equation 6-4). Thus this reaction is thermodynamically favorable under

$$\text{pyruvate} + \text{ATP} \rightarrow \text{phosphoenolpyruvate} + \text{AMP} + P_i \qquad (6\text{-}4)$$

physiological conditions. As is appropriate for an enzyme catalyzing a reaction that commits product to anabolic uses, phosphoenolpyruvate synthase is facilitated by a high value of the adenylate energy charge (*34*). A number of compounds were observed to be negative modifiers for phosphoenolpyruvate synthase. As seen in Figure 6-10, all of these negative modifiers are key compounds in biosynthetic or storage sequences, and thus are appropriate regulators of the reaction in which carbon atoms derived from the growth substrate become committed to biosynthesis or storage.

SUMMARY

Metabolic sequences are typically regulated by several inputs. For an amphibolic sequence these will include at least the energy charge as an indication of the cell's need to regenerate ATP and one or more modifiers that indicate the need for the production of biosynthetic starting materials. Biosynthetic sequences will be regulated at least by the energy charge as an indication of the energy status of the cell and by the end product or end products of the sequence as an indication of the need for the synthesis. Other signals reflecting such information as the availability of nitrogen or the levels of glycolytic or other intermediates affect the rates of many sequences.

Although the energy charge response of each sequence will be modulated by individual and specific inputs, there must be at any time a weighted-average curve representing the sum of ATP-regenerating activity and a weighted-average curve representing the sum of ATP-utilizing sequences. The interaction of these average curves will regulate the overall balance between catabolic and anabolic metabolism and stabilize the energy charge, while the shapes of curves for individual sequences can vary freely in response to momentary metabolic needs.

There must be a hierarchy among ATP-utilizing sequences, with essential maintenance metabolism and membrane activities, growth, and storage of fat or polysaccharide being increasingly dispensable in that order. Although in higher organisms it is subject to modulation by hormone effects, this hierarchy is probably established at the cellular level by the shapes of responses of appropriate enzymes to the energy charge and to other regulatory parameters. Enzymes that regulate storage sequences should have the steepest response curves with midpoints at the highest values of energy charge; enzymes regulating essential intermediary metabolism should have somewhat less steep slopes and midpoints at somewhat lower values of energy charge; and enzymes regulating growth should be intermediate. The limited information, from experiments *in vitro*, relevant to this expectation is consistent with it. It is suggested that use of GTP, UTP, and CTP in the synthesis of macromolecules is an evolutionary adaptation to allow energy for such syntheses to be funneled through a single reaction—that catalyzed by nucleoside diphosphate kinase—and thus allow for regulation at a single reaction of the partitioning of energy between macromolecular synthesis and other ATP-consuming activities of the cell.

Partitioning of carbon between oxidation, leading to regeneration of ATP, and biosynthesis occurs at many branchpoints. A major junction of this type, and one of the cleanest, is at pyruvate in aerobic eukaryotes and at phosphoenolpyruvate in aerobic prokaryotes. A start has been made toward elucidation of the roles of energy charge and other regulatory parameters at this branchpoint by means of kinetic experiments *in vitro*. The results are consistent among themselves and with expectations based on known metabolic needs and interactions.

7

The Adenylate Energy Charge
in Intact Cells

The most characteristic feature of an organism is organization. The functional correlations that are involved in any aspect of the life of an organism are many and complex. The cellular controls that are the main subject of this book operate within single cells and are not, at a fundamental level, strikingly different in mammalian cells of various types than in single-celled eukaryotes, such as yeast or protozoa, or in bacteria. Even in a unicellular organism, centralization of the control of reaction rates in order to stabilize the concentrations of a thousand or more compounds would be totally infeasible; centralized control of a thousand or more reactions in each of several billion cells in a mammal would be even more impossible. Fortunately we do not need to use our central nervous systems for this task. The only possible arrangement is the one that has evolved, in which the features needed for control are built into the operating elements themselves.

The observation that organisms can maintain themselves, and in the process maintain the concentrations of most metabolites within rather narrow limits, proves the existence of highly effective interacting regulatory systems. The properties of regulatory enzymes that have been observed *in vitro*, some of which have been discussed earlier in this book, provide a beginning toward understanding how some of these controls operate. But a detailed picture of regulatory interactions within an intact functioning cell must come in part from observation on such cells. It seems probable that new methods, not now available, will be needed.

STABILITY OF CONCENTRATIONS
AND CONCENTRATION RATIOS

It has long been known that the concentrations of biosynthetic building-block metabolites, such as amino acids, are reasonably constant in cells of a given type. Within somewhat wider limits, the same can be said of the concentrations of metabolites generally. It has been known for 20 years that feedback regulation of the enzyme catalyzing the first reaction in each biosynthetic sequence by the end product of the sequence is an important factor contributing to the stabilization of concentrations. These facts have by now been incorporated into all serious textbooks of biochemistry, and need not be documented here. We will be concerned primarily with evidence from intact cells for the stabilization of the adenylate energy charge and with attempts to observe the effects of variation of the value of the charge in intact cells.

Stability of the Adenylate Energy Charge

As has been noted earlier, the value of the adenylate energy charge in metabolizing cells seems to be very similar for all cell types, and also to change very little with changes in metabolic conditions. The narrowness of the range of normal fluctuations in the value of the charge has become apparent only during the last few years, and we do not yet have the final precise picture.

Evaluation of the energy charge in intact cells depends of course on accurate estimation of the relative concentrations of ATP, ADP, and AMP. Those estimations depend in turn not only on the sensitivity and accuracy of the analytical methods but equally on the adequacy of the sampling techniques. Because of the rapid turnover of the adenylate pool, fast killing and simultaneous inactivation of all enzymes that catalyze reactions in which the adenine nucleotides are consumed, produced, or interconverted are necessary. This necessity was not generally appreciated until fairly recently. Many determinations of adenine nucleotides, as well as of other metabolites, have been performed on bacteria or yeast cells that had been harvested by centrifugation and washed by one or more cycles of resuspension and recentrifugation. Even when the analytical techniques were excellent, results obtained in this way are worse than useless because they are actively misleading. They reflect the situation in cells at some point in a sequence of alternate anaerobic packing in a pellet and aerobic or anaerobic metabolism in nutrient-free buffer, but they are not likely to bear any meaningful relationship to concentrations in cells in the culture from which the samples were obtained.

Energy charge values were calculated from all concentrations of adenine nucleotides that were found in a literature survey in 1971. The results of these calculations are shown in Figure 7-1. The survey was not exhaustive, but there is no reason to doubt that the values tabulated are representative. If taken literally, the figure shows that after perhaps three billion years of evolutionary experimentation the energy charge has finally stabilized within a

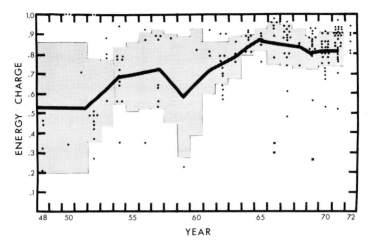

Figure 7-1. Values of the adenylate energy charge, calculated from the determinations of ATP, ADP, and AMP tabulated by Chapman *et al.* (*30*), plotted against the year in which the analysis was reported. The line is a 3-year moving average of the energy charge values. The shaded region covers one apparent standard deviation on each side of the line. Since the error is of course not homogeneous for analyses performed in different laboratories on different cells or tissues, employing different methods, the shaded area is only a rough indication of the relative spread of the results that were published at a given time. The three reports shown by square symbols, all from the same laboratory, are not included in the averages.

narrow range, in organisms of all types, within the past 30 years. If anyone were so naive as to accept this view, it would seem indeed fortunate that metabolic biochemistry developed during the last few decades and not 50, 100, or 1000 years earlier, when regulation of the adenine nucleotides was in a state of chaos. An alternative and considerably more likely explanation is that scientists all too often publish results before suitable methods are available by which reliable results might be obtained, or without giving much thought to sampling and processing. Methods for determination of nucleotides have improved since the 1950s, but it seems likely that the inaccuracy of most of the earlier reports stemmed to a greater extent from inadequate sampling than from errors in the determinations themselves. Treatment of samples during processing in preparation for analysis is another source of potential error. Thus we and others, after disrupting cells and inactivating enzymes by rapid transfer of bacterial cells to perchloric acid, routinely precipitated most of the perchlorate by neutralization with potassium hydroxide and removed potassium perchlorate along with protein by centrifugation. Some enzyme activity or activities that act on ATP recover on neutralization, however, leading to calculation of energy charge values lower than the values in the initial sample. It is thus necessary to remove precipitated protein by

centrifugation before neutralization. This simple change in processing caused
an increase of about 0.1 in the energy charge values calculated for *E. coli*
(*114*) and a larger increase in the ATP values determined for *Bacillus brevis*
(*44*).

So many papers reporting estimates of nucleotide concentrations *in vivo*
have been published in the past few years that it does not seem worthwhile
to add them to Figure 7-1. When the procedures used and the apparent care
with which the values were obtained are taken into account, the apparently
best recent values are found to correspond to a slightly higher average value
and a narrower range than is indicated even at the right-hand edge of the
figure. It seems a reasonable hypothesis at present that the adenylate energy
charge values for all or nearly all cells under all or nearly all conditions of
steady metabolism are within the range of 0.87 to 0.94.

In addition to indicating changes in the results of estimations of the adenine nucleotides, Figure 7-1 illustrates a more general point, and one of
special importance to graduate students and others relatively new to research: one should never be intimidated by the weight of published evidence.
The old adage that the most attractive hypothesis can be destroyed by one
stubborn little fact should be accepted only with considerable reserve. First,
the fact may not destroy the hypothesis but merely show the need for rethink-
ing and modifying it. Second, a sizable portion of the facts that may be re-
trieved from the scientific literature, however stubborn they may appear, are
simply not true. Stabilization of the ATP/ADP concentration ratio, or of
the ATP mole fraction, or of the energy charge, might well have been proposed any time after 1956 on the basis of simple reasoning concerning metabolic function, using the analogy of biosynthetic feedback regulation as a
starting point. But anyone who originated such a proposal and who then
went to the biochemical literature and believed what he found there would
have abandoned the hypothesis forthwith.

The Adenylate Energy Charge in Various Organisms

Adenylate energy charge values, calculated from levels of the adenine nucleotides reported in the biochemical literature, have been tabulated (*29, 30*).
Methods of sampling and significance of the results are also briefly discussed.

The earliest and still one of the most convincing demonstrations of how
strongly the energy charge is stabilized in mammalian cells comes from the
careful determinations by Williamson of concentrations of adenine nucleotides in rat liver perfused with various materials (*122–124*). Values of energy
charge that may be calculated from results obtained with control livers average 0.88. In liver perfused with a variety of metabolites, 13 out of 14 energy
charge values were between 0.8 and 0.9; the only exception was a value of
0.72 resulting from perfusion with fructose.

In *E. coli* cells growing under conditions of energy limitation, the energy charge remained at 0.85 or above even at a generation time of 15 hours, which is 10 to 12 times the generation time under the same conditions but with adequate glucose (R. J. Sedo and D. E. Atkinson, unpublished results).

Transient Decrease and Recovery of the Energy Charge

Once the value of the energy charge has been found to have virtually the same value in cells of many, and perhaps all, types under most or all conditions of active steady metabolism, little is to be gained by further measurements of the same kind. As with man-made devices, study of transient phenomena may supply types of information that cannot be obtained with steady-state systems. The simplest question that can be approached in this way is how fast the charge returns to its steady state after the system has been perturbed. From the results of the few experiments of this type that have been performed, it is evident that when an energy source is available the energy charge recovers quite rapidly after being forced to an abnormally low level.

One way of causing a decrease in the value of the energy charge is momentarily to increase the rate of utilization of ATP by addition of a substrate for a kinase. If the phosphorylated product can be metabolized to lead to regeneration of ATP, the energy charge can be expected to recover promptly. An early and careful experiment of this type was reported in 1966 by Coe (*39*), who worked with Ehrlich ascites cells. The energy charge, calculated from the concentrations of ATP and ADP found by Coe, is shown in Figure 7-2

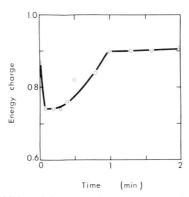

Time   (min)

Figure 7-2. Effect of addition of glucose on the energy charge of Ehrlich ascites tumor cells. Ascites cells were suspended in phosphate buffer (pH 7.3–7.4). One minute after suspension, glucose was added to 0.77 mM. At the times indicated on the abscissa the cells were killed with perchloric acid, and ATP and ADP were assayed enzymically (*39*). The energy charge values presented here were calculated from the ATP and ADP levels plotted in Figure 6 of Coe (*39*) on the assumption that the adenylate kinase reaction was at equilibrium.

to fall rapidly on the addition of 0.77 mM glucose but to regain its steady-state value within 1 minute. Several such experiments have been recorded with test systems ranging from cell suspensions to intact mammals. Over-gaard-Hanson (88), in an experiment similar to Coe's except that the concentration of glucose added was 5 mM, observed a response [plotted in Chapman et al. (31)] that was very similar to Coe's but longer lasting. Perfusion of rat liver with fructose (126) or intravenous injection of fructose (96) caused the energy charge to fall to about 0.65. The pattern was very similar to that shown in Figure 7-2, except that recovery required about 10 minutes in both cases.

When glucose is exhausted in E. coli cultures, the energy charge falls by 0.1 to 0.2 units, and is stabilized at this new value for some time. If glucose is added to such starving cultures, the energy charge rises to the value characteristic of growth within a minute or two (30).

The response of yeast to starvation depends on the enzymatic capabilities of the cells. When cells of a respiration-deficient mutant were filtered and resuspended in medium lacking glucose the energy charge fell to below 0.1 within 1 minute. When glucose was added, the charge recovered fully within 2 minutes (115). When wild-type yeast was grown anaerobically on glucose, the energy charge on starvation fell rapidly to 0.4 to 0.5 and rose to the normal value for growing cells very rapidly when glucose was supplied (15). Cells grown aerobically on glucose and harvested before exhaustion of the substrate behaved similarly. In contrast, cells grown on ethanol and cells grown on glucose but allowed to pass through the normal adaptation to use of ethanol after exhaustion of glucose maintained a high value of the energy charge for a day or more. When a nitrogen source was available in the medium after exhaustion of ethanol, the charge was stabilized at about 0.7. When cells that had used glucose and ethanol sequentially were resuspended in a medium containing neither a source of energy nor of nitrogen, the charge remained at the level characteristic of growth, about 0.9. Although the point was not definitively tested, it seems likely that the presence of available nitrogen in the former case allowed a small amount of biosynthesis to occur until the charge fell enough to stop it. In any case, although these two cultures behaved somewhat differently, both of them maintained relatively high values of the charge during starvation, and in that respect resembled each other and differed from the other cultures described. Yeast does not produce functional mitochondria when grown anaerobically or in the presence of glucose. The results thus suggest that cells that contain mitochondria (those grown on the nonfermentable substrate ethanol, or on glucose but harvested after adaptation to oxidation of the ethanol that had accumulated during the initial fermentative phase) maintain a high value of energy charge during starvation, but that those lacking mitochondria (the respiration-deficient mutant or wild-type cells grown anaerobically or harvested from aerobic cultures before exhaustion of glucose) do not. The regulatory basis for this distinction is not known, but of course cells containing mitochondria may be expected to utilize endogenous reserves more effectively than those incapable of respiration.

Possible Oscillations or Other Periodic Variation of the Energy Charge

Any regulated parameter must vary, at least slightly, around its regulated value, and it is these variations to which the regulatory system responds. Thus our repeated assertion that the energy charge is essentially constant in an intact cell under conditions of normal steady metabolism does not imply absolute constancy. There is no doubt that the energy charge fluctuates or oscillates around its average value. The question of interest here is whether these fluctuations are extremely small, serve no metabolic purpose, and are merely the result of the impossibility of attaining perfection in regulation or whether they constitute part of the evolutionary functional design, and are of relatively large magnitude. The rather extensive literature on oscillations, usually of the oxidation states of the pyridine nucleotide cofactors, that have been recorded for enzyme systems *in vitro* and for intact cells and even populations of cells in suspension will not be discussed here, since no meaningful brief discussion seems possible. If such oscillations are ultimately established as valid and general, they must of course be taken into account in future discussions of metabolic regulation. A finding that the energy charge in typical cells constantly oscillates with considerable amplitude would not change the basic points made in this book concerning the thermodynamics and kinetics of metabolism and the interactions between sequences, but it would require an extensive change in viewpoint as to the details of the interactions and would introduce a time scale as an important aspect of those interactions. It seems to me that at present our information concerning metabolism is more compatible with a steady value of energy charge than with one that oscillates over a relatively wide range. This opinion is based in part on the damping that it seems would be exerted by the interactions of the adenylate system with a very large number of metabolic sequences (it seems unlikely that the time constants that would be important in potential oscillation would be equal for all these sequences) and on the short period (crest-to-crest time) that would be necessary if the amplitude of the oscillation were great enough to nearly turn off ATP regeneration at the peak and ATP utilization at the minimum (see below).

Other types of periodic variation of energy charge besides sinusoidal oscillation might be possible. For example, Goldbetter (52) proposed that the charge remains at a constant high level most of the time, but drops periodically to a very low level from which it returns rapidly. In a graph based on a computer simulation, the charge is at 0.945 most of the time, but drops every 200 seconds to 0.55. The total period of drop and recovery is about 30 to 45 seconds. The model used to generate the graph was a simulation only of the behavior of isolated phosphofructokinase in an open system, so it could have no direct relevance to regulation of the energy charge *in vivo*, which depends on interaction between ATP-regenerating and ATP-utilizing sequences. But regardless of the basis for the suggestion, the question arises whether a pattern of this general type might be found in the real world. As Goldbetter points out, it has attractive features. If ATP could be produced during short intervals when the charge is so low that reactions using ATP are nearly totally prevented, and if a supply of ATP were then available most of the time without the need for simultaneous regeneration of ATP, the regulation of pseudocycles would seem to be facilitated. Metabolism at any given instant would be cleanly catabolic or cleanly anabolic; the apparent steady-state value of the energy charge would be a time-weighted average of a parameter that actually fluctuated widely; and the balance between catabolism and anabolism (R-type and U-type sequences) would be maintained by variation of the fraction of time occupied by each type of metabolism rather than, as we have assumed, by simultaneous regulation of the relative rates of catabolic and anabolic sequences.

But however attractive alternating on-or-off metabolic control may seem, the small size of the adenylate pool, as compared with the rate of use of ATP, seems to make such a pattern quite untenable. At an energy charge of 0.945 the adenylate pool is about 90% ATP; at a charge of 0.55 this has fallen to about 40%. Thus use of approximately half of the ATP present at the beginning of the proposed plateau would cause the charge to fall from the plateau value to the bottom of the proposed dip. But the turnover time of ATP is probably of the order of 1 second for some types of cells, and considerably less for others (*29*), so in well under a second after the beginning of the "plateau," the charge would reach its lowest value. A plateau in the sense, for example, of constancy of the energy charge within 10% thus could not last for more than perhaps 5 to 100 msec (depending on the type of cell) in the absence of ATP regeneration. If oscillations of considerable magnitude in the value of the energy charge are indeed a feature of metabolic regulation, the period of oscillation must be only a few milliseconds at most. Oscillation at such frequencies seems unlikely. Arguments from unlikelihood cannot prove anything rigorously, but in the absence of compelling evidence to the contrary it seems reasonable to consider the apparent constancy of the energy charge to be real, rather than to represent merely the average value of an oscillating parameter.

ENERGY CHARGE, ADENYLATE POOL, AND FUNCTIONAL CAPACITIES

Covariation of Energy Charge and Adenylate Pool

Conditions of stress that cause a decrease in the value of the energy charge usually also cause the total adenylate pool level to decrease, sometimes by a much larger factor (*29*). The chemistry of the system provides no basis for predicting or rationalizing this correlation; ordinary metabolic uses of ATP generate equimolar amounts of ADP or AMP, so that no change in the total adenylate concentration would be expected. A clue was provided by the observation that IMP or its degradation products are produced when the adenylate pool falls concomitantly with the energy charge in liver (*126*) or in ascites tumor cells (*76*, *82*). This observation suggests that the decrease in total adenylate level results from deamination of AMP, with production of IMP. Removal of AMP would obviously tend to raise the energy charge, since the concentration of AMP occurs only in the denominator of the expression for energy charge; thus activation of adenylate deaminase when the energy charge falls might be a useful means of limiting the extent of sudden drops in the energy charge. Because of the action of adenylate kinase (equation 7-1), removal of AMP will tend to raise the ATP/ADP concentration

$$ADP + ADP \rightleftharpoons ATP + AMP \qquad (7\text{-}1)$$

ratio. The reaction will be pulled to the right as written, increasing the concentration of ATP and decreasing that of ADP. Thus whichever of the related regulatory parameters is considered—energy charge, ATP/ADP ratio, or ATP/AMP ratio—activation of adenylate deaminase when the energy charge falls would limit the extent of a transient negative peak caused by sudden metabolic stress.

The activity of adenylate deaminase does, as predicted, increase strongly with decrease in energy charge *in vitro* (*28*, *31*). The response of the enzyme from Ehrlich ascites tumor is seen in Figure 7-3. The increase in the rate of the reaction as the energy charge falls from its physiological value of 0.9 to around 0.65 is striking. (Values below about 0.65 can be ignored because energy charges in that range seem not to have been observed in surviving mammalian cells.) It is clear that, if these results reflect the behavior of the enzyme *in vivo*, a tendency for the energy charge to fall will be strongly resisted by removal of AMP from the pool. Such protection can be of use only for a very short period, because of the relatively small size of the adenylate pool and the rapid rate of ATP turnover; thus this response pattern probably has evolved merely to round off the negative peak of the severe drop in energy charge (or ATP/ADP ratio) that may occur in acute energy emergencies. This

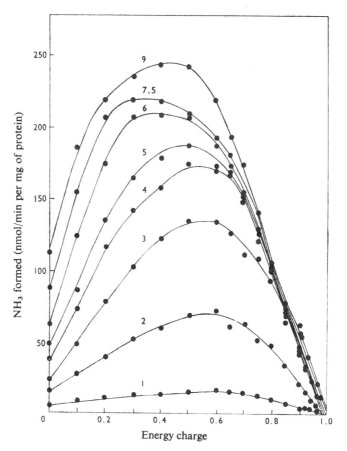

Figure 7-3. Response of AMP deaminase from ascites tumor cells to variations in adenylate energy charge at different adenine nucleotide pool sizes. Reaction mixtures contained 1–9 mM total adenine nucleotides, as indicated by the numbers identifying the curves, at energy charge values specified on the abscissa. NH$_3$ produced was measured by coupling with the glutamate dehydrogenase reaction. From Chapman *et al.* (*31*).

protection is obtained at the expense of loss of much of the cell's supply of adenine nucleotide. Obviously the extent of such protection must somehow be limited. Loss of all of a cell's adenine nucleotides would almost certainly be lethal, and the usefulness of a mechanism that killed a cell while protecting it would not be great. The strong and nonlinear response of the enzyme to variation in the total adenylate pool level, seen in Figure 7-3, appears to provide the needed protection. If the charge falls, for example, to 0.7, AMP will be deaminated at a rapid rate at any pool value above 4 mM. As further deamination reduces the pool below this level, the rate of the reaction will diminish rapidly. At a charge of 0.7 and a pool level of about 1.5 mM, the reaction rate would be about equal to that under normal physiological conditions (charge, 0.9; pool level 4–5 mM). Probably the actual rate *in vivo* is slower, because of other constraints that are lost on destruction of the cells, and return to the steady-state level probably indicates cessation of pool depletion. It is of interest that the conditions indicated by the experiments of Figure 7-3 for return to basal levels correspond reasonably well with the lowest values of energy charge and of pool observed in liver following injection of fructose (*96*) or perfusion of liver with fructose (*126*).

Bacteria do not contain AMP deaminase, but Schramm and colleagues (*105*) have shown that an enzyme that catalyzes cleavage of the nucleoside bond in AMP, producing adenine and ribose 5-phosphate, has very similar properties. The observation of similar unusual behavior in two enzymes that catalyze reactions that are chemically dissimilar and produce different products, having in common only the fact that they remove AMP, adds significantly to the confidence that may be placed in functional interpretation of those properties as providing for protection of the energy charge by removal of AMP.

If this interpretation of the properties of adenylate deaminase shown in Figure 7-3 is correct, it and AMP nucleosidase are the first enzymes playing a protective role in metabolic regulation that have been observed to have a built-in self limitation as a second level of metabolic protection. It will be interesting to see whether other enzymes are found to show similar patterns.

The properties of adenylate deaminase probably go far toward explaining the tendency for the sum of concentrations of the adenylate nucleotides to fall when the energy charge falls. However, this enzyme cannot be responsible for all of the facts that have been reported. For example, Chagoya de Sánchez *et al.* (*26*) showed that intraperitoneal injection of adenosine into rats caused an increase in both the total adenylate pool in liver and the energy charge. The basis for this interesting increase in energy charge is not known. Relative slopes of enzyme response curves and differences in the degrees of saturation of adenylate-binding sites may be involved, but any detailed speculation here would be premature.

Shift-up Experiments

When a culture of *E. coli* that has been growing with ammonia as the nitrogen source, and which has therefore been synthesizing amino acids, is suddenly supplied all of the amino acids in excess, the rate of growth increases. During the transition period the first change that has been observed is an increase in the rate of ribosomal RNA production, followed by increases in the rates of biosynthesis of DNA and protein and in the rate of cell division

(79). Presumably because of the heavy demand for them as building blocks
in the synthesis of RNA, the nucleoside triphosphates decrease in concentration during the transition (22). The extent of decrease in the concentration
of ATP varies among strains of E. coli. In a strain in which the ATP concentration fell by about 50%, the energy charge decreased from about 0.93 to
about 0.86 (J. S. Swedes and D. E. Atkinson, unpublished results). This
decrease was small in comparison with the change in ATP concentration
and was short lived; the value returned to normal in 30 to 40 minutes, which
is less than the generation time. Nevertheless, it is of interest that during the
transition time the energy charge was lower than the value corresponding to
steady growth, but macromolecules were being synthesized more rapidly
than during the preceding steady growth period. This situation illustrates
the fact that no single parameter controls metabolic processes by itself. As
we have discussed earlier, the adenylate energy charge is of special importance among regulatory parameters because it appears to correlate all metabolic sequences, but for any single reaction or sequence it is only one of
several regulatory inputs. Under conditions of balanced steady growth, the
value of the charge appears never to deviate far from 0.9. Other regulatory
parameters (concentrations and concentration ratios) are presumably also
held within relatively narrow limits under these conditions. But in any system
controlled by two or more inputs, if one is displaced from its normal range
the others may be caused to vary in the functionally opposed direction. Thus
when amino acids suddenly become available to cells that have been producing them, it may be expected that the intracellular concentrations of amino
acids will initially rise. Both because amino acids are precursors of protein
synthesis and because of their poorly understood but well-established role
in regulation of RNA synthesis, this increase in concentration will lead to an
increase in the rate of macromolecular synthesis. The resulting more rapid
rate of utilization of nucleoside triphosphates will tend to decrease the concentrations of the nucleotide pool; through the action of end product negative feedback controls the rates of synthesis of nucleotides will be increased
to bring them into balance with the rates of utilization.

The overall changes to be expected during a nutritional shift-up are illustrated in a schematic and highly simplified manner in Figure 7-4. During
steady growth before the shift, curves R and U represent, respectively, the
weighted averages of the responses to energy charge of regulatory enzymes
in sequences that regenerate ATP and in sequences that utilize ATP. As discussed in Chapter 6, the response to energy charge of each individual enzyme
is modulated by other regulatory parameters, so that the response must be
represented by a family of curves within a fan-shaped envelope, rather than
by a single line. When the energy charge response of one ATP-requiring
sequence is altered by a change in the value of another regulatory parameter

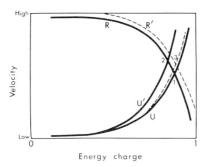

Figure 7-4. Suggested changes in metabolic energy charge responses during an amino acid shift-up experiment. See text for discussion.

such as the concentration of an end product, the effect on weighted-average responses, such as are represented by curve U in Figure 7-4, is negligible. But when the concentrations of all amino acids suddenly increase, many ATP-utilizing response curves will be shifted upward within their modulatory ranges. As discussed in the preceding paragraph, this may be in some cases because of increase in the concentrations of amino acids as precursors of proteins, in others because amino acids are, directly or indirectly, positive modifiers for RNA synthesis, and in still others because a tendency for nucleotide pools to fall leads to a decrease of end product inhibition. So many processes that are heavy consumers of ATP will be affected that the weighted-average curve must be shifted upward, as is illustrated by curve U' in Figure 7-4. As a result, the intersection of the two curves will move from point 1, characteristic of normal steady metabolism, to point 2. This point corresponds to higher fluxes through both catabolic (R-type) and anabolic (U-type) sequences than normal, as shown by the vertical coordinate, and a lower value of energy charge.

The situation represented by point 2 is abnormal, and is seen only during the metabolic imbalance that exists at the beginning of a transition such as that produced by amino acid shift-up. Immediately after falling, the energy charge begins to recover, and has reestablished its initial value of about 0.9, characteristic of steady growth, within a few minutes. Presumably the normal controls of amino acid synthesis and amino acid uptake cause the levels of amino acid pools to decline toward the initial values, so that curve U' moves back toward curve U. The process is not merely returned to point 1, however, since the rate of steady growth after completion of a transition is higher than the rate before addition of amino acids. Probably both the R and U weighted-average curves are somewhat displaced after the shift-up from their initial position. The U curve may reasonably be expected to move toward, but not to reach, its initial position. This is illustrated by the broken line between

curves U′ and U. The position of curve R after the shift-up is more difficult
to predict. The rates of synthesis of amino acids will decrease nearly to zero,
but the rates of all other syntheses will increase. It is impossible at our present
state of knowledge to predict whether the result of these two effects will be
an increase or a decrease in the concentrations of compounds, such as citrate,
that seem to serve in the regulation of glycolysis as indicators of levels of biosynthetic starting materials for biosynthesis and thus change the shapes of
R-type curves (Chapter 6). But one change is certain: of the material that
moves down the glycolytic sequence, a larger portion will be oxidized to
lead to the regeneration of ATP than before the shift-up. This is necessarily
true, because the synthesis of amino acids, which formerly consumed a very
significant fraction of the carbon processed by glycolysis, virtually ceases
when amino acids become available exogenously. Thus even if the actual rate
of glycolysis returns to the preshift value, the rate of ATP regeneration will be
higher. In consequence, the R curve, as a measure of ATP regeneration, will
move upward as illustrated by curve R′. In the new steady-growth condition,
curve R′ will intersect a slightly changed curve U at point 3. The value of the
energy charge at this point will be expected to be, and is experimentally
found to be, very near that of point 1.

Energy Charge and Rates of Metabolism and Growth

It is evident from our uncertainties as to the exact change in positions and
slopes of weighted-average R and U curves that accompany various changes
in environmental conditions that we cannot suggest any general relation between growth rate and energy charge. Point 3 of Figure 7-4, for example,
might be at a slightly higher or slightly lower value of energy charge than is
point 1. It seems likely, indeed, that no general relation exists, and that under
various conditions, allowing for different rates of steady growth, there may
be small differences in energy charge and that the value of energy charge, if
measurable to the necessary three or four significant figures, would not be
found to correlate with the rate of growth. But what seems certain is that the
range of these variations is very narrow, and that after transient perturbation
by changes such as nutritional shift-up or shift-down, the charge returns to
a value very close to its previous level. During steady growth, when the values
of other regulatory parameters are also at normal steady states, the energy
charge is very close to 0.9.

Considerations similar to those of Figure 7-4 help in understanding how,
even if the value of the energy charge is so important in metabolic regulation,
the same value of energy charge nevertheless can be compatible with very
different rates of metabolism and growth. First it must be realized that response curves of both the R and U types, such as those of Figure 4-2 (which

are reproduced as broken lines in Figure 7-5) are actually more complex than was discussed in Chapter 4. The vertical coordinate of Figure 4-2 was labeled "Velocity" to simplify the discussion at that level. Such curves do in fact represent reaction velocities and metabolic fluxes, since it is total flux rates that are being held in balance. But at another level, R and U curves represent enzyme responses, which usually take the form of changes in affinity for substrates. The velocity of an enzyme-catalyzed reaction is dependent on the ratio $(S)/(S)_{0.5}$. Thus when substrate concentrations are essentially constant the reaction velocity is proportional to the affinity of the catalytic site for substrate (assuming that the catalytic site is rather far from saturation), so that the same pair of curves can represent both enzyme response and velocity of flux. However, reaction velocities depend also on the substrate concentration, the numerator in the ratio $(S)/(S)_{0.5}$. As discussed in Chapter 5, in the regulatory range where an enzyme responds to the concentration of a modifier metabolite, variation in the concentration of substrate must always be at least as important in the determination of the reaction velocity as is variation in the concentration of modifier. Thus when substrates are in limited supply the curves illustrating the response of an enzyme to the value of the energy charge and the curves for metabolic flux as a function of energy charge will not necessarily be the same.

The types of changes in metabolic flux curves that seem likely to occur during an amino acid shift-up were illustrated in Figure 7-4. Figure 7-5 shows, in a general and schematic way, the changes that might accompany severe limitation in the availability of the carbon and energy source. The basic responses of the enzymes to the value of the energy charge are shown by the broken lines labeled R_{resp} and U_{resp}. As assumed in our earlier discussion, enzymes of ATP-regenerating sequences will be essentially maximally active at energy charge values below about 0.7 or 0.75. However, if

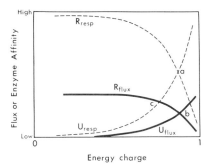

Figure 7-5. Suggested changes in metabolic energy charge responses resulting from severe limitation of carbon and energy source. See text for discussion.

the substrate (glucose, for example) is present at a very low level, the concentration of substrate will limit the first step in glycolysis and all subsequent steps as well. Thus the flux as a function of energy charge will be represented by a curve like that labeled R_{flux}. This curve has the same general shape as curve R_{resp}, but the flux, even at low values of energy charge, is much lower than it would be if the supply of glucose were adequate. Similarly, the concentrations of intermediates in biosynthetic sequences will be lower than normal, so that fluxes through such sequences will also be lower, for any given value of the energy charge, than they would be when the carbon supply was adequate. This depression of biosynthetic rates is indicated by the position of curve U_{flux} relative to U_{resp} in Figure 7-5. At the intersection of curve R_{flux} and U_{flux} (point b), the fluxes through all sequences, and hence growth and all metabolism-related functions, are much slower than they would be if the carbon and energy supply were present in excess (point a), but the value of the energy charge is about the same. Because of the large number of reactions involved and the still larger number of regulatory inputs, the exact shapes of curves R_{flux} and U_{flux} relative to R_{resp} and U_{resp} cannot be predicted, and thus it is impossible to predict whether the energy charge at point b will be slightly higher or slightly lower than at point a. Probably no general prediction could be valid; the situation may vary with the precise circumstances of the nutritional limitation. Both point a and point b really represent small ranges rather than points, and it seems likely that the range of possible energy charge values around a and that around b may overlap, so that rapid metabolic fluxes and growth rates might occur under some circumstances at lower values of energy charge than those that, under different conditions, are associated with slower fluxes and growth rates. The point to be emphasized, as before, is that the range of energy charge values that are compatible with steady metabolism and growth is very narrow.

It might be felt that Figure 7-5 arbitrarily stacks the deck in favor of an essentially constant energy charge, in that both flux curves are decreased by about the same amount from the enzyme response curves. If the R_{flux} curve were far below the R_{resp} curve while the U_{flux} curve remained high, for example, the curves would intersect at a point, like c, corresponding to an energy charge markedly lower than normal. However, the indication of a similar degree of depression of both flux curves was not arbitrary. Intersections away from the usual energy charge range may occur transiently, as seen in the amino acid shift-up experiment discussed in the preceding section, but such abnormal energy charge values will be short lived as was observed experimentally to be true in that case. For example, if the oxygen supply for an organism growing aerobically were suddenly depleted (or removed by the experimenter), the dependence of ATP regeneration on the value of the energy charge might be expected to change from that shown by a curve similar to R_{resp} to one similar to R_{flux} in Figure 7-5. Initially there would be little change in the U curve. In consequence the energy charge would drop from point a to point c. If the organism were facultative (able to grow either aerobically or anaerobically), a period would follow during which concentrations of metabolites and probably levels of key enzymes would adjust to the values characteristic of anaerobic metabolism. With this shift the curve of ATP regeneration would rise toward R_{resp}, the energy charge would increase into the normal range, and growth would resume. Such a transient decrease in the energy charge has been observed to follow a shift from aerobic to anaerobic conditions in *E. coli* (*30*) and in yeast (*16*).

Not only is the nearly equal change in the R and U curves of Figure 7-5 not arbitrary, but it is a necessary consequence of the patterns of metabolic regulation. At such important branchpoints as pyruvate or phosphoenolpyruvate where, as discussed in Chapter 4, metabolites are partitioned between pathways leading to regeneration of ATP and those leading to biosynthesis, the energy charge is a major regulatory input, and partition is usually controlled by alteration of the relative affinities of competing enzymes for their common substrate. With this type of regulation, the partition of the branchpoint metabolite between the competing pathways is relatively independent of the concentration of that metabolite (Figure 5-8). Therefore, a change in the relative affinities $[(S)_{0.5}]_A/[(S)_{0.5}]_B$ will have approximately the same effect on the partition ratio whatever the concentration of substrate.

We noted in Chapter 4 that control of partition by regulation of the affinities of coupling metabolites allowed for especially sensitive control. Now we see another and perhaps even more important advantage of that pattern of control: it insulates the partitioning mechanism from the effects of fluctuation in availability of energy and carbon sources. The regulatory effects of the adenylate system are exerted at the same points and in the same way in feast as in famine. Thus ATP-regenerating and ATP-utilizing sequences must come into balance, at almost exactly the same value of energy charge, whether the carbon and energy source is present in excess (point a in Figure 7-5) or is severely limiting (point b). The metabolic role of the adenine nucleotides and of the adenylate energy charge is not regulation of the growth rate; the role is more fundamental and more essential to life than that. It is the correlation of all metabolic sequences and the regulation of the partitioning of resources among them. This correlation and controlled partitioning is a primary cause of the metabolic homeostasis that is essential for life and hence for growth, whether fast or slow.

Energy Charge and Functional Capacities

From what has been learned about the adenylate energy charge *in vivo* and about its effect on enzyme behavior *in vitro*, it seems that the rates of many or most ATP-requiring processes must be sharply reduced when the energy charge falls slightly below its normal range. It seems likely that there is a hierarchy of such processes in terms of their responses to the value of the energy charge. Energy-storing sequences, such as the syntheses of polysaccharide or fat, should be most sensitive to decrease in energy charge. Biosyntheses of structural macromolecules should be next, and activities that are essential for maintenance of life should be able to function at lower values of charge. Metabolic hierarchy of this type was discussed in Chapter 6. Its existence is evident from common observation, and is exploited in animal husbandry. Rapid growth and deposition of fat is obtained in domesticated animals grown for food by inducing consumption of a maximal amount of feed under conditions that discourage exercise. An extreme example is the fatty liver that is induced in geese in France (to be used in production of the fatty liver paste that in some circles is considered a delicacy) by forced feeding. Beginning with overfeeding at that extreme and rather disgusting level, decreases in food intake lead in turn to cessation of pathological fatty deposition in the liver, then to decrease and to cessation of deposition of fat in normal storage depots, then to decrease of growth rate, and finally to emaciation and death. Clearly fat deposition occurs only when energy is available in excess, growth only when it is available at an adequate level, and life only when it is above an irreducible threshold.

Because the concentrations of metabolic intermediates and biosynthetic starting materials will ordinarily decrease, with decreasing food intake, in parallel with decrease in the ability to regenerate ATP, it is impossible on the basis of present evidence to estimate to what extent the hierarchy of metabolic capabilities depends on the adenylate system. However, some observations on enzyme responses *in vitro* are compatible with an important role for energy charge in this regard. In *E. coli* the predominant storage compound is not fat, but glycogen, and the step at which the rate of synthesis of glycogen is regulated was shown by Preiss (*94*) to be the synthesis of ADP-glucose. The response to energy charge of the enzyme that catalyzes this step is the steepest yet observed, and the steep portion of the curve is at the upper edge of the physiological range of energy charge values (*109*); this response is obviously consistent with the expectation that storage materials should be made to a significant degree only when the energy state of the cell is unusually favorable. The next steepest response to energy charge that has been observed *in vitro* is that of nucleoside diphosphate kinase. As discussed in Chapter 6, this enzyme may be a master control element regulating the flow of energy into channels where it is available for the macromolecular syntheses that are necessary for growth. Responses observed for enzymes that participate in the metabolism of compounds of low molecular weight are all considerably less steep than the two just described.

When *E. coli* is grown in a medium containing a limiting level of glucose, the energy charge falls by about 0.1 unit when the glucose is exhausted, and rises for a short period about three hours later (*111, 119*). The rise results from metabolism of an exogenous substrate that had been lost from the cells during growth, as can be demonstrated by the lack of any such increase in energy charge when cells are centrifuged after exhaustion of glucose and re-suspended in medium lacking any carbon source. The major excretion product of *E. coli* growing on glucose is acetate (*100*), and on the addition of low levels of acetate to centrifuged and resuspended cells the secondary rise in energy charge value was duplicated almost exactly. Small samples were removed from cultures at intervals and exposed to isopropyl thiogalactoside. This compound is widely used as an inducer for β-galactosidase. The amount of β-galactosidase produced paralleled the value of energy charge quite closely, falling when the supply of glucose was exhausted, rising about three hours later, and then declining when the energy charge fell again.

Because isopropyl thiogalactoside is not hydrolyzed by β-galactosidase, it may be used to study the capacity of cells to produce the enzyme; the induction of enzyme does not alter the energy state of the cell because no substrate is available for it. The situation is of course very different when induction is caused by the presence of lactose. If lactose is present during growth on glucose, it has long been known that growth ceases briefly when glucose is exhausted and then resumes. The resumption of growth is parallel with, and dependent on, the production of β-galactosidase, which allows lactose to serve as an energy and carbon source. When the energy charge was followed during this transition from growth on glucose to growth on lactose, it was found to drop as in the cultures containing no alternate substrate except excreted acetate, but to rise much more rapidly and to remain high, of course, during growth on lactose (*119*). The rise in energy charge coincided with the induction of β-galactosidase. In this case there is evidently a mutual rein-forcement—when a small amount of β-galactosidase is produced the resulting metabolism of lactose tends to raise the energy charge (and the availability of metabolic intermediates and building blocks), resulting in an increased rate of synthesis of β-galactosidase, and so on. For our purposes the significant observation was that, although energy charge cannot of course be the sole determinant of the rate at which β-galactosidase is produced in induced cells, the rate of production of the enzyme paralleled the energy charge both when the nonmetabolizable inducer was employed and when lactose was used.

In correlations of functional capacities with the energy charge in *E. coli*, the charge has always been in or below the usual range; no conditions that would lead to a sustained elevation in the value of the charge have been discovered. As noted earlier, Chagoya de Sánchez and colleagues (26) were able to increase the energy charge in rat liver transiently by about 0.04 to 0.05 units by intraperitoneal injection of adenosine. There was a simultaneous enhancement of glycogen biosynthesis and a decrease in the rate of fatty acid catabolism. These changes are obviously in the direction that would be expected to follow from an increase in the energy charge.

Uncoupling of Variations in Energy Charge and in the Size of the Adenylate Pool

In an earlier section of this chapter we described the general observation that the energy charge and the adenylate pool tend to vary together, and the suggestion that this correlation may be caused at least in part by the activation of AMP deaminase in eukaryotic cells, and of AMP nucleosidase in bacteria, when the energy charge falls. Because of this covariance, it is difficult in normal cells to obtain a clean comparison of the relative importances of the energy charge (and the ATP/ADP and ATP/AMP ratios) and of the absolute concentration of ATP. Considerations discussed in Chapter 4 logically make it nearly inescapable that the charge and its component ratios must be much more metabolically relevant than are individual concentrations, but direct demonstration in intact cells was obviously desirable. This demonstration was achieved by use of a mutant strain of *E. coli* lacking the enzyme for conversion of IMP to succinyl-AMP, and thus unable to synthesize adenylates.

When the adenine-requiring strain was grown in batch culture containing limiting amounts of adenine, the concentrations of ATP, ADP, and AMP began to fall on the exhaustion of adenine. The energy charge remained at about 0.9 until the concentrations of the adenylates had fallen to approximately 30% of their normal values, and then began to decline. The ability of the cells to incorporate isotopically labeled leucine into protein (the mutant strain also requires leucine, which facilitates this measurement) remained high while the energy charge value was normal, in spite of the decrease of about 70% in the concentration of ATP, and decreased approximately in parallel with the energy charge (114).

When the cells of the mutant were centrifuged and resuspended in medium lacking both glucose and adenine, the charge was stable at about 0.8 which, as previously shown in experiments with wild-type *E. coli*, is typical of cells in a nongrowing state that are not yet severely energy-starved. The concentrations of the adenylates were stable and near their normal values. This stability presumably resulted from the absence of RNA synthesis under these conditions. When glucose was added, the energy charge rose immediately to its normal growth value of about 0.9 and the adenylate pool level began to fall, probably because ATP was being consumed in RNA synthesis. As in the batch culture described above, the energy charge remained at about 0.9 until the pool had fallen to about 30% of its normal value, and then declined. The ability of the cells to incorporate labeled leucine into protein was very low during the initial period when the cells were starved for both glucose and adenine, rose when the energy charge rose (while the concentration of ATP was falling) to nearly the level characteristic of growing cells, and then declined with the energy charge. The fact that the rate of protein synthesis rose when energy charge rose, even though the concentration of ATP was decreasing, does not of course constitute a rigorous test of the relative importances of energy charge and the ATP concentration, since the concentrations of numerous metabolic intermediates and precursors for synthesis of other amino acids must also have increased after addition of glucose. However, the fact that the ability to synthesize protein remained high while the charge was high, showing no tendency to change in response to the decrease in the concentration of ATP, and then fell roughly in parallel with the energy charge, is striking evidence that such an integrated process as protein synthesis is more sensitive to changes in energy charge than to variation, over a wide range, in the absolute concentrations of ATP, ADP, and AMP.

Growth, since it requires the properly correlated action of nearly all of the biochemical capacities of a cell, would seem to supply the most rigorous test of the relative metabolic importance of energy charge and of absolute concentrations of nucleotides. Accordingly, the adenine-requiring mutant was grown in continuous culture in a chemostat with adenine as the limiting nutrient. The results are shown in Figure 7-6. Moving from right to left in the figure corresponds to a steadily decreasing rate of growth as adenine becomes progressively more limiting. Each point in this figure was obtained at a steady state of growth where the cell density had been constant for at least three hours. The two points on the right correspond to cultures growing nearly at the rate characteristic of this strain in minimally supplemented medium. That is, the adenine supply was not significantly limiting. When adenine became limiting (third point from the right) the concentration of ATP and the total adenylate pool level fell by nearly 50%, but there was no detectable change in the energy charge and only a very small decrease in growth rate. With more stringent limitation of the adenine supply the concentration of ATP and the adenylate pool level fell further to about 30% of the normal value. At these lower levels of the pool, the cells were capable of sustained steady growth, although at a reduced rate. There was no observable change in the energy charge. These results show that growth rate is nearly

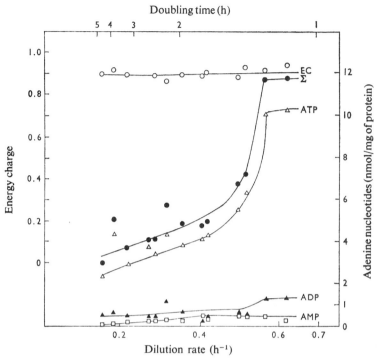

Figure 7-6. Adenine nucleotide concentrations and energy charge in adenine-limited cultures of an adenine-requiring strain of *Escherichia coli* (strain PC 0294). Growth rate in an adenine-limited chemostat culture was varied by the rate of medium addition. Each point represents the mean of three samples taken at hourly intervals after the cell density had reached a steady state. Curve identifications: EC, adenylate energy charge; Σ, adenylate pool (sum of ATP, ADP, and AMP). From Swedes *et al.* (*114*).

insensitive to the concentration of ATP over a twofold range, and that growth is possible even when the ATP concentration is decreased by a factor of 3. In contrast, steady growth has not been observed when the energy charge is as much as 10% below its normal value. In the experiments summarized in Figure 7-6, even more severe limitation of adenine led to a decrease in energy charge, but this was always associated with a decrease in cell density as growth ceased and the cells leaving the culture in the effluent were not replaced by growth. In other words, as soon as the energy charge fell detectably there was no steady growth and thus no point for plotting in the figure.

To summarize the findings shown in Figure 7-6: When adenine was slightly limiting, the intracellular concentration of the adenine nucleotides decreased by 50% before there was any marked effect on growth. When limitation was made more severe, both the rate of growth and the intracellular concentrations of the adenine nucleotides decreased, but the energy charge remained constant. When the energy charge decreased by a detectable amount, growth ceased and steady-state continuous culture became impossible. The conclusion is inescapable that growth is far more sensitive to variation in energy charge than to change in the concentration of ATP or of the other adenine nucleotides.

The inability of E. coli cells of this strain to maintain a normal value of the energy charge when the adenylate pool level falls below about 30% of its normal value, seen both in the suspensions of cells starved for adenine and in the adenine-limited steady-state cultures, is interesting. Many explanations could be suggested, but there is no basis at present for any choice among them. It is of interest, however, that we have never observed the adenylate pool to fall by more than about 50% in wild-type E. coli under a variety of stress conditions. Only in the abnormal case of genetic dependence on adenine has the pool been forced below that level. As seen in Figure 7-6, a 50% decrease has little effect on growth. Thus it appears that, as a consequence of the regulation of the adenylate pool size, the systems that regulate the energy charge seldom if ever are confronted by a decrease of more than 50% in the concentrations of AMP, ADP, and ATP, and that they are perfectly capable of coping with changes of that magnitude. Whatever the reason for collapse of the ability to maintain the energy charge when the pool falls below 30%, this situation probably never occurs in a normal E. coli cell.

For functional reasons very similar to those described for the adenine nucleotides, we would expect that the ratios or mole fractions of the pyridine nucleotide coupling systems would be more strongly stabilized than the absolute concentrations of the individual nucleotides. (As noted in Chapter 4, several enzymes have been shown to respond in vitro to the degree of reduction of the NAD or NADP system and to be insensitive, over a reasonable range, to the size of the pool.) The expected behavior was observed in Neurospora crassa by Brody, who, by using mutant strains and varying growth conditions, was able to cause both the total NAD and the total NADP pools to vary by a factor of nearly 3. In all cases the mole fractions of NADH and NADPH remained constant within experimental error (25).

SUMMARY

The mole fraction of ATP in the adenine nucleotide pool and the closely related parameter, the adenylate energy charge, are strongly stabilized in the intact metabolizing cell. It seems probable that the energy charge varies less than the actual concentrations of most or all metabolites.

As predicted from the underlying principles of chemical energy transduction, as well as from the behavior of enzymes *in vitro*, functional capacities *in vivo* are much more sensitive to variation in energy charge than to variation in the absolute concentration of ATP. This relationship has been illustrated by protein synthesis (followed by incorporation of labeled leucine or by synthesis of β-galactosidase in induced cells), and by growth experiments. Growth of *Escherichia coli* is nearly insensitive to a 50% decrease in the concentration of ATP, but steady growth has not been observed when the charge is outside its normal narrow range. Under special conditions, such as abrupt changes in the concentrations of other metabolites, the energy charge may be transiently displaced from its normal value, but if an energy source is available, recovery is always rapid.

Because metabolic regulation, whether by the energy charge or by other parameters, is usually exerted on the substrate affinities of enzymes that compete for branchpoint metabolites, the end result of regulation by the adenine nucleotides is balance among catabolic and anabolic conversions along with stabilization of the immediate energy supply of the cell, the adenylate system. The energy charge does not regulate the rate of metabolism or growth, but rather the relative rates of ATP-regenerating and ATP-utilizing sequences. Therefore, the normal value of energy charge is compatible with a wide range of rates of metabolism or growth, whereas (except for transient displacements during brief periods of metabolic adjustment to changed conditions). a value only slightly lower seems not to be compatible with growth at all.

8

General Summary and Discussion

The pattern that emerges from any extensive consideration of the properties of organisms is one of an exceedingly complex and sophisticated design. Individual species can easily be observed to change in response to changes in environmental conditions, as a consequence of heritable variation and differential survival and reproduction. There is no reason to doubt that similar changes were responsible for the designs themselves, and thus for speciation. Of course the heritable variations may have included extensive reshuffling, amalgamation, and redistribution of DNA and need not have been limited to simple point mutations and gene duplication. The inference that biological complexity has been achieved by the mindless processes of mutation and selection need not disturb us. The old theological slogan "no design without a designer," however reasonable it may seem on the basis of everyday human activity, cannot stand when the facts of biology are considered. It has become clear that the capacity for conscious design is merely one of the latest biological properties to be achieved by evolution. The mind that is capable of design, itself far more complex than anything it has yet designed, is a product of mindless design.

In urging that metabolic and molecular aspects of living organisms be considered as functionally interrelated products of evolutionary design, it would be difficult to improve on Darwin's words in one of the greatest and most personal passages in "The Origin of Species," written, of course, when virtually nothing was known of metabolism or the molecular constitution of organisms: "When we no longer look at an organic being as a savage looks at a ship, as something wholly beyond his comprehension; when we regard every production of nature as one which has had a long history; when we contemplate every complex structure and instinct as the summing up of many contrivances, each useful to the possessor, in the same way as any great mechanical invention is the summing up of the labour, the experience, the reason, and even the blunders of numerous workmen; when we thus view each organic being, how far more interesting—I speak from experience— does the study of natural history become!'' When living things are considered in this light, the study of biology generally, and of biochemistry in particular, becomes a matter of attempting to unravel the functional interrelationships of a very intricately engineered mechanism. As suggested in Chapter 1, the approaches to be employed are necessarily quite different in philosophy from those appropriate to the study of such products of inanimate processes as rocks, weather patterns, or stars. Both types of study demand the highest intellectual standards and the best logic of which the investigator is capable and they employ many of the same methods and tactics of research, but their premises and indeed the intellectual frameworks within which they are carried out differ. Our view of the nature of the system we are investigating must affect not only the types of experiments we do, but our evaluation of the results.

The first question to be considered is what inferences regarding regulation may be drawn from the degree of variation in an observed parameter. The logic is obvious when the object under study is a product of human design such as a thermostated water bath. The temperature of a sample of water in a container would be expected to approximate that of the surroundings, and to follow changes in ambient temperature with a time constant dependent on the heat capacity of the sample and the efficiency of heat exchange with the surroundings. If instead the water is observed to be maintained at a temperature significantly different from that of the surroundings and to be essentially independent of changes in ambient temperature, and if it can be seen that the heat capacity of the sample is not extremely large or its thermal insulation from the environment nearly perfect, no one would doubt the conclusion that the temperature of the water is regulated. The more sensitive and effective the regulation, the smaller will be the fluctuations in temperature. If the control system turns the current through the heating elements on when the temperature falls to a specified value, and off when it rises to some other specified value, the temperature of the bath will fluctuate between the two set points, and may overshoot slightly at both. The closer the set points, the better the regulation, as measured by the range of fluctuation of bath temperature. Better regulation can be achieved if the heater current, instead of being switched on and off, is varied as necessary over a narrow range around the time-average value. No one would question the conclusion that the regulation is better the less the temperature varies. That conclusion requires no knowledge of the mechanism of the regulatory system; the only relevant observation is the range of temperature fluctuations. And no one would deny that dynamic regulation (as opposed to passive isolation from the environment, for example) demands that the parameter to be regulated (in this case temperature) must be sensed and must be an input into the regulatory system.

Somehow this relationship between fluctuation and regulation, so self-evident when we consider technological objects, is frequently lost sight of when cellular events are under discussion. Several metabolic papers have said that the concentration of some metabolite is unlikely to be important as a regulatory input because it varies so little. Of course the valid conclusion is exactly opposite: if, in spite of changes in environment, metabolic flux rates, and other factors, the concentration of a metabolite remains nearly constant, that constancy is convincing proof that the concentration of the metabolite is sensed, directly or indirectly, and that fluxes are regulated in such a way as to minimize fluctuations in the sensed concentration.

A striking example of this flaw in regulatory logic is the construction of elaborate computer-simulation models of glycolysis and the citrate cycle that ignore the regulatory effects of the adenine nucleotides. The developer of the models has said that there is no reason why these compounds need be taken into account; since their concentrations are so nearly constant in the cell he feels that they would not significantly affect the operation of the model. That fact, if true, indicates how far the simulation is from being in any meaningful sense a model of glycolysis in a real cell. Since glycolysis is a major pathway leading to regeneration of ATP, the composition of the adenine nucleotide pool would necessarily fluctuate widely if it were not sensed and stabilized by regulation of the flux through the glycolytic pathway. Thus a simulation of the regulation of glycolysis that begins by postulating that the concentrations of ATP, ADP, and AMP are constant has ignored what on quantitative grounds must be the major control input, and, however many man years and computer hours have gone into this development, cannot be even a useful first approximation to reality. The metabolic system is of course enormously more complex than a water bath, but such a simulation has no greater probability of relevance than a detailed study of a water bath that began with the assumption that the temperature of the water, since it is virtually constant, may be ignored.

A different but perhaps related fallacy is that of thinking of a proposed regulatory input as if it were the only factor affecting the control system. This fallacy, too, may be illustrated by a technological analogy. The speed of a vehicle is one of the inputs into the control system of an automobile automatic transmission. However, the transmission may sometimes be in second gear when the car is traveling at 35 miles per hour, and sometimes in third gear at the same speed. It is impossible to predict response of the transmission from knowledge of vehicle speed alone. No informed person would conclude that this impossibility proves that vehicle speed has no effect on the response of the transmission. Other factors, such as the position of the accelerator pedal and the degree of vacuum in the input manifold, are also sensed, and the response of the system depends on all inputs. Even knowledge of the direction of change in vehicle speed does not allow prediction of the response of the transmission. As the car slows in going up a hill, the transmission will shift down from third to second gear. But when the accelerator pedal is pushed all the way down for rapid acceleration, the same downshift will occur as the speed of the car increases.

The fact that when a system or process is regulated by several inputs there can be no one-to-one relationship between the response and any one input (unless all others are fixed) has escaped the attention of some metabolic chemists. For example, the pronounced effect of citrate on the kinetic properties of phosphofructokinase *in vitro* leads to the suggestion that citrate may be a negative modifier of glycolytic flux *in vivo*. However, at least one worker has observed the rate of glycolysis and the concentration of citrate to vary in the same direction during a metabolic transition, and has concluded that this observation proves that citrate does not function as a negative modifier. The relation of this conclusion to the automatic transmission analogy is obvious. All that the observation proves is that the concentration of citrate is not the only factor regulating the rate of glycolysis, and no one would have ever imagined that it could be.

When many factors contribute to an end result, it is possible to draw spurious general conclusions on the basis of specific and trivial experiments. Thus a biologist interested in the reasons why migratory birds in the Northern Hemisphere fly south in autumn might consider day length, altitude of the sun above the horizon at noon, temperature, availability of food, hormonal and other physiological factors, interactions with other birds, and so on. Several of these, and many other factors at different levels, may be involved. Another worker, impatient with all that preliminary speculation, might clip the wings of a few birds, leaving others as controls, and prove conclusively that birds fly south because their wings have not been clipped. Similar logic is not difficult to find in the biochemical literature. For example, mitochondrial electron transport phosphorylation must require at least the four reactants in the equation for the process: oxygen, NADH or $FADH_2$ as the electron source, ADP, and orthophosphate. Depletion of any one must prevent regeneration of ATP. The observation that when mitochondria are carefully prepared the rate of oxygen consumption decreases sharply when ADP is exhausted was important in demonstrating a tight stoichiometric coupling between electron transport and phosphorylation of ADP in these mitochondria, and thus presumably also *in vivo*. However, that observation had no relation to regulation *in vivo* of the rate either of oxygen uptake or of phosphorylation. Exhaustion of any of the four reactants must prevent the overall process; thus in terms of regulation the result was trivial. Nevertheless, several textbooks use it as the basis for the statement that availability of ADP has been shown to be the factor regulating electron transport phosphorylation *in vivo*.

The pronounced effects of energy charge on key enzymes of the catabolic processes support the suggestion that glycolysis and the citrate cycle, and hence the transfer of electrons to NAD^+, are regulated in response to the value of the energy charge. If so, the level of NADH or, more likely, the $NADH/NAD^+$ concentration ratio or the NADH mole fraction, is probably an important limiting factor in electron transport phosphorylation in the intact cell. There may also be direct effects of the energy charge and of many other parameters. In any case, simplistic proposals based on the inability of any process to proceed *in vitro* in the absence of one of its reactants cannot be relevant to the real problems of metabolic control.

Literature references are not given in the preceding paragraphs because the point of the discussion is not polemic. The objective of the enumeration of examples of faulty logic in relating biochemical observations to conclusions is not to disparage the papers that contain them, but to make readers aware of them and to urge that such reasoning be avoided in the future. It should be noted, however, that the illustrations are neither imaginary straw men set up to be knocked over nor gleanings from the ancient literature. All can be found in relatively recent publications.

Some of the points made in the preceding discussion have more positive aspects when viewed, as it were, from the opposite direction. Thus, as has been noted at several points in this book, the fact that the value of the adenylate energy charge is nearly constant in spite of the rapid turnover of ATP and the participation of ATP in virtually all metabolic sequences proves, by the same reasoning as that used in the water bath analogy, that the energy charge or an equivalent parameter is a general input into the regulation of metabolic sequences. The responses of enzymes *in vitro* to variation in energy charge supply insight into how this control may be exerted, and many types of experiments *in vivo*, including probably types yet not developed, will be necessary before we have an understanding of the operational details. But neither type of experiment is necessary to establish the reality of the regulation—that is established unequivocally by the observation that fluctuations are small.

A number of similarly general conclusions follow from well-known features of metabolism. From the facts that glycolysis serves at least two functions essential to growth—the provision of electrons to be used in regeneration of ATP and the supply of starting materials for biosynthesis—and that growth can occur under a variety of conditions, it follows that glycolysis must be effectively regulated by at least two inputs, one reflecting the need for ATP and the other the need for starting materials. Much work will be needed to establish how many feedback loops actually link the concentration of biosynthetic intermediates to the rate of glycolysis and how they relate to each other and to the adenylate energy charge. Such research is not needed, however, to establish the reality of interaction between intermediate concentrations and energy charge in regulation of glycolysis; that is established by the general pattern of metabolic organization.

Biochemists as a group have tended historically to be suspicious of general conclusions based on general features of organisms or of metabolism, and to favor what is often seen as the more definite testing of specific hypotheses by specific experiments. But when an organism is considered as a designed mechanism, and amenable to the kinds of reasoning that would be used in investigating a technological device, the validity of the general approach is evident. When general relationships can be established on the basis of known features, a great deal of unfocused experimentation can be avoided and investigators can concentrate on problems at the next level.

When we speak of an organism as an energy-transducing system, we usually are thinking of such obvious relationships as those between catabolic and biosynthetic sequences, where the conversion of ADP to ATP in one set of reactions is coupled with the conversion of ATP to ADP in the other in such a way as to produce favorable equilibrium constants for biosynthetic sequences. But energy flow, or what can be considered energy expenditure, is involved in every aspect of an organism's activities. Free energy can in a general way, and within limits, be equated with order, as entropy is in a general sense related to disorder. Thus order (a state of high free energy) can be produced in one system or subsystem only at the expense of a coupled decrease in order (free energy) in another. In a dynamic system such as a living cell, all component subsystems have a tendency to move towards states of lower free energy, and expenditure of energy is needed not only to produce order but also to maintain it. As one obvious example, proteins are constantly undergoing degradation and must be replaced. Protein turnover may play a useful biological role in some cases, but on the basis of present knowledge it seems likely that most protein replacement can be compared to the constant repairs that are necessary to keep a house in good condition. That is, it is a process of repair or replacement of cell components that, in terms of biological advantage, should last indefinitely but simply are not that durable. In principle, if enzymes and other proteins were highly stable, the cell, once having synthesized them, would not need to expend energy further on their maintenance or replacement. In contrast to such structural and rather stable types of order, much of the order of a cell is dynamic, relating to concentrations and fluxes. Even in principle, a constant expenditure of energy is required for maintenance of this kind of order.

Perhaps the most general feature of dynamic order in an organism is the arrangement of its metabolic processes into paired unidirectional sequences or pseudocycles, as discussed in Chapter 3. We might reasonably suggest that this relationship, which is schematically illustrated in Figure 8-1, is the basic functional design element of metabolism. It is universal, in the sense that virtually every metabolic sequence is a member of such a pair, and it is an essential feature of biological design, since it underlies and is prerequisite to the functional control of the chemical activities of the cell. The essential features are that x is greater than y, and that kinetic controls hold the ATP/ADP concentration ratio far from the equilibrium ratio for hydrolysis. Such organization allows for separation in time of the two reaction sequences, and for kinetic selection between them on the basis of momentary need. The cost in free energy of this separation in time is considerable, and is proportional to the difference between x and y. This was discussed earlier, with examples. Thus when fat is respired the yield of ATP is about 80% of the number of ATP equivalents that are required for synthesis of the fat. The other 20% represents free energy expenditure in maintaining this particular aspect of dynamic order. Similar expenditures are involved as inevitable design features of every pseudocycle. In addition, it cannot be expected that kinetic control will absolutely prevent nonproductive cycling; to the extent that cycling exists, it is another drain on the cell's free energy that is necessary for maintenance of dynamic order.

ATP is used in maintenance of the order of the cell at many levels, and probably at many not yet recognized. A number of regulatory systems that involve covalent modification of enzymes have been found, and it is reasonable to expect that there may be many other such cases. In order for the modification to serve a useful regulatory role, the group that is attached must

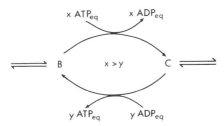

Figure 8-1.   The basic design element of metabolism: a pair of oppositely directed unidirectional reaction sequences. The coefficients x and y are number of ATP equivalents in the sense defined in Chapter 3, and are not necessarily the actual numbers of ATP molecules as such that are used or regenerated.

of course be removed when it is to the cell's advantage to revert to its previous state. For example, the regulatory effects on glycogen breakdown that are provided by phosphorylation of phosphorylase kinase and of phosphorylase *b* must be capable of reversal by removal of the phosphoryl groups. Each such enzyme that is phosphorylated or adenylylated under certain conditions, with the added group being removed under other conditions, obviously participates in a sort of miniature pseudocycle, with ATP being expended in each cycle. Thus in these cases again, ATP is used in regulatory systems that aid in the maintenance of dynamic chemical order in the cell. Most such covalent enzyme modifications that have been discovered involve ATP directly, but in the cascade system of glutamine synthase regulation, studied by Stadtman and colleagues (*50, 51*) the enzyme responsible for the addition and removal of the adenylyl group is in turn modulated by the addition and removal of a uridylyl group, so that here one molecule of ATP is used directly and one indirectly.

Maintenance of a cell or multicellular organism as an island of organization in a relatively disorganized environment places severe demands on the bounding membranes through which materials pass into and out of the cell. Not only must energy be expended in active transport of materials across the membrane against concentration gradients to establish the ordered composition of the cell, but additional energy is needed to maintain this order against inevitable leakage. It has been estimated that about 30% of the total energy expenditure of a bacterial cell may be related to membrane function. The cycles of membrane polarization and depolarization in brain may be responsible for the very high rate of energy metabolism in this tissue.

When biosynthesis and growth are considered as processes of making more ordered molecules or structures out of less ordered ones, it seems valid to say that most expenditures of ATP are related in one way or another to the production or maintenance of chemical order. All of the discussion in the preceding few paragraphs could be paraphrased in terms of information, and expenditure of ATP could then be related to the conservation and use of biological information. It may be expected that more sophisticated examples of this relationship between ATP and order or information will be found at each level of study. One possible example was proposed by Hopfield (*59*): the very small error rate of DNA replication may be achieved by kinetic means through the use of ATP. Briefly, he suggested that the association rates of C, the correct base, and of D, an incorrect competitor for the recognition site, are about equal, and that the greater affinity of the site for C arises from the greater dissociation rate of the complex containing D. If this is true, and if both the C complex and the D complex can be converted to a high energy form from which D again has a much greater tendency to dissociate than does C, the effective overall degree of discrimination between

C and D would be greatly increased. If such kinetic editing actually occurs, ATP is presumably used in the generation of the high-energy form. Hopfield suggested that this same general mechanism might be involved also in such other information-transfer reactions as the synthesis of RNA or of protein.

Chemical energy is always a matter of concentration ratios. It is thus only because the ratios ATP/ADP and ATP/AMP are held in the living cell far from their hydrolytic equilibrium values that ATP can play the roles in energy transduction, maintenance of structure, and conservation and use of biological information that have been ascribed to it. Ratios can be stabilized at values far from equilibrium only by kinetic control, and it is thus necessary that metabolic processes, both those that use ATP and those in which it is regenerated, be regulated in response to fluctuations of ratios of the adenine nucleotides from their normal values. This is a logical necessity; once the central role of ATP in energy transduction was recognized, the need for stability of the ATP/ADP and ATP/AMP ratios, and hence the need for regulation of at least all important metabolic sequences by these ratios, could have been deduced. The logical necessity for stabilization of the adenylate concentration ratios by regulation of metabolic sequences is in no way weakened by the fact that the existence of such regulation was not in fact deduced, but rather discovered by experiment. Key enzymes have been shown to respond *in vitro* to ratios of adenylate concentrations rather than to absolute concentrations, the ratios have been found to be strongly stabilized *in vivo*, and growth has been shown to be highly sensitive to small changes in the values of the ratios but relatively insensitive to changes in absolute concentrations of the adenine nucleotides. It would be extremely difficult, if not impossible, to rationalize the metabolic roles of ATP if any one of these observations had come out otherwise. Thus the organization of metabolism and metabolic regulation around the adenine nucleotides, including the control of all metabolic sequences by the ratios (or mole fractions) of these coupling agents, is not an unsubstantiated hypothesis or merely one way to rationalize certain experimental results; rather these concepts are part of a package of correlated relationships, every one of which is essential if ATP is to function in metabolism in the ways that it is known to do.

In metabolism as in other contexts in which concentration ratios are important, it is often more convenient to convert ratios to mole fractions. There is a one-to-one relationship between concentration ratios and mole fractions, so that any effect of ratios may be expressed in terms of mole fractions or vice versa. However, the relationship is not linear, so the form of the dependence of a reaction velocity or other parameter on a mole fraction will be different from the form of its dependence on the corresponding concentration ratio. It is because mole fractions are stoichiometric, and thus linearly related to events of chemical interest, that relationships are frequently seen much more clearly through the use of mole fractions than they could be if ratios were used. All of the references to concentration ratios in the preceding paragraphs could be restated in terms of mole fractions. At the level of this discussion, such a restatement would not make any difference, but when calculations are to be done or experiments planned or their results interpreted, the stoichiometric character of mole fractions makes them much to be preferred. Because there are three adenine nucleotides, the simple mole fraction of ATP is not an appropriate parameter. The interconvertibility of AMP, ADP, and ATP by means of the adenylate kinase reaction, however, simplifies the situation. As discussed in Chapter 4, the energy charge is merely the metabolically effective mole fraction of ATP. Thus all of the statements concerning the logical necessity of stabilization of adenine nucleotide concentration ratios and of regulation of all major sequences by these ratios may be restated in terms of the adenylate energy charge.

It has been recognized since Lipmann's 1941 review (74) that, because the adenylate system stoichiometrically couples metabolic sequences, metabolic energy is quantized. The discussion of the costs of compounds and of metabolic conversions in terms of ATP equivalents in Chapter 3 is a formal expression of this quantization, and the whole organization of metabolism into oppositely directed pairs of sequences, which is a necessary condition for kinetic control of metabolic conversions, depends on it. It might seem that there is some inconsistency between the statements (a) that energy metabolism is quantized, with the actual number of ATP molecules used or regenerated in each sequence being important, as discussed in Chapter 3, and (b) that nucleotide ratios and mole fractions, rather than absolute concentrations, are important in stabilization and control, as discussed in Chapter 4. But there is no real difficulty here. Two related but different aspects of metabolism are being considered. The amount of an electrochemical conversion is strictly stoichiometric with the amount of current that flows through the reaction cell, but the ability of a battery to supply current depends on the ratio of its oxidized to its reduced components. Similarly in metabolism, strictly stoichiometric coupling between the adenine nucleotide pool and all metabolic sequences coexists with the kinetic effects of the adenylate energy charge. Both, as discussed above and elsewhere in this book, are essential; neither would serve any biological function without the other.

The fact that metabolism is organized around the adenine nucleotides, both in terms of stoichiometric coupling and of kinetic control, does not, of course, mean that the energy charge alone can control all aspects of the chemical activity of a living cell. As discussed in Chapter 6, for any given reaction or reaction sequence the energy charge will be only one of several regulatory inputs, and in the context of that single reaction or sequence it is no more important than the others. The unique importance of the adenylate energy charge is that it affects all sequences and thus is more responsible than any other single parameter for biochemical homeostasis. Because of this central role of the adenine nucleotides, we may reasonably consider the effects of many other metabolite modifiers to be modulations of the energy charge response of the target enzyme. A similar idea is expressed in the statement that a stable energy charge maintains regulatory enzymes in a proper state to respond to variation in concentrations of modifier metabolites. Thus energy charge regulation may be said to provide the stable basis for action of other regulatory compounds.

In a broader sense, the combined action of the adenine nucleotides and other regulators of primary energy metabolism may be considered to provide the stable chemical background against which the programmed changes in the life of the cell or organism can occur. Homeostasis is essential to life, but it is not the whole story. Even a bacterial cell goes through a cell division cycle, and in higher organisms there are very complex patterns of development and differentiation, which necessarily involve initiation, acceleration, slowing, or termination of many chemical processes. So a cell or organism does not by any means remain in a strictly homeostatic state with regard to all of its components and all of its chemical activities, merely growing at a uniform rate and with all chemical processes proceeding at constant velocity. But it seems likely that the sort of homeostasis that we have discussed in this book must be a necessary condition for orderly development. If the central pathways of intermediary metabolism (glycolysis, respiration, and the biosynthesis of building blocks such as amino acids and nucleotides) are regulated in such a way as to hold the adenylate energy charge and the concentrations of the building blocks essentially constant and independent of the momentary demands for energy or for building blocks, cells will be able to respond consistently to the signals, mostly unknown to us, that cause the events of differentiation to occur to just the right degree and in precisely the correct sequence. The responses must be finely graded, and it seems evident that a cell will be able to respond correctly to a developmental trigger only if, at the time of exposure to the stimulus, the cell is in a standard metabolic state.

The basis for all kinetic effects of enzymes, from catalysis itself to the modulation of catalytic properties in response to modifiers, must be conformational change. The conformational changes of substrates that convert them to the transition state must be accompanied by, and in an important sense caused by, conformational changes in the enzyme. The changes in affinity for a substrate that are caused by binding of substrate or modifier molecules at other sites must also result from conformational change, which in this case must be transmitted from one site to another and, since the sites are usually on different subunits, from one subunit to another.

Electronic control circuits, which supply the closest analogy to metabolic control systems, function by modulating an external source of electrical power. In contrast, metabolic control systems must be selfpowered. The only apparent source of energy for the conformational changes on which catalysis and metabolic regulation depend is the free energy of binding of ligands to enzymes. Not only must the association between an enzyme and its substrate and modifiers be extremely specific, it must be strong enough to cause changes in conformation of the enzyme—changes that, taken alone, would entail an increase in free energy and so would not occur. These conformational changes must be very specific and must lead to consequences, such as catalysis or precise modulation of catalysis, that are advantageous to the organism. The fact that linear chains of amino acids can form themselves into globular proteins with all of these capabilities is one of the most incredible of the many incredible aspects of life.

A book such as this must leave both the author and the reader with the feeling that we are only beginning to recognize some of the basic generalizations of biochemistry. It is as true as it has always been that each advance producing an answer at one level raises several questions at a more fundamental level. To take an example from a field very close to that discussed in this book, since the discovery of hormones the question of how the target cell recognizes the appropriate hormone has been of evident importance. With the discovery of cyclic AMP and its role as a second messenger, that problem may be said to have been solved for many hormones. The target cell has in its membrane an adenylate cyclase that is specifically activated by the appropriate hormone, and cyclic AMP, when produced on the inner side of the membrane, specifically activates the right enzymes to lead to the functionally proper response to the hormone. But of course that answer, as is typical of answers to scientific questions, only allows the problem to be phrased at another level—that of differentiation and differential gene expression. How does it happen that the target cells and no others produce an adenylate cyclase specific for a given hormone, and why does cyclic AMP activate one process in cells of a given type and lead to totally different responses in cells of other types?

If not universally, it is at least usually true that answering a scientific question merely means rephrasing it at a more fundamental level. It is not yet clear whether this process has an end, but if it does we are certainly not yet within sight of it, nor can we imagine it. Whether science is ultimately an Endless Frontier or not, the horizon is still receding from us with no apparent end. Each discovery, like each hill topped in a geographical exploration, discloses more unknown territory and allows us to ask questions that could not have occurred to us before. There have always been scientists who have seemed capable of considering only questions that were recognized in their youth, and who are blind to the excitement of new problems. The most frequently quoted example is the physicist who commented, shortly before Becquerel's discovery of radioactivity, that physics had become a mature science with nothing remaining but determination of the fundamental constants to higher precision. In our own field, a professor of physiology at Cambridge advised Hopkins in 1907 to give up biochemistry because the subject was already played out (*33*). The most conspicuous recent statement of this type took the form of a highly erudite book (*112*) rather than a passing comment, but it is based on the same myopic view of the nature of science and on apparent inability to see the fundamental unanswered questions that surround every current generalization.

It is in the nature of scientific research that, as long as it receives reasonable support and is pursued by able and dedicated people, some of the problems being considered at any time will be more fundamental or more sophisticated, or both, than those studied at earlier times. Thus scientists are always, and rightly, impressed by the importance of recent advances. We may reasonably feel that progress in biology in the past 50 years is one of the greatest intellectual achievements of human history. It is difficult for us to realize that 50 years ago scientists also felt that the recent past had been marked by advances of unprecedented importance. The physiologist Starling is quoted as having said in 1923 "When I compare our present knowledge of the workings of the body . . . with the ignorance and the despairing impotence of my student days, I feel that I have had the good fortune to see the sun rise on a darkened world." We should not doubt that there were good reasons for that statement. Yet it is difficult for us today to see the state of biochemistry and physiology in 1923 as anything but appallingly primitive and unsatisfying, with very little fundamental information available and virtually no unifying generalizations. It seems certain that in 25 or 50 years, if research is not seriously impeded by political constraints or lack of support, scientists will look back on the 1970s much as we do on the 1920s, and wonder how an intelligent scientist could have written a book proclaiming the imminent end of meaningful scientific research because soon no fundamental problems would remain.

Our present store of information in biology and our inferences and generalizations, including those discussed in this book, are so evidently incomplete, tentative, and provisional as to make it clear that immensely more remains to be discovered about the evolved functional interactions that constitute life than has yet been learned. Many of the important advances of the next decades will be relatively unsurprising developments and extensions of present knowledge, but we may expect that, as in the past, there will also be new directions and new insights quite different from anything that we can now imagine. The one prediction that seems safe is that an evolutionary approach stressing the functionality both of individual features and of the interrelationships between them will continue to be the best guide to the understanding of life at increasingly more fundamental levels.

APPENDIX A

Some Elementary Aspects of Thermodynamics

One of the striking characteristics of living systems is chemical mobility. The high rates of reactions in living cells necessarily involve high rates of energy conversions—from radiant to chemical energy, from chemical energy to mechanical energy and to heat; and particularly interconversions of chemical energy in the synthesis of complex compounds at the expense of the degradation of others. Organisms have been aptly termed energy conversion systems. It must thus be obvious that metabolism can be intelligently discussed only within the framework of thermodynamics, the science of energy conversions. This appendix is included in the hope that it will be helpful to readers with little or no background in physical chemistry or to those whose formal course work in thermodynamics dealt with the gas phase to the exclusion of liquids and liquid solutions. It would be unrealistic to attempt a thorough coverage of thermodynamics in a few pages, and a digest of postulates and equations would probably be of little value. Accordingly the approach will be descriptive and illustrative with no pretensions of rigor. Such concepts as heat and temperature, for example, will not be defined; although they are not as simple as they seem, their intuitive meanings will suffice for our purposes. The topics suggested are those that seem most relevant to discussions in this book and it is hoped that careful reading of this appendix will supply a minimal understanding of free energy relations and of equilibrium and steady-state conditions. It should be obvious, however, that anyone planning to work in metabolism or enzyme chemistry will need a much more extensive and rigorous preparation in thermodynamics than can be obtained from a discussion such as this.

Thermodynamics deals with processes involving the transformation of energy in a system or the exchange of energy between a system and its surroundings. The *system* is merely the sample of matter in which the observer is interested, and it is often in textbook examples (much less often in real cases) isolated from the surroundings by some sort of wall, which may or may not conduct heat. In the absence of actual boundaries, there must of course be some definite way of specifying just what is included in the system. The *surroundings* comprise all other matter with which the system can interact to a significant degree. Usually the surroundings, defined in this way, include only matter in the immediate vicinity of the system, but this is not always true. For a photosynthesizing plant the surroundings must include the sun.

THE FIRST LAW OF THERMODYNAMICS

The first law of thermodynamics, or the principle of the conservation of energy, is merely the statement that if a system exchanges no energy with the surroundings its energy content will remain constant. If there is exchange, the change in energy content of the system will be equal to the energy gained from the surroundings minus that lost to the surroundings. This law or principle seems self evident, and it gives no trouble. Using the customary symbols, the law may be expressed in the form of equation A-1, where q is

$$\Delta E = q - w \qquad (A-1)$$

the net heat flow *into* the system (heat gained from the surroundings minus heat lost to the surroundings) and w is the net work done *by* the system (work done by the system on the surroundings minus work done by the surroundings on the system). It is obvious that both q and w may be either positive or negative, and so, of course, may ΔE, the change in energy of the system.

The letters q and w are used for either large or small amounts of heat and work while the symbols Δ (for large changes) and d (for infinitesimal changes) are used in the usual way for other thermodynamic functions. Thus, $\Delta E = q - w$ for large changes and $dE = q - w$ for infinitesimal changes in E. This treatment of q and w is usual in thermodynamics because the heat absorbed and work done are not perfect differentials—that is, they depend not only on the initial and final states of the system but also on the pathway by which the change occurs. The notation dq would thus be misleading, as it implies a differential that is capable of integration—in other words, it implies that the change in q for any process should be determined by the initial and final states of the system. This, however, is not true for q (or for w) in most physical and chemical processes; the change in E, and thus the difference between q and w, is fixed by the initial and final states, but the actual values of q and w depend on the path. Of course if we know the initial and final states of a system and the value of either q or w, we can calculate the other. The minus sign in equation A-1 is a consequence of the rather unfortunate convention that w is work done *by* the system on the surroundings. If the opposite and more consistent definition had been adopted—if w were work done *on* the system, as q is heat absorbed by the system, the equation would be $\Delta E = q + w$ and it might be more obvious that ΔE is the net energy put into the system either as heat or as work and that, although the total energy change is determined by the initial and final states (is independent of the path) the partitioning between work and heat is variable.

Changes in E and in the other thermodynamic functions to be introduced in the next section depend only on the overall process and not on how it is carried out. Such terms as dE are thus straightforward differentials, since they may be integrated to give definite values that are independent of the way in which a process occurs.

These statements may seem rather abstract, but they may be illustrated by very simple processes, for example, by expansion of a gas to twice its volume with no change in temperature. Choosing two from the infinite number of possible paths for the expansion, we will consider (a) expansion into an evacuated chamber; that is, expansion against zero external pressure; and (b) very slow expansion against a piston with an opposing force on the piston that is essentially equal to the force of the gas on the piston at all times during the expansion. The values of ΔE for the two cases must be equal, since the initial and final states are the same. For an "ideal gas"—one with no interaction between molecules—ΔE would be zero for this process; for a real gas ΔE will be positive, but independent of the way in which the change was carried out. (In the real gas, molecular motion is somewhat constrained by interaction between molecules; thus when the gas expands, weakening the interactions, the same temperature will correspond to greater molecular motion, and energy must be put into the system to maintain the temperature. In many real cases heat does not flow into the expanding gas fast enough to hold the temperature constant; thus the temperature of an expanding gas tends to fall to a degree proportional to the strengths of the interactions between molecules.) However, the values of q and w would be very different in the two cases. In (a) no work is done—the system has nothing to work against—so $w = 0$ and $q = \Delta E$ [hence $q = 0$ for a perfect gas and $q > 0$ (there is absorption of heat) for a real gas]. In (b) the system performs work on the surroundings (the piston); in fact the hypothetical pathway described allows the maximal performance of work that is possible for this process, as is shown in the next paragraph. So w is positive and rather large, and $q = \Delta E + w$ (in this case $q = w$ for an ideal gas and q is slightly greater than w for a real gas). Between these two pathways are infinitely many possibilities, allowing all values of w and q between the extremes illustrated. The value of ΔE would, however, be identical in each case.

Work is a product of a force times the distance over which it is exerted. In the example just considered, the comparison may be clarified if simple expansion into a vacuum is replaced by expansion against an imaginary weightless, frictionless piston, with a vacuum on the other side. Now in comparing the two types of expansion (against an unloaded or against a loaded piston) we see that the travel of the piston (the distance term in the work equation) is the same in both cases. In the first case, however, no force is required to move the piston; zero force times a finite distance is zero work. Introduction of the hypothetical piston does not change the fact that expansion into a vacuum entails no work. In the second case, the opposing force exerted by the piston is at all times equal to the force that the system can exert on the piston. The product of force times distance thus has its highest possible value. A process occurring under such conditions, with opposing forces balanced, is said to be carried out *reversibly*, because an infinitesimal change in conditions would cause a reversal in the direction of the process. The reversible pathway always results in the maximal value of heat absorption, q, and, if work is involved, also in the maximal amount of work.

It will be obvious, however, that there are no reversible processes in nature. If the external pressure is exactly equal to that of the system, the piston will not move; in a chemical reaction system exactly at equilibrium there is no net reaction; when solid and liquid phases of a substance are exactly at the melting point there is no net melting; and so on. In other words, any reversible process requires infinite time for completion; therefore it does not occur. In many real processes it is possible to approach reversibility very closely, but this condition is not common in biological systems. Nevertheless the concept of reversibility is useful in setting upper limits for q and w: we know that for any *real*—that is, irreversible—process both w and q must be less than the values calculated for the same process carried out reversibly.

THE SECOND LAW OF THERMODYNAMICS

The second law has been anticipated to some extent in the last few paragraphs. This law may be expressed in many ways. We shall take it as the concept that any system not at a temperature of absolute zero has an irreducible minimum amount of energy that is an inevitable property of that system at that temperature. That is, a system requires a certain amount of internal energy just to be at any specified temperature. We may attribute this energy to thermal motions of the molecules, including the various types of oscillations of their component atoms. This particular energy is termed the *isothermally unavailable* energy, since it is obvious that none of it can be given up isothermally (unless there is a chemical or physical change in the system) because any decrease in this kind of energy must necessarily mean a decrease in temperature. It is also obvious that the isothermally unavailable energy of any system will increase with an increase in temperature, since the energy of the molecular and atomic motions must increase with an increase in temperature. Isothermally unavailable energy is represented in thermodynamics by the term ST, where S is the *entropy* of the system and T is the absolute temperature. We thus define entropy as isothermally unavailable energy divided by the absolute temperature.

One other relationship should be intuitively apparent: in general, the larger and more complex the molecule, the more types of vibrations are possible, and hence the more energy is stored in them at any given temperature. That is, compounds of complex structure will usually have higher contents of isothermally unavailable energy (per mole) than most simpler compounds. However, the bonding in even a large and "floppy" molecule will decrease the susceptibility of the component parts to thermal agitation; hence the entropy of a compound with such molecules, although high per mole, will usually be lower than the sum of the entropies of the smaller compounds into which it may dissociate. In a qualitative way it will be apparent that the amount of energy stored in the thermal motions of a system will be diminished by any restrictions placed on free motion. Thus entropy will increase in any process in which such restrictions are decreased, for example, in the melting of a solid or the vaporization of a liquid. It follows that entropy will also increase in any process, including a chemical reaction, that results in less restriction due to chemical bonding or similar interactions. Such decrease in restriction may result either from a weakening of bonds or from a decrease in the number of bonds. For example, the dissociation of one compound into two or more will usually reduce the number of bonds in the system and thus, as noted above, increase its entropy. By extension of these relations, it can be seen that the system of highest entropy would be one with no restrictions on thermal motion, that is, one in which each atom moved independently and could assume any position in the system. In other words, entropy would be maximal in a completely random or disordered system. At the other extreme, entropy is low in a highly ordered system such as a crystal. Of course, the more energy is stored in thermal motion, the more energy will be needed to raise the temperature of the system by one degree. It thus follows that entropy, defined on the basis of the ratio of heat absorbed to temperature increase, is synonymous with randomness or disorder provided that these terms are appropriately defined.

The relation between entropy and randomness may be summarized by the equation defining entropy increment in terms of heat capacity and temperature. When a system is warmed by absorption of heat from its surroundings, the change in entropy is given by equation A-2, where C is the heat capacity

$$dS = q_{max}/T = C \, dT/T \qquad \text{(A-2)}$$

of the system (the amount of heat required to raise the temperature of the system by one degree). Increasing randomness on a molecular or atomic scale will, by increasing the amount of energy in random thermal agitation, increase C and thus increase the entropy. It can be seen qualitatively that this reasoning extends to any process in which there is a decrease in restrictions on thermal motion. Thus if two gases occupying equal volumes separated by a membrane are mixed by rupture of the membrane, the entropy of the system will increase because of the increased space available to each molecule. In the case of ideal gases (with no interaction between molecules) the increase of entropy resulting from mixing would be exactly equal to the sum of the entropies of expansion of the gases separately into evacuated chambers of the same volume as the initial chamber (thus doubling the volume). For real gases, mixing will lead to a decrease in interaction between like molecules (because of dilution) and also to the appearance of interactions between unlike molecules, so that the entropy of mixing will not depend solely on expansion.

Like most simplified illustrations of mathematical concepts, the foregoing discussion is by no means rigorous. For example, equation A-2 shows that if any two systems are compared, the one with the higher heat capacity must have the greater rate of change of entropy with temperature, dS/dT. We implicitly assumed that this system with the higher value of C and of dS/dT will also have the higher entropy, S. This relation would necessarily be true if C were constant over the temperature range from absolute zero to the temperature at which we observe the system; in that case integration of equation A-2 would give $S = C \ln T$.

In fact, heat capacities vary with temperature, and a higher value of S does not necessarily accompany a higher value of dS/dT. But for most processes of interest in chemistry or biology the initial and final states are quite similar, and for such processes S and dS/dT will usually vary in the same direction; hence our discussion, although not rigorous, will usually give the right qualitative results, that is, will allow a correct prediction as to whether the entropy of the system will increase or decrease in a given process. The treatment given here may help the reader with little background in thermodynamics to form a reasonable mental picture of entropy in relation to randomness and may allow him to predict the direction of the entropy changes accompanying many types of chemical reactions or physical processes.

It might be mentioned in passing that in chemical thermodynamics we speak of order or disorder in rather specialized terms. Many extrapolations of the concept of entropy as equivalent to disorder in other contexts seem ambiguous or misleading. In everyday systems, order is a highly subjective concept. For example, a library might contain a million books arranged alphabetically on the basis of the 3rd word (and when necessary succeeding words) in the 17th line of the 41st page. To anyone knowing the system, this library would represent total order; any book that had been removed could be replaced in its precise position. To anyone not having the code, the library would represent total disorder, and the sequence of books along the shelves would make no sense in terms of content, author, date of publication, or any other likely basis of classification. The entropy of the system would not, however, change in any meaningful sense because of the observer's knowledge or lack of knowledge of the system.

Energy Functions

The energy designated by the symbol E is the energy that is characteristic of the system as such. Although this is the total energy of the system, it is sometimes termed *internal energy* to emphasize its independence of the external environment. In addition to their internal energies, all real systems possess various other types of potential energy by virtue of interaction with their surroundings. For example, after a boulder rolls down a mountainside its internal energy may be unchanged, but its total potential energy will have decreased because of its changed position relative to the gravitational field of the earth. Electrostatic, magnetic, and other forces may also contribute to interaction energies. The energy of air flow moved travelers and cargo at sea for thousands of years. But the type of interaction energy most likely to be relevant to chemical or physical changes in systems on or near the earth's surface is the energy associated with the mere occupancy of space and its defense, as it were, against the encroachment of the surroundings. It will be clear that this space energy must be proportional to the volume of the space occupied and to the external pressure against which it is defended. That is, this energy term is merely PV, where V is the volume *of the system* and P is the *external* pressure.

The two distinctions that we have discussed—isothermally available versus isothermally unavailable, and energy of the system itself ("internal" energy) versus energy of interactions with the surroundings—are the basis for distinguishing the thermodynamic categories of energy. The symbols used are defined in equations A-3 to A-6. "Available" in this listing means "isothermally available." Because gravitational, magnetic, and similar interactions have no significant effect on most chemical or biological processes, the term X will be omitted in the remainder of this chapter.

$$H \;=\; E \;+\; PV \;+\; X \tag{A-3}$$

total   internal   interaction   all other
energy   energy   energy   interaction
(space occupancy)   energy

$$H \;=\; G \;+\; ST \tag{A-4}$$

total   available   unavailable
energy   energy   energy
(internal)

$$E \;=\; A \;+\; ST \tag{A-5}$$

internal   internal   unavailable
energy   available   energy
energy   (internal)

$$G \;=\; A \;+\; PV \;+\; X \tag{A-6}$$

available   internal   interaction   all other
energy   available   energy   interaction
energy   (space occupancy)   energy

The names commonly used for these functions are: H, enthalpy or heat content; E, energy or internal energy; G, free energy or Gibbs free energy; and A, work function or Helmholtz free energy. Thermodynamics deals with the changes in these functions as a consequence of physical and chemical processes rather than with their absolute values. Hence, H, E, G, and A are rarely used; the terms of interest are ΔH, ΔE, ΔG, ΔA, and ΔS, where Δ has its usual meaning of "the change in . . . ." In fact, H, E, G, and A have no quantitative meaning, since only *changes* in these properties can be measured. The situation is analogous to the height of a mountain, which can be expressed only in relative terms (with reference to a neighboring mountain, to a nearby plain, to sea level, etc.). Any convention as to reference or standard states could be used in defining a scale for ΔH, ΔE, ΔG, and ΔA, since the reference value obviously will cancel out in the application of these functions to any process. The convention that has been adopted because of its convenience is that H, E, G, and A will be taken as zero for any pure element in its stable form at any temperature. The relative value of each function can then be assigned to any compound on the basis of the real or imaginary process of converting the free elements to the compound. The relative values so obtained are termed values "of formation" and are usually indicated by the abbreviation "form" as a subscript. Thus for CO_2, ΔH_{form}, the heat of formation, is the heat absorbed when one gram-atom of graphite and one mole of gaseous oxygen combine to form one mole of carbon dioxide gas. At 18°C, this property has the value of -94.05 kcal, the negative sign indicating that heat is evolved, rather than absorbed, in the process. The other values, ΔE_{form}, ΔG^0_{form}, and ΔA^0_{form}, similarly refer to the formation of the compound from its elements at the same temperature. These functions are usually expressed in kcal/mole. Of the four properties, only ΔH_{form} and ΔG^0_{form} are often used in biochemistry.

The heat of formation, ΔH_{form}, of a compound depends on the temperature and the physical state of the compound (solid, liquid, gas, solute in aqueous solution, etc.), but to a first approximation it is independent of concentration. For example, ΔH_{form} of water vapor at 30°C is greater than ΔH_{form} of liquid water at the same temperature by the heat absorbed in the evaporation of 1 mole of water at 30°C; but ΔH_{form} of the vapor will be nearly independent of the partial pressure of the water vapor (thus, for example, ΔH_{form} is independent of the extent to which the vapor is diluted by air). Correspondingly ΔH_{form} for a compound dissolved in water may be nearly independent of concentration. Free energy, on the other hand, varies with concentration. In dealing with free energy terms (ΔG or ΔA) it is thus necessary to define reference concentrations. Any appropriate reference state could be chosen for a particular problem, but as an aid in the tabulation of data it is helpful to have a generally accepted set of standard states. For solids, pure liquids, or solvents, the pure material is usually taken as the standard state; for gases, the pure gas at 1 atm, corrected for molecular interations; and for solutes, a 1 M solution (again corrected for interactions). For any material in the standard state, the *activity* (effective concentration) is given the value of 1. These conventions should be familiar from elementary chemistry courses, where equilibria are expressed in terms of molarity with the solvent being assigned the "concentration" of 1 (or being "omitted because its concentration does not change appreciably").

Free Energy and Work

From equations A-3 through A-6, we may obtain physical meanings for ΔG and ΔA. We may subdivide w into two types of work: work of expansion against an external pressure ($P\,dV$) and all other types of work (mechanical, electrical, etc.), which we will indicate by w'. Then equation A-1 becomes

$$dE = q - P\,dV - w' \qquad (\text{A-7})$$

Omitting the term X from equation A-3, we obtain $H = E + PV$, and by differentiation

$$dH = dE + P\,dV + V\,dP$$

Substituting the value of dE from equation A-7, we obtain

$$dH = q - P\,dV - w' + P\,dV + V\,dP$$

or

$$dH = q - w' + V\,dP \qquad\qquad (A-8)$$

Differentiating equation A-4, we obtain

$$dG = dH - S\,dT - T\,dS$$

Substituting the value of dH from equation A-8, we obtain

$$dG = q - w' + V\,dP - S\,dT - T\,dS \qquad\qquad (A-9)$$

For a reversible process, $q = T\,dS$, so these terms in equation A-9 cancel out. We have seen that in a reversible process the work obtained is the greatest amount of work that could be obtained, and we will designate this reversible work w'_{max}. Then

$$dG = -w'_{max} + V\,dP - S\,dT \qquad\qquad (A-10)$$

For any process occurring at constant temperature and pressure the last two terms equal zero, and thus

$$dG = -w'_{max} \qquad\qquad (A-11)$$

For a finite process,

$$\Delta G = -w'_{max} \qquad\qquad (A-12)$$

For any process at constant temperature and pressure, then, $-\Delta G$ indicates the theoretical maximum amount of work that could be done as a consequence of the process. The work actually available from any real (irreversible) process must be less than $-\Delta G$, but may approach that value very closely when the process is carried out nearly reversibly.

Since a system at equilibrium can do no work, $dG = 0$ for any process at equilibrium at constant temperature and pressure. (No net process occurs in a system exactly at equilibrium, but no work would be done even if the process did occur.) Any process going toward equilibrium could in principle do work, and hence $\Delta G < 0$ for such processes, which are termed *exergonic*, or energy releasing. For a process imagined to move away from equilibrium, $\Delta G > 0$. Such processes would be *endergonic*. Actually all processes move toward equilibrium, so for all real processes at constant temperature and pressure, $\Delta G < 0$. This is probably the most important relationship of thermodynamics as applied to biochemistry. Calculation or estimation of the free energy change for any process allows us to predict the direction in which the process must go, if it goes at all. To repeat, *the value of ΔG is negative for all real processes at constant temperature and pressure.* By nearly identical reasoning it can be shown that for a process at constant volume and temperature, the maximum obtainable work is given by $-\Delta A$, so that under these conditions $\Delta A = 0$ at equilibrium and $\Delta A < 0$ for any real process. For many biological processes, ΔG and ΔA will be identical, since pressure, temperature, and volume are all essentially constant. Where evolution or absorption of gas is involved, however, it may be necessary to distinguish between constant volume and constant pressure. Since nearly all biochemical reactions, *in vivo* or *in vitro*, are observed at constant pressure, ΔG is the function of interest.

Entropy and Heat Transfer

For a reversible process $\Delta S = q_{max}/T$ and for any real process $\Delta S > q/T$. It follows that $\Delta S > 0$ for any real process in an isolated system (since there is no heat exchange, $q = 0$). The entropy of the system thus increases in any process in such a system, and equilibrium is the condition of maximum entropy in an isolated system. If "the universe" is taken as an isolated system, the relationships just stated lead to the statement, "In any real process the entropy of the universe increases." It is seldom if ever useful, however, to consider the universe as our system. In most cases, appreciable amounts of energy are exchanged with only a very limited nearby portion of the universe. If, as before, we define the surroundings of the system as all other matter with which the system interacts to a significant degree, we see that the system plus surroundings may be considered a sort of isolated supersystem (since our process involves no energy exchange beyond the surroundings). We may then say that in any real process the entropy of the *system plus surroundings* is increased. It is emphatically not true, however, that in a real process the entropy of any *system* necessarily increases (unless it is an isolated system). When ice melts, its entropy increases; when water freezes, its entropy decreases. Nevertheless in both cases the entropy of system plus surroundings increases; that is, the sum of the entropy change for the system and that for the surroundings is always positive.

In the case of the ice-water system, the explanation of the entropy changes is very simple. Ice can melt only if the surroundings is warmer than $273°K$ —thus warmer than the ice. We will denote the temperature of the surroundings by T_s. In the melting of a definite quantity of ice, a definite amount of heat, which we will indicate by q, must be absorbed by the system—the ice—and thus must be lost by the surroundings. So the entropy change for the ice-water system is $q/273$—an increase—and the entropy change for the surroundings is $-q/T_s$—a decrease. Since T_s must be greater than $273°K$ if the ice is to melt, the overall entropy change for system plus surroundings,

$$\Delta S_{total} = q/273 - q/T_s$$

must be a positive value. When the temperature of the surroundings is less than $273°$K, the direction of heat flow is reversed and some water freezes. Now the entropy of the system increases, that of the surroundings decreases, and

$$\Delta S_{total} = -q/273 + q/T_s$$

Since T_s is now less than $273°$K, the total entropy change again must be positive.

Freezing and melting, because of their large and obvious changes in entropy, help to clarify the relationship between heat transfer and entropy change. However, it should be evident that exactly similar considerations show that any transfer of heat from a warmer to a cooler body must entail an increase in the entropy of the cooler body, and a numerically smaller decrease in the entropy of the warmer, so that the net change is always positive. It can also be seen that the net entropy change approaches zero as the difference between the two temperatures approaches zero. That is, when the two bodies are at very nearly the same temperature the entropy increase per unit of heat exchanged is very low. In the extreme case when the two temperatures are exactly equal the entropy change accompanying heat transfer is zero—but under these conditions there is no net heat flow anyway. This simple case illustrates the generalizations that all real processes go toward equilibrium, that the entropy of system plus surroundings increases in any real process, and that this entropy change becomes smaller as the process approaches equilibrium, finally becoming zero in the imaginary case of a process proceeding exactly at equilibrium.

Entropy, Metabolism, and Evolution

It is mainly the failure to understand the distinction between the system and the system plus surroundings that has led to the erroneous ideas on the relationship of entropy to metabolism, growth, and evolution that are still sometimes encountered. Since an organism is a low-entropy system, some authors have suggested that the second law of thermodynamics does not apply to organisms. Of course that suggestion is not valid. The entropy of the portion of the substrate that is assimilated into the cell may decrease, but the entropy of the cell plus surroundings always increases as a consequence of metabolism. In fact, the rate of entropy increase associated with metabolizing tissue is high, as would be expected of any sample of matter made up of rapidly reacting systems far from equilibrium.

The statement that evolution proceeds contrary to predictions derived from the second law (because complex organisms are descended from simpler ones) is also readily seen to be completely unfounded. Evolutionary changes are slow, and in one generation any decrease in entropy attributable to greater complexity of the offspring is utterly negligible compared to the entropy increases involved in the metabolic processes by which the offspring is produced and by which it grows. The situation is as if a small droplet of spray, rising a few inches from the foot of Niagara Falls, were to cause an observer to doubt the validity of the second law as applied to water in a gravitational field.

One other misconception regarding entropy and evolution is sometimes expressed. A large amount of carbon now exists in the relatively low-entropy form of organic matter (both living and dead). At some time in the past, this carbon must have existed in much higher-entropy forms, such as carbon dioxide, bicarbonates, carbonates, or perhaps methane. Surely, then, the development of life and the production of all of this organic matter were accompanied by massive entropy decreases, and this is sometimes said to demonstrate that life does not "obey" the second law. The answer to this argument is obvious from the preceding discussion. The net production of organic matter on the earth does not occur by a simple reshuffling of energy and entropy among the compounds involved, but is a consequence of the absorption of enormous amounts of radiant energy from the sun. As noted previously, where photosynthesis is concerned an isolated system must include the sun. And as we have seen, it is only in an isolated system that the second law predicts that entropy must increase.

For convenience, we will take as our system all living matter and all non-living matter on the earth with which it interacts significantly. This system is not isolated. If we consider that biological processes generally occur essentially at constant temperature and pressure, it follows that what the second law in fact predicts is that the free energy of the system should decrease as a result of every physical or chemical process that occurs in it. But there is a steady and very large flow of free energy *into* the system in the form of the sunlight absorbed by parts of the system. (When a molecule absorbs a photon and is excited to a more reactive state its free energy is increased.) Thus the free energy of the earth's surface is constantly tending to increase because of absorption of radiant energy (much of it by chlorophyll) and constantly tending to decrease because of the chemical reactions going on (mostly in living organisms). The world system is now approximately at a steady state, with a high rate of energy absorption and conversion but with little or no net change in the total amount of living matter. Over the whole history of the earth, however, there has been a conversion of nonliving matter to organisms, characterized by much lower entropy, with radiant energy as the driving force:

$$\text{photons} + CO_2 + H_2O + NH_3 \rightarrow \text{organisms}$$

Free Energy and Concentration

As we have seen, the symbol ΔG^0_{form} is used for t. free energy of formation of a mole of a substance at its arbitrary standard state. In order to apply free energy values to real problems, however, we need values for free energies at *any* concentration. As with most thermodynamic relationships, the calculations involved in obtaining such values are easily illustrated in the case of an ideal gas. Concentration in this case is equivalent to the partial pressure of the gas, and is thus especially easy to deal with.

We will consider a change in pressure of an ideal gas that occurs at constant temperature and does no work other than work of expansion. From equation A-10, $dG = -w'_{\text{max}} + V\,dP - S\,dT$, it follows that for the process described

$$dG = V\,dP \qquad (A\text{-}13)$$

For 1 mole of a perfect gas $PV = RT$, hence $V = RT/P$. Substituting into equation A-13,

$$dG = \frac{RT\,dP}{P}$$

from which

$$\Delta G = RT \int \frac{dP}{P} = RT \ln \frac{P}{P_0} \qquad (A\text{-}14)$$

where P_0 is the initial pressure and P the final pressure of the gas. For the special case where P_0 equals 1 atm (the usual standard state for an ideal gas), we have then

$$\Delta G = RT \ln P$$

which gives the change in free energy per mole of an ideal gas in going from the standard state to any pressure P. Since, as we have seen, the usual free energy scale is based on free energies of formation from the elements, we may express the free energy of 1 mole of an ideal gas at pressure P by equation A-15. Here ΔG^0_{form}, as previously described, is the free energy of forma-

$$\Delta G = \Delta G^0_{\text{form}} + RT \ln P \qquad (A\text{-}15)$$

tion of 1 mole of the gas at its standard state from the free elements at the same temperature. This relation can be quite easily extended to solutions. Each component of an ideal solution exerts a vapor pressure that is the product of its mole fraction and the vapor pressure of the pure material at the same temperature; thus the vapor pressure of each component is proportional to its concentration. That is, for a change in concentration of any component, the change in vapor pressure is given by

$$\frac{c}{c_0} = \frac{P}{P_0}$$

Substituting into equation A-14, we obtain equation A-16. As before, we

$$\Delta G = RT \ln \frac{c}{c_0} \qquad (A\text{-}16)$$

set $c_0 = 1$ at the standard state and thus have for the difference in free energy between the standard state and a solution of concentration c

$$\Delta G = RT \ln c$$

Then the free energy of the component will be given by equation A-17.

$$\Delta G = \Delta G^0_{\text{form}} + RT \ln c \qquad (A\text{-}17)$$

Of course the standard states used in equations A-15 and A-17 are different. This is of no concern, since the choice of standard states to be used in any problem is a matter of convenience so long as the usage is consistent. If it becomes necessary to convert from one standard state to another, the free energy difference between the standard states is merely calculated from equation A-14. Thus to convert from a standard state of a gas at a pressure of 1 atm to a standard state of a 1 M solution we merely add $\Delta G = RT \ln(P_s/P_0)$, where P_0 is 1 and P_s is the partial pressure in equilibrium with the 1 M solution.

Activity Coefficients

The discussion so far has applied only to ideal gases, ideal gas mixtures, and ideal solutions. In an ideal gas or gas mixture there is no interaction between either like or unlike molecules; in a solution a solute will behave ideally if all of its interactions are equal. Ideality in a solution may be approached in either of two ways: (a) the components may be so similar, as in a benzene-toluene mixture, that interactions between like and unlike molecules are essentially equal; or (b) the solution may be so dilute that virtually all interactions of solute molecules are with solvent molecules (and, of course, virtually all interactions of solvent molecules are with solvent molecules). In either of these cases the activity of the solute will be very nearly proportional to its molar concentration, as is true of the components of an ideal gas mixture. Thus for ideal gas mixtures and ideal liquid solutions, a straight line results when nearly any property of a component of the mixture is plotted against the mole fraction of the component. For practically all biochemical substances, the only nearly ideal solution is a highly dilute solution. In accurate work with actual solutions, it is thus necessary to use a corrected or idealized 1 M solution, rather than the real thing, as the standard state. This ideal solution is said to have an *activity* of 1. Activity has the units of concentration (usually moles per liter). However, the actual concentration of a solution of unit activity may be either greater or less than 1 M, and sometimes by considerable amounts.

Experimental determination of the activity-concentration relationship for a given solution is in principle extremely simple. One merely measures any property that would be a linear function of concentration in an ideal solution at various concentrations and plots the results. Useful properties are partial pressure of the solute, freezing point depression, boiling point elevation, osmotic pressure, and electrochemical behavior. In general such plots are linear at low concentrations, but diverge from a straight line as the concentration is increased. The linear portion of the line is extrapolated, and for any solution the activity is the idealized concentration read from the extrapolated curve. The activity coefficient, f, is the factor by which concentration must be multiplied to yield activity:

$$a = fc \qquad \text{or} \qquad f = a/c$$

The quantitative relationships of thermodynamics apply to activities rather than to actual concentrations; thus for example equation A-17 is more accurately written as A-18.

$$\Delta G = \Delta G^0_{\text{form}} + RT \ln a \qquad\qquad (A\text{-}18)$$

If every solution contained only one solute, the determination of activity coefficients would be straightforward. It will be obvious, however, that for solutions containing a number of solutes the direct method will not suffice. The number of possible interactions becomes large and the activity coefficient of each solute changes not only with its own concentration, but with all of the others as well. The interactions are especially strong in solutions of electrolytes, where electrostatic attractions and repulsions are involved. The development of methods for the prediction of activity coefficients has been an important part of classical physical chemistry. The most widely used first approximation, the Debye-Hückel equation, can be found in any handbook or text in physical chemistry or chemical thermodynamics.

Since biological solutions contain not only many types of small ions but also large molecules each carrying many positive and negative charges, interactions are strong and complex. It would be expected, then, that in such solutions the use of activities rather than concentrations would be especially important. In fact, however, concentrations are used in nearly all biochemical work. There are several reasons for this, but the most important one is simple necessity. We do not use activities because we cannot. The complexity of the system makes accurate estimation of the activity coefficients difficult or impossible. (It must be remembered that in most cases little is known of the concentrations and still less of the physical natures of the macromolecules involved—how many of what species are present, how many positive and negative charges each bears, and so on.) Little is gained by the use of a correction factor when the factor itself is grossly incorrect.

It may thus appear that nearly all biochemical work dealing with equilibria or with rates of reactions (this includes most biochemical research) is hopelessly inaccurate and hardly worthy of serious consideration. Fortunately the situation is by no means that bad. One reason often given is that most of the substrates and products of biochemical reactions are present at low concentrations, so that their activities are essentially equal to concentrations. Unfortunately this statement is less valid than it may first appear; even though substrate and product concentrations are low, in the presence of buffer and other ions and of proteins and other multiply charged macromolecules, the activities of substrates and products may differ greatly from their concentrations. The real reason that metabolic and enzymic biochemistry is worth going on with even though few of the results in the field have much quantitative thermodynamic significance is that the objectives of most biochemical work do not depend critically on such quantitative significance. In evolving the coupling stoichiometries that make pairs of oppositely directed unidirectional pathways possible (Chapter 3), organisms have established such large values for the free energy changes (or the overall equilibrium constants) of nearly all metabolic sequences that even considerable uncertainty as to the exact values does not affect our understanding of the functional relationships.

The lack of rigor in most of our thermodynamic and kinetic data should not be taken as evidence that physical chemistry is unimportant in biochemical research. Physical chemical concepts supply an indispensable base for investigation and understanding of biological processes. The lack of precision in many of our applications is an unfortunate but by no means fatal shortcoming of enzyme and metabolic chemistry at the present time. It does not seriously impede our use of thermodynamics as an aid to rationalization and understanding.

Free Energy and Chemical Equilibrium

The chemical equation A-19 specifies a process in which 1 mole of C and

$$A + B \rightleftharpoons C + D \qquad (A\text{-}19)$$

1 mole of D are produced and 1 mole each of A and B disappear. The change in free energy accompanying the reaction can obviously be calculated by

adding up the free energies of the products formed and subtracting the free energies of the reactants that are used up. If we consider first the special case where all reactants and products are present at their standard states (the idealized 1 M solution; activity $= 1$), the change in free energy for the reaction can be calculated directly from the standard free energies of formation. Since the symbol ΔG^0_{form} is somewhat unwieldy, we will designate standard free energies of formation by the abbreviations $G_A{}^0$, $G_B{}^0$, $G_C{}^0$, and $G_D{}^0$. The change in standard free energy, ΔG^0, for reaction A-19 is then given by equation A-20. For the general case, when reactants and products are not

$$\Delta G^0 = G_C{}^0 + G_D{}^0 - G_A{}^0 - G_D{}^0 \tag{A-20}$$

all at unit activity, we use equation A-18, which expresses the free energy of formation of one mole of compound A at activity a_A

$$\Delta G_{form} = G_A{}^0 + RT \ln a_A$$

Equations for the other components of the reaction are of course similar. The change in free energy for reaction A-19 at any activities of reactants and products can now be obtained by adding the free energies of products formed and subtracting the free energies of reactants used:

$$\Delta G = (G_C{}^0 + RT \ln a_C) + (G_D{}^0 + RT \ln a_D)$$
$$- (G_A{}^0 + RT \ln a_A) - (G_B{}^0 + RT \ln a_B)$$

On rearrangement, this becomes

$$\Delta G = G_C{}^0 + G_D{}^0 - G_A{}^0 - G_B{}^0 + RT \ln\left(\frac{a_C a_D}{a_A a_B}\right) \tag{A-21}$$

We see by comparison with equation A-20 that the first four terms of equation A-21 equal the standard free energy of reaction. Thus

$$\Delta G = \Delta G^0 + RT \ln\left(\frac{a_C a_D}{a_A a_B}\right) \tag{A-22}$$

We can evaluate ΔG^0 in terms of activities by considering the special case of equilibrium (at constant temperature and pressure). Since $\Delta G = 0$ at equilibrium, for a system at equilibrium we have equation A-23. By equa-

$$\Delta G^\circ = -RT \ln\left(\frac{a_C a_D}{a_A a_B}\right)_{eq} \tag{A-23}$$

tion A-20 ΔG^0 is constant; thus the term $(a_C a_D/a_A a_B)$ must also be constant. In fact it is the familar equilibrium constant of elementary chemistry. Equation A-23 may then be written

$$\Delta G^0 = -RT \ln K \tag{A-24}$$

and equation A-22 becomes

$$\Delta G^0 = -RT \ln K + RT \ln\left(\frac{a_C a_D}{a_A a_B}\right) \tag{A-25}$$

For convenience in computation, the natural logarithms are converted to the base 10 (equation A-26):

$$\Delta G = -2.30 \, RT \ln K + 2.30 \, RT \ln\left(\frac{a_C a_D}{a_A a_B}\right) \tag{A-26}$$

If the activity ratio $(a_C a_D/a_A a_B)$ is designated by Q, we obtain equation A-27, which was introduced in Chapter 3 as equation 3-12.

$$\Delta G = 2.30 \, RT \log Q/K \tag{A-27}$$

The great majority of applications of thermodynamics in metabolic chemistry involve only simple manipulations of equations A-20, A-22, A-24, A-25, and A-27. For example, if the appropriate standard free energies of formation are available, ΔG^0 for a reaction is obtained by the use of equation A-20. The equilibrium constant is found from equation A-22, or the free energy change at any specified activities of reactants and products from equation A-25. As previously discussed, activities are usually unknown, so that concentrations must nearly always be used in biochemical applications of these equations.

All processes move toward equilibrium and, as we saw earlier in this chapter, ΔG is less than zero for all real processes at constant temperature and pressure. Thus to establish in which direction a reaction can be expected to go, it is merely necessary to calculate the value of ΔG from equation A-22 (or A-27). If the value obtained is negative, the reaction, if it occurs at all, will go in the direction written. A positive value of ΔG shows that the reaction as written cannot occur, but that it may occur in the opposite direction. It is intuitively obvious, and may easily be seen from equation A-21, or any of those derived from it, that the free energy for a reverse process is numerically equal but opposite in sign to that for the forward direction. Any chemical system not at equilibrium is potentially capable of reaction toward equilibrium, and the sign of ΔG tells us in which direction equilibrium lies.

The quantities ΔG and ΔG^0 are sometimes confused in biochemistry. Because ΔG^0 is relatively easily estimated, it is sometimes used as a measure of the tendency of a reaction to proceed. Actually, of course, ΔG^0 indicates the direction of potential reaction only in the special case where the reaction parameter Q has the value of 1. Under any other conditions, the appropriate value of ΔG must be used. For conditions that differ considerably from the standard state, ΔG and ΔG^0 will frequently differ in sign. In such cases the use of ΔG^0 for ΔG will necessarily lead to erroneous predictions as to reaction direction.

The relationships between ΔG, ΔG^0, K_{eq}, and the direction of reaction are illustrated in Figures A-1 and A-2. The curves of both figures were calculated for the simplest case of a reaction with a single reactant and a single product, $A \rightleftharpoons B$. The abscissa shows the mole fraction of B in the mixture and the vertical scale indicates the free energy of a system containing A and B in the total amount of one mole. Thus the curve shows the relative free energy of such a system as a function of varying mole fractions of the components. The slope of the curve at any point is dG/dn_B, where n_B is the number of moles of B. This slope is thus ΔG, in kilocalories per mole, for the reaction $A \rightarrow B$. The reaction may be represented by a ball on such curves of G versus extent of reaction. The ball will always roll toward equilibrium (the minimum of the slope), and the strength of its tendency to roll will increase with distance from equilibrium, as shown by the constantly increasing slope of the curve.

In Figure A-1, $K_{eq} = 1$. ΔG^0, which is merely the slope of the curve when the reaction parameter Q has the value of 1, is 0 in this case because at

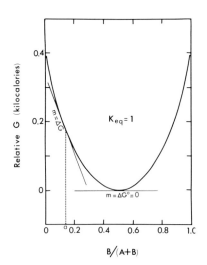

Figure A-1. Relative Gibbs free energy of a system containing compounds A and B in a total amount of one mole, plotted as a function of the mole fraction of B. For the conversion $A \rightleftharpoons B$, $K_{eq} = 1$. ΔG, the molar change in free energy for the reaction at any composition of the A-B pool, is the slope of the curve corresponding to that composition as illustrated for composition a.

equilibrium the concentrations of reactant and product are equal so that $Q = 1$. The tangent drawn at the arbitrary mole fraction indicated by point a on the abscissa merely illustrates the fact that the slope of the curve at any point is the molar free energy change of the reaction at that composition of the reaction mixture.

Curves for reactions with values of the equilibrium constant other than 1 are illustrated in Figure A-2. When $K_{eq} = 4$, the system is at equilibrium when the mole fraction of B is 0.8. When the mole fraction of B is less than 0.8, the slope of the curve will be negative, and the conversion of A to B will be thermodynamically feasible. The standard free energy, ΔG^0, is merely the slope at a mole fraction of 0.5, where $Q = 1$. The other curve of Figure A-2 shows the reciprocal case of a reaction for which $K_{eq} = 0.25$ and ΔG^0 is positive.

Because the relation between the reaction parameter Q and the free energy charge associated with the reaction has only one degree of freedom, specification of the slope at any mole fraction of B (or at any value of Q in the more general case of a reaction with more than one reactant and one product) specifies the whole curve. It is for that reason that ΔG^0 values are useful. The magnitude of ΔG^0 is of no importance in itself, but from it one may calculate the position of equilibrium (the minimum of the curve), as well as the value of ΔG (the slope of the curve) at any value of Q. The farther the standard state happens to be from equilibrium, the greater is the slope at that point (the value of ΔG^0). It should be remembered that G has no absolute value,

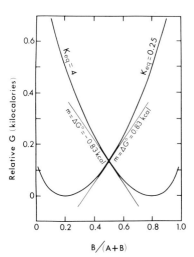

$B / (A + B)$

Figure A-2. Same as Figure A-1, except that curves of relative free energy are shown for cases where $K_{eq} = 0.25$ and $K_{eq} = 4$. The standard molar free energy change, ΔG^0, is the slope of the curve at the composition corresponding to a value of 1 for the reaction parameter Q.

so that the position of zero on the vertical scale is arbitrary. For convenience in comparing the curves, the relative free energy of the equilibrium mixture was given the value of zero in each case.

Free Energy "Efficiencies"

This book discusses interrelations between metabolic sequences as stoichiometric relationships, and expresses them usually in terms of coupling coefficients based on ATP equivalents. Because metabolic interactions have been frequently discussed in another framework, that of free-energy efficiency, the reasons why that approach is not used here should be indicated.

Free-energy efficiency calculations are based on division of the ΔG^0 for one reaction or sequence by ΔG^0 for another. This operation, which may seem superficially plausible, is seldom, if ever, justified. Equilibrium constants are ratios, and they may appropriately be multiplied or divided. The definition of an equilibrium constant leads directly to the fact that K_{eq} for a sequence of reactions is the product of the K_{eq} values for the individual reactions. What seems to be overlooked in many discussions of metabolic energetics is that ΔG^0 is the logarithm of K_{eq}. (The constant by which log K_{eq} is multiplied to obtain ΔG^0 is merely a scale factor taking units into account.) Whenever it is appropriate to multiply or divide numbers, it is appropriate to add or subtract their logarithms. Thus ΔG^0 for a sequence of reactions is the sum of the ΔG^0 values for the individual reactions. Multiplication or division of logarithms is appropriate only in special cases, and the free energy of chemical reactions is not one of those cases. Multiplying the logarithms of two numbers is equivalent to using the logarithm of either number as the exponent of the other; thus if

$$\Delta G_1{}^0 = -RT \ln K_1$$

and

$$\Delta G_2{}^0 = -RT \ln K_1$$

then

$$\Delta G_1{}^0 \Delta G_2{}^0 = R^2 T^2 \ln(K_1)^{\ln K_2} = R^2 T^2 \ln(K_2)^{\ln K_1}$$

and

$$\Delta G_1{}^0 / \Delta G_2{}^0 = \ln(K_1)^{1/\ln K_2}$$

It seems self-evident that there is no chemical justification for using one equilibrium constant in an exponential term for another, and that the results of such an operation can have no meaning.

Perhaps the commonest of such errors deals with the "efficiencies" of sequences in terms of ATP yield. Thus, if ΔG^0 for the oxidation of glucose $= -677$ kcal/mole, if 38 moles of ATP are produced, and if ΔG^0 for phosphorylation of ADP is 8 kcal/mole, it is often said that the efficiency of glycolysis is $(8 \times 38)/677 = 45\%$. What this calculation really implies is merely that the metabolic yield of ATP is 45% of the yield that would correspond to a K_{eq} value of 1 for the overall process. This is equivalent to saying that K_{eq} for the actual process is very large. As is discussed in Chapter 3, that is a very important aspect of metabolism, but it is not a measure of efficiency. The efficiency of a device is its energy output (for example, as electrical or mechanical energy) divided by the energy input (for example, as heat). The lack of relevance of this concept to the discussion of ATP yields should be obvious.

Another example of this misunderstanding of the meaning of ΔG^0 values is still found in some textbooks. In the most frequently encountered specific case, the standard free energy of hydrolysis of a phosphorylated metabolite is divided by the standard free energy of hydrolysis of ATP and the result is said to be the efficiency of the kinase that catalyzes the phosphorylation. Thus if ΔG^0 for hydrolysis of glucose 6-P is taken as -3 kcal/mole and that for hydrolysis of ATP as -8 kcal/mole, it is said that 8 kcal of energy is "used" and only 3 kcal "conserved" in the hexokinase reaction so that its efficiency is 3/8, or 37%. This statement is false in every part. Energy is neither used nor conserved in any meaningful sense in this reaction, the standard free energy changes do not necessarily apply under physiological conditions, and the concept of efficiency is totally inapplicable to a ratio of free energies.

As discussed earlier in this chapter, a process may be written, for the purposes of thermodynamic analysis, as a sum of any series of steps, real or hypothetical, that add up to the process in question. Thus the hexokinase reaction (equation A-28) may, for some purposes, be written as the sum of

$$\text{ATP} + \text{glucose} \rightarrow \text{glucose 6-P} + \text{ADP} \qquad \Delta G^0 = -5 \text{ kcal/mole} \qquad \text{(A-28)}$$

the hydrolysis of ATP and the phosphorylation of glucose at the expense of inorganic phosphate (equations A-29 and A-30). If we know ΔG^0 values

$$\text{ATP} + \text{H}_2\text{O} \rightarrow \text{ADP} + \text{P}_i \qquad \Delta G^0 = -8 \text{ kcal/mole} \qquad \text{(A-29)}$$

$$\text{glucose} + \text{P}_i \rightarrow \text{glucose 6-P} + \text{H}_2\text{O} \qquad \Delta G^0 = 3 \text{ kcal/mole} \qquad \text{(A-30)}$$

corresponding to equations A-29 and A-30, we obtain the value for equation

A. Some Elementary Aspects of Thermodynamics

A-28 by addition. It does not matter that equations A-29 and A-30 are introduced purely for the sake of analysis, and that the reaction does not go in this way. The free energy change for any process is independent of pathway, so we are free to invent an unlikely imaginary pathway if it is convenient. This is true, of course, because the free energy changes for all steps will be added, and the *sum* of such changes must be identical for any real or imagined path that effects the same conversion. But this is not true for the *product* or *quotient* of free energy changes, and it is the quotient that is often referred to as a measure of efficiency. The absurdity of such calculations is illustrated by considering a man on a mountainside at an elevation of 10,005 ft who walks down to 10,000 ft. Since he has merely walked down a gentle slope, the question of energy efficiency or of conservation of altitude would never occur to him. A man with a surveyor's transit at an elevation of 9997 ft might measure the altitudes of the hiker's initial and final positions relative to his own position and report that the hiker started at 8 ft of altitude and ended at only 3 ft; thus his change of position conserved altitude only to the extent of 37%. This is the kind of reasoning that is employed in the evaluation of "efficiency" of the hexokinase reaction. Of course the number obtained by the surveyor has no real meaning, and its value depends on his own position. If he were at 9000 ft, he would consider the walker to start at 1005 ft of altitude, and to end at 1000 ft for a very commendable efficiency of 99.5%. And if he used sea level as his base point, the corresponding values of altitude sacrificed and conserved would be 10,005 and 10,000, and the efficiency would be an amazing 99.95%. Yet the process (the walk) is identical in all three cases and if our surveyor realized (as all real surveyors of course do) that relative altitudes may be added or subtracted, but not multiplied or divided, he would reach the same value of -5 feet for the vertical component of the walk in every case. In the hexokinase reaction, the path by way of inorganic phosphate (equations A-29 and A-30) is a useful fiction. The actual reaction no more goes by way of inorganic phosphate than the hiker necessarily goes down to whatever level is used as a point of reference for the calculation of altitude.

Although evaluations of free energy "efficiencies" are erroneous, knowledge of the free energy change accompanying a reaction does, of course, give us information of value in the analysis of metabolism. Thus if ΔG^0 for the hexokinase reaction is -5 kcal/mole, K_{eq} for this reaction is about 3600. This leads to the useful fact that, at the physiological ATP/ADP concentration ratio of about 5, hexokinase could in principle maintain a concentration of glucose 6-P more than 15,000 times that of free glucose in the cell. Thus the large negative value of ΔG^0 for this reaction, far from indicating an undesirable degree of inefficiency, actually is one of the bases for the very desirable ability of the cell to use glucose at low concentrations. In a more general context, the high values of equilibrium constants for metabolic sequences, which correspond to low values of the fictitious "free energy efficiency," are necessary for the establishment of unidirectional pairs of reaction sequences as described in Chapter 3, and are thus essential to life.

APPENDIX B

"High-Energy Bonds," Thermodynamics, and Open Systems

Lipmann's suggestion in 1941 (74) of the symbol ∼ (usually termed "squiggle") for weak bonds that are broken relatively easily has been misunderstood and perverted in a number of ways. Such concepts as the storage of energy in a peculiar type of bond, the release of energy on breaking a bond, and the movement of a phosphoryl group, complete with a squiggle bond, to another site have no chemical meaning. They and related statements have been presented in textbooks and reviews, and have had the unfortunate effect of confining metabolic chemistry behind a jargon curtain that has tended to isolate it from simple and direct chemical considerations, and to confuse and confound the relations between thermodynamics and metabolic processes in the minds of many students. Generations of students in all fields of biology have been taught that the energy needed for vital processes is liberated by the breaking of high-energy bonds. (It is, however, obvious that bonds hold atoms together, and that energy is required, not liberated, when bonds are broken.) The question of what kind of latch or superbond kept the atoms together until the squiggle bond was allowed to relax and flick them apart with release of energy was never confronted. These concepts were consistent neither with common sense nor with what these same students were learning about bonds in first-year chemistry courses, and their widespread acceptance is a tribute to the ability of the human mind to compartmentalize concepts. This compartmentalization has served as a block to rational consideration of the simple thermodynamic aspects of metabolism. Discussions of high-energy bonds, at least in their worst forms, are not found in the better of the current biochemical texts, but they have spread into elementary biology textbooks, at both the college and the high-school level, and now pervade the treatment of metabolism in most such books. Thus for years to come students will continue to learn in biology classes about a very important class of bonds that release energy on breaking, while learning in chemistry that a bond is an abstraction for the forces that hold atoms together (and must, of course, be overcome if the bond is to be broken).

A concept can become widely accepted and can survive for a long time only if it is, or seems to be, useful. The squiggle-bond concept was, if one stayed behind the jargon curtain and avoided consideration of what the words meant, very useful. It led biochemists to think stoichiometrically about metabolism and to recognize the quantization of metabolic energy. When an investigator's real meaning was the number of moles of ATP produced or consumed in a sequence, this meaning in the immediate context was not seriously blurred if he spoke of the number of high-energy bonds produced or broken. And it is easily understandable that many workers, having learned about metabolism in terms of high-energy bonds, respond negatively, and sometimes emotionally, to suggestions that the concept of such bonds should be abandoned.

It should be emphasized that the ambiguities and errors that the squiggle-bond approach has introduced into metabolism were not inherent in Lipmann's review. That review, one of the most important papers in the history of biochemistry, first clearly stated two of the fundamental generalizations of biological chemistry: the great importance of activation in metabolism and the existence of stoichiometric coupling between all metabolic sequences. With regard to the first point, Lipmann said:

> Groups, such as phospho-, acetyl-, and amino- are brought by metabolic mechanisms intermediately into the positions from where they easily can be carried into desired paths. More or less energy is lost or better used up because of special paths adopted in forming these groups. These biologically interesting linkages designed to transfer groups with loss of energy will be called "weak linkages" based on the usual chemical nomenclature with respect to cleavage processes.

Because of the special metabolic interest that he correctly felt these chemically activated groups to have for metabolism, Lipmann suggested the squiggle as a convenient symbol to indicate them. It is clear from the passage quoted above that the symbol was not intended to indicate a peculiar bond that somehow differed qualitatively from other bonds; that misinterpretation was due to later authors. The squiggle was proposed as a symbol for bonds that differed from others not in kind but only in degree; that is, they are easily broken in displacement reactions. There is nothing specifically biological in such bonds, and Lipmann's original discussion does not suggest any such specificity. The concept of a "good leaving group," developed by physical organic chemists, is essentially equivalent to the original meaning of a group symbolized by attachment through a squiggle bond. Had Lipmann persisted in his description of these important bonds as "weak linkages" or, perhaps, "labile bonds," an incalculable amount of later ambiguities might have been avoided. But, in order to emphasize the importance of activation of this type in metabolic energetics, Lipmann also suggested the term "high-energy bond" for these labile linkages, and that term was the one that caught on. Those who took the name literally without understanding its valid meaning were responsible for the unfortunate notions that have prevailed in much of the literature on metabolic energetics during the past 30 years.

The invalidity of the concept of a bond that liberates energy on breaking is discussed by Banks and Vernon (*19*). Their paper also includes, however, some statements that are not compatible with the views on metabolism presented in this book. It thus seems desirable to explain why I do not feel that their discussion shows the treatment of metabolism given here, and especially in Chapter 3, to be incorrect.

Banks and Vernon maintain that thermodynamics is not relevant to the study of metabolism, and that only kinetic factors need be considered. A major point in their argument is that organisms are open systems, and that, therefore, simple thermodynamic considerations, which were developed for closed systems, do not apply to them. Similar statements have been made by several other authors. These statements apparently arise from the preoccupation of some teachers and thermodynamics texts with perfect gas systems doing pressure-volume work on the surroundings, and with the attempt to refine the subject to the maximal level of mathematical austerity. In this process of refinement, there has often been more emphasis on what thermodynamics cannot do than on what it is good for. Some thermodynamicists seem to feel that their scientific purity is somehow dependent on lack of contact between their subject and the real world. But such attitudes should not be allowed to come between us and the situations that we are studying. Thermodynamics is an extremely useful body of relationships derived from experience. It is not a set of disembodied postulates, and the mathematical austerity and remoteness from reality that are sometimes imposed on it are neither necessary nor in keeping with its origins and its wide applicability. In its application to chemical processes, including those occurring in organisms, we may well consider thermodynamics to be a set of generalizations crystallized from common sense, and there is no reason to separate them from their mother liquor.

Although an analogy can never prove anything, it may very usefully illuminate an argument and, if chosen with care and used to illustrate rather than to persuade, may be valuable. The movement of water in a gravitational field supplies a close and useful analogy to many aspects of a chemical re-action. Of course there are possible pitfalls—for example, flowing water has momentum and a chemical reaction does not—but these are easily avoided. Such an analogy will be used to illustrate the applicability of thermodynamics to an open system.

Consider two reservoirs of water (tanks or lakes), with the water level in reservoir B being b cm above some reference point, and the water level in C being c cm above the same reference point. The difference in water levels, $b - c$, will be termed h, and we will assume that b is greater than c. Consider that water is flowing from B to C and driving a water wheel in the process. (The water wheel is not essential to the argument, since the change in free energy of water in flowing from B to C depends only on h, and is independent of whether any work is done; the wheel is only to give focus to the analogy.) We can imagine four situations:

1. B and C are reservoirs of finite size, and there is no movement of water into or out of either except for the flow from B to C. Thus the two reservoirs and the connector between them constitute a closed system in the thermodynamic sense. The water levels are changing, b decreasing and c increasing, so that the value of h decreases at a rate proportional to the rate of flow.

2. Same as (1), but reservoir C has very sensitive automatic instrumen-tation that senses the water level and pumps water back to B by a different pathway to maintain b, c, and h constant. Any error in the system can be negligibly small compared to the value of h. (Whether the system is open or closed depends on details of the definitions used, but there is clearly an input of energy from the outside to run the pump.)

3. B and C are pools in a flowing stream. The system is at steady state; the values of b, c, and h are constant.

4. B and C are infinitely large reservoirs, so that in the finite time of observation there is no change in the values of b, c, and h. The system may be said to be closed, but an infinitely large system is of course an abstraction.

It is clear that an observer stationed at the hub of the water wheel cannot distinguish between situations (2), (3), and (4). All that matters thermody-namically is the head of water h, and this is constant in all three cases. Since h is constant, these systems are more convenient for consideration of h and its relationships to other parameters of a system than is situation (1).

The analogy with the chemical conversion of B to C is, I think, exact as regards the aspects relevant to our discussion. The corresponding situations are:

1. A simple closed system; a reaction occurring in a reaction vessel.

2. A case where the product is converted to reactant by other processes

at such a rate as to keep the concentration ratio (product)/(reactant) constant. This situation is approximated closely in the case of the (ATP)/(ADP) ratio *in vivo*, as discussed in Chapter 4.

3. A chemical steady-state system. This is approximated very closely by most metabolic sequences *in vivo*, where there is continuous flux through a sequence of intermediates, but no change in concentrations.

4. The abstraction of infinite reservoirs of reactants and products, so that concentration will not change as a consequence of reaction.

There is nothing especially "proper" about situation (1), and it is not true that simple thermodynamic considerations apply only to that situation. On the contrary, elementary texts often invoke infinite reservoirs of reactants and products, as in situation (4), in discussing the meaning of ΔG and other thermodynamic functions. As conventionally defined, ΔG is the change in free energy that accompanies the conversion of a mole of B to a mole of C without change in the concentration, activity, or chemical potential of either. In more specific terms, ΔG must be related to a specified equation, and signifies the change in free energy when the numbers of moles of reactants shown in the equation are converted to the corresponding numbers of moles of products, all at constant chemical activity. Since the abstraction of situation (4) is often used to explain the meaning of ΔG, it can hardly be seriously maintained that ΔG values do not apply in a simple and direct way to that situation, or to situations (2) and (3), which are real situations, met with in metabolism, that are equivalent to abstraction (4). Far from not applying to open systems, thermodynamics at this simple level applies more simply to steady-state systems than to closed systems. The total change in free energy in a reaction occurring at steady state can be determined merely by multiplying ΔG in kcal/mole by the number of moles that have reacted. In a closed system, the same calculation requires integration between initial and final states in which the chemical activities of all reaction components may be different.

It should be stressed that in situations (2), (3), and (4) there is no change with time in the concentration, activity, or chemical potential of B or C, and that in the situations that are attainable in the real world, (2) and (3), there is also no change in the amount of either. Yet water is flowing from B to C (and work may be done because of the turning wheel). This is important because it has been suggested that unless there is a change in the amount, or the concentration, or the chemical potential of the reactants and products, a reaction can be ignored:

The only reactions of relevance are those in which a net change in *amount* of a reactant occurs. ATP does not, therefore, act as an energy source for muscle contraction (*17*).

The breakdown of ATP, even though it may be, e.g., in muscle contraction, the final chemical process before the mechanical changes, does not enter into the thermodynamic account since the chemical potential of ATP remains constant. To interpret the function of ATP in energetic terms is, in these circumstances, therefore, meaningless (19).

In any energetic (i.e., thermodynamic) accounting only those substances whose chemical potential changes need be considered. It follows that if, during normal contraction, the concentration of ATP does not change then the thermodynamic parameters associated with its formation and breakdown, such as the standard free energy of hydrolysis, are totally irrelevant (19).

ATP . . . cannot then be regarded as a universal source of energy. Its chemical potential remains constant and it therefore does not enter into any simple thermodynamic considerations (19).

The last three statements are especially surprising. The chemical potential of component A of a system, symbolized as μ_A, is defined as $\partial G/\partial n_A$, where ∂G is change of free energy of the system and ∂n_A is change in number of moles of component A. That is, the chemical potential of a substance is simply the increase in the free energy of the total system that would result from addition of one mole of that substance with no other change in the system. Since a chemical reaction can be visualized as the removal of a reactant and the addition of a product, the change in free energy accompanying the conversion of A and B to C and D is given by Equation B-1 where Δn

$$\Delta G = \Delta n_C \mu_C + \Delta n_D \mu_D + \Delta n_A \mu_A + \Delta n_B \mu_B \qquad (B\text{-}1)$$

terms represent the numbers of moles of components that are added (Δn_A and Δn_B will be negative, since A and B are removed). These terms are merely the coefficients in the balanced chemical equation. Thus for the reaction $2A + B \rightarrow 3C + D$, the change in free energy of the system is given by Eq. B-2.

$$\Delta G = 3\mu_C + \mu_D - 2\mu_A - \mu_B \qquad (B\text{-}2)$$

Equation B-1 is a widely used relationship. It is obviously most easily applied to cases where all chemical potentials remain constant. It is by no means true that the compounds and their reactions in such cases enter into no simple thermodynamic considerations. For example, the chemical potential of gasoline in the tank and of oxygen in the air remain constant, but an automobile moves as a consequence of reaction between gasoline and oxygen. Chemical potential is itself a slope or derivative—the rate at which free energy changes with addition of the component. There is no reason, in logic or in chemistry, why a change in the slope should be necessary for a reaction to be regarded as a source of energy.

Perhaps the point really at issue here is the meaning of a chemical equation. An equation should, I think, be taken as representing a process or event, either potential or real. Banks and Vernon seem to consider an equation to result in principle from an inventory of reactants and products; that is, to represent obligately the actual changes in amounts of reactants and products in the system (although that view does not seem to lead to the statements regarding the necessity of change in chemical potential that were quoted above). Different views as to the significance to be attached to a chemical equation lead to differences in the meaning of equation B-1. If the chemical equation to which it refers signifies an event or process, this equation gives the change in free energy of the system that results from that event. It does not matter in how many other reactions A, B, C, or D may participate; equation B-1 shows the change in free energy of the system that results *from the specific reaction to which it applies.* The presence or absence of other reactions, including a reaction that reconverts the product to reactants at exactly the same rate as our reaction, thus holding amounts and concentrations constant, has no effect on the equation, since it does not pretend to deal with all free energy changes, but only with those that result from the reaction under consideration. Summation of the ΔG values from such equations for all reactions occurring in the system would give the total change in free energy.

If, on the other hand, the equation implies an inventory of the system, as Banks and Vernon seem to imply, it is only the net change in amounts of compound that count (again overlooking the comments about change in chemical potential), and nothing of thermodynamic interest is admitted to have occurred if the products are cycled back to reactants at the same rate as they are produced. This assumption that ΔG in equation B-1 refers to the total change in free energy of the system, rather than to that resulting from a specific reaction, leads to serious difficulties, however. The coefficients (Δn values) in equation B-1 must relate to a specific chemical equation, but it is difficult to see what stoichiometric coefficients can mean if a whole system is somehow to be dealt with in one equation. If A is reacting with six compounds in six reactions going at different and perhaps changing rates, there is no overall stoichiometry. Each reaction must be dealt with individually. If the value of ΔG over some time interval can be calculated for each, the sum of these values gives the overall free energy change for the system. The appropriate application of equation B-1, I think, is to a specific chemical reaction, considered individually. These comments apply equally, of course, to other equations that define ΔG, such as B-3.

$$\Delta G = \Delta G^0 + RT \ln Q \qquad \text{(B-3)}$$

This ambiguity as to how equations B-1 and B-3 should be applied, as well as the concern over the fact that living organisms are open systems, may arise from the dictum, found in many textbooks, that for thermodynamic consideration we must divide the universe into system and surroundings. As long as we deal only with perfect gases, Carnot cycles, ideal heat engines, and all of the related paraphernalia that usually keep students from realizing that thermodynamics provides simple and straightforward methods for dealing with real systems of interest, we can speak of *the* system and *the* surroundings. But there is no inherent reason why we need be so rigid, and in dealing with real situations we should be perfectly free to deal with systems (or subsystems) within systems in whatever way will best suit our purposes. There is no reason why these subsystems need be physically distinct in the sense of spatial separation; several reactions occurring simultaneously in the same solution can each be treated independently, as noted above, even though they occupy the same space.

The main conclusion that Banks and Vernon reach is that ATP and ADP cannot be involved in energy coupling to muscle contraction or to metabolic reactions if their concentrations are essentially constant. Thus they say (*18*):

> When a muscle operates *in vivo* as an open system in which the ATP concentration is held constant by transphosphorylation from phosphorylcreatine to ATP and/or by oxidative phosphorylation, the free energy of hydrolysis of ATP vanishes from any thermodynamic account since it is not obvious how to calculate the free energy change for a reaction which *shows no change*.

This last quotation seems clearly to be based on a definition of a chemical equation in terms of an inventory. The alternative view, on which the concepts presented in this book are based, is that the free energy change that is of interest corresponds to the flux through the system (the rate of conversion of ATP to ADP) and that this change is real and meaningful quite independently of whether the product ADP is recycled by other reactions to regenerate ATP. It is in fact only this recycling that allows for continuing utilization of ATP and hence a continuing decrease in free energy associated with the reactions in which ATP is used.

We know that energy flow occurs through cyclic transducing systems. Our aim should be to understand these systems and their functional integration in metabolic chemistry as well as possible. If this is our goal, it seems probable that we can agree that the conversion of ATP to ADP is not the ultimate energy source for any biological process (ATP is regenerated at the expense of various chemical reactions of metabolites, and the ultimate source of free energy in organisms is sunlight), but that this conversion serves as the immediate energy source for muscle contraction and for most chemical activities of a cell. It makes no difference if anyone wishes to substitute "energy conduit" or "energy transducing system" or any other similar phrase for "immediate energy source"; the meaning is the same. And we should be clear on one point: this role of the ATP/ADP couple as energy transducer is a strictly thermodynamic role. The adenylate system exerts very important kinetic effects on metabolism, which have been the main subject of my own research during the past decade and are discussed in this book, but those effects are superposed on, and mutually interdependent with, the thermodynamic functions of these compounds in energy transduction.

One final point should be discussed. Banks (*17*) says that ΔG^0 for hydrolysis of ATP is "an almost irrelevant parameter." Banks and Vernon make similar comments, and end their paper with the sentence "One thing would appear certain: The standard free energy of hydrolysis of ATP is its least interesting property" (*19*). I believe that consideration of the function of the adenylates in energy metabolism shows these statements to be incorrect. As discussed in Chapter 3, the thermodynamic consequence of stoichiometric coupling of the conversion of ATP to ADP with another reaction is to cause a large increase in the equilibrium ratio of product to reactant for the other reaction and thus to allow conversions to proceed that would be thermodynamically unfavorable if not coupled. It is true that this function does not depend solely on the equilibrium constant for hydrolysis of ATP. The immediately important point is that the concentration ratio (ATP)/(ADP) is held in the cell at a value of about 10^8 times its equilibrium ratio. It is this difference that makes the ATP/ADP couple a useful energy transducing system. In principle the same effect could be obtained if a different coupling system, consisting of X-P and X, were used, even if the equilibrium concentration ratio (X-P)/(X) were one. However, to obtain the same effect that is exerted by the ATP/ADP system, the physiological ratio (X-P)/(X) would need to be maintained at 10^8. This would not be feasible. First, there would be kinetic difficulties. If the concentration of X-P were 10 mM (which is somewhat higher than the normal ATP concentration), the concentration of X would be only 10^{-10} M. At this level, the average amount of X in a bacterial cell of typical size would be less than one molecule, and it would be impossible on kinetic grounds to phosphorylate X fast enough to regenerate X-P to meet the energy needs of the cell. Second, even aside from this difficulty it would be extremely hard to regulate a ratio such as 10^8. If only one millionth of the cell's supply of X-P were used without immediate regeneration, the (X-P)/(X) ratio would be changed by a factor of 100. Ratios are most easily stabilized when they are near 1, and the actual physiological (ATP)/(ADP) ratio is about 5. Reasons for a value of 5 rather than 1 are discussed in Chapter 4, but the important point here is that the ratio *in vivo* is in fact not far from 1. If the components of the energy transducing system are to have a physiological concentration ratio near 1, but must also be very far from equilibrium, it follows that the equilibrium constant must be far from 1. The equilibrium constant, and hence the standard free energy, of the hydrolysis of ATP is, according to this view, a very interesting and important property. Any compound thought of as a possible replacement for ATP would necessarily have a large equilibrium constant for hydrolysis.

APPENDIX C

The Briggs-Haldane Treatment

The discussion in Chapter 5 was based on the assumption that association and dissociation steps are rapid in comparison with the actual catalyzed reaction, in which bonds are broken and formed, and that therefore the free enzyme and the enzyme-substrate and enzyme-product complexes are virtually in equilibrium with the free reactants and products during steady-state catalysis. This, the assumption suggested by Henri and Brown and accepted by Michaelis, is generally termed the Michaelis assumption. It leads to the conclusion that the Michaelis constant (the concentration of substrate at which the reaction velocity is half of the velocity at a saturating concentration of substrate) should be a close approximation to the equilibrium constant for dissociation of the enzyme-substrate complex to free enzyme and free substrate. Using the nomenclature of equation C-1, which is identical with equation 5-1, the equilibrium constant for dissociation of the enzyme-substrate complex is k_2/k_1. If the Michaelis treatment is valid, the reciprocal of the Michaelis constant is the equilibrium constant for association of substrate with enzyme, and kinetically determined Michaelis constants give valuable information concerning affinities of enzymes for their substrates. Most textbooks say, however, that the Michaelis constant

$$E + S \underset{k_2}{\overset{k_1}{\rightleftharpoons}} ES \underset{k_4}{\overset{k_3}{\rightleftharpoons}} EP \underset{k_6}{\overset{k_5}{\rightleftharpoons}} E + P \qquad (C\text{-}1)$$

is $(k_2 + k_3)/k_1$ in general, and that it equals k_2/k_1 only in a special case of no particular importance. If that statement and the Briggs-Haldane treatment (107) on which it is based are valid, the kinetically determined Michaelis constants supply no valid information concerning enzyme-substrate affinities. A typical statement to that effect was quoted in Chapter 5.

We saw in Chapter 5 that the properties of typical regulatory enzymes seem to show clearly that quasiequilibrium between enzymes, ligands, and the enzyme-ligand complex is the usual situation. If the Briggs-Haldane treatment were valid, we would conclude that the Michaelis condition of quasiequilibrium, although a special case, must have been selected for in the evolution of regulatory enzymes. Actually, as we will show, the Briggs-Haldane treatment is not significantly more general than the Michaelis treatment.

The relationship between the two treatments may be deduced intuitively by consideration of activation energy profiles, as illustrated by the schematic formalized profiles shown in Figure C-1. The energy barriers to be surmounted in each step are given the same numbers in the figure as the corresponding velocity constants in equation C-1. The classical Michaelis treatment corresponds to profile A. Here the energy barriers in association and dissociation steps are low compared with the barrier in the conversion of substrate to product (or vice versa) on the enzyme. Association and dissociation are in consequence so much faster than the S to P conversion that the E, S, ES and E, P, EP systems are virtually at equilibrium. An equivalent statement is that the high barrier $EX^{\ddagger}$ kinetically isolates the E, S, ES system, from the E_r, P_r, EP system, allowing each to equilibrate.

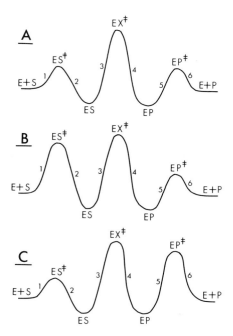

Figure C-1.   Energy profiles for enzyme-catalyzed reactions. See discussion in text.

Both the Michaelis and Briggs-Haldane treatments are derived for initial velocities—the reaction velocities that occur as soon after initiation of the reaction as the quasi-steady-state is established, while the concentration of product is still negligible. For the case illustrated by profile A, when the concentration of product is essentially zero, the rate of formation of EP from E + P may be taken as zero. The complex EP is thus produced only by step 3, and is consumed by steps 4 and 5. Reaction 5 is, in the initial states that we are considering, essentially irreversible since reaction 6 can be ignored. Because of the relative heights of the relevant energy barriers, the chance of EP being irreversibly removed is very large compared to the chance of its being converted to ES (the velocity of step 5 is very large compared to that of step 4), and the effective concentration of EP is therefore zero. It should be remembered that reaction velocities are exponential rather than linear functions of activation energies; if, for example, the height of barrier 5 were 10 kcal and that of barrier 4 were 20 kcal, the velocity ratio k_5/k_4 would be given by the expression

$$\exp(\Delta G_4^{\ddagger} - \Delta G_5^{\ddagger})/RT = \exp(10{,}000/600) = 1.7 \times 10^7$$

So this degree of difference in energy barriers, which does not seem unreasonably large, would allow E, P, and EP to remain at equilibrium within less than one part in a million during the course of the reaction. The same considerations apply in just the same way to the relative velocities of steps 2 and 3. Of course such an emphatic velocity difference is not necessary for Michaelis kinetics; equilibrium within a few percent would lead to essentially Michaelis behavior.

Since it is frequently said that the Briggs-Haldane treatment is general, with the Michaelis treatment being only a special case of it, we might expect that there are many profiles that are adequately described by Briggs-Haldane but not by Michaelis. When we try to visualize such profiles, however, it soon becomes obvious that there is only one. This is shown as B in Figure C-1. If the ES‡ barrier is nearly as high as, or higher than, EX‡, the enzyme, substrate, and enzyme-substrate complexes will no longer be at virtual equilibrium. The net velocity of the forward reaction will still be equal to the velocity of step 3 as long as barrier EP‡ is sufficiently lower than EX‡. Thus ES will be partitioned between step 2 and step 3, but will be produced only by step 1, and it is obvious without algebraic analysis that the Michaelis constant in this case will be equal to $(k_2 + k_3)/k_1$.

The lack of generality of the Briggs-Haldane treatment is seen when we attempt to apply it even to the reversal of case B. To avoid confusion in referring to individual steps, the right-to-left reaction of profile B has been rewritten as the left-to-right reaction of profile C, with designation of S and P exchanged. In this case, when EP‡ is nearly as high as or higher than EX‡, the EP complex will no longer be at virtual equilibrium with free enzyme and free product. It will partition between steps 5 and 4. Thus ES is formed by both reaction 1 and reaction 4, and the net velocity of the forward reaction is no longer equal to the velocity of step 3, but instead to the velocity of step 3 minus that of step 4. It is clear that in this case no function of k_1, k_2, and k_3 can define the kinetic Michaelis constant; k_4 and k_5 must also be taken into account.

Sketching of schematic energy profiles thus demonstrates the relationship between the Michaelis and the Briggs-Haldane treatments: the Briggs-Haldane expression, $K_m = (k_2 + k_3)/k_1$, is valid when $EP^{\ddagger}$ is low relative to $EX^{\ddagger}$, and the Michaelis expression, $K_m = k_2/k_1$, is valid when both $ES^{\ddagger}$ and $EP^{\ddagger}$ are low relative to $EX^{\ddagger}$. (The other barriers need not be much lower than $EX^{\ddagger}$. A difference of about 2.7 kcal/mole in the heights of $ES^{\ddagger}$ and $EX^{\ddagger}$ would cause the velocity of step 2 to be 100 times that of step 3, and thus would allow steps 1 and 2 to be within about 1% of equilibrium during steady-state catalysis of the reaction.) Because $ES^{\ddagger}$ and $EP^{\ddagger}$ interchange when the reverse reaction is considered, it is clear that there is no reaction for which the Briggs-Haldane treatment is valid in both directions but for which the Michaelis treatment is not valid. The supposed greater generality of the Briggs-Haldane treatment is thus reduced to its applicability to one special case, and even then in one direction only.

The Briggs-Haldane expression was obtained by an erroneous derivation from equation C-2. From this equation, it is easy to show that at the steady

$$E + S \underset{k_2}{\overset{k_1}{\rightleftharpoons}} ES \overset{k_3}{\to} E + P \tag{C-2}$$

state equation C-3 applies.

$$\frac{(ES)}{(E)(S)} = \frac{k_1}{k_2 + k_3} \tag{C-3}$$

If we assume that $(EP) = 0$, so that $(E) + (ES) = (E)_T$, as in the Michaelis treatment, equation C-3 may be converted to equation C-4, from which it was concluded that the Michaelis constant is given in general by the ex-

$$\frac{v}{V_m} = \frac{(S)}{[(k_2 + k_3)/k_1] + (S)} \tag{C-4}$$

pression $(k_2 + k_3)/k_1$. The error introduced by Briggs and Haldane and perpetuated in numerous textbooks was the failure to realize that the concentration of EP will not approach zero in the general case, but only when $EP^{\ddagger}$ is low relative to $EX^{\ddagger}$. Consequently it is not generally true that $(E) + (ES) = (E)_T$, and the conversion of equation C-3 to equation C-4 is not valid in any

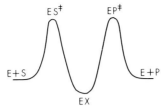

Figure C-2. Energy profile for a hypothetical enzyme-catalyzed reaction with only one enzyme-ligand complex. See discussion in text.

general sense. The Briggs-Haldane treatment will, of course, apply to a reaction that is described adequately by equation C-5; that is, one in which

$$E + S \underset{k_2}{\overset{k_1}{\rightleftharpoons}} EX \underset{k_4}{\overset{k_3}{\rightleftharpoons}} E + P \qquad \text{(C-5)}$$

there is only one enzyme-ligand complex, which must then be reached in a single step from either free substrate or free product. The corresponding energy profile would be that shown in Figure C-2. But such a reaction seems so unlikely that it may be disregarded. In addition, this profile would not lend itself to expansion to provide for reactions with more than one substrate and one product.

The relationship between the two treatments may also of course be demonstrated algebraically, although it would be a mistake to believe that demonstrations of the type given above are less rigorous than more formal mathematical approaches. From equation C-1 we can write the steady-state conditions C-6 and C-7.

$$d(ES)/dt = k_1(E)(S) + k_4(EP) - k_2(ES) - k_3(ES) = 0 \qquad \text{(C-6)}$$

$$d(EP)/dt = k_3(ES) + k_6(E)(P) - k_4(EP) - k_5(EP) = 0 \qquad \text{(C-7)}$$

Initially, when $(P) = 0$, it follows from C-7 that

$$(ES)/(EP) = (k_4 + k_5)/k_3 \qquad \text{(C-8)}$$

Still assuming that $(P) = 0$, the reaction velocity must be given by equation C-9 and the maximal velocity at a saturating level of substrate by equation C-10, regardless of what step is rate limiting.

$$v = d(P)/dt = k_5(EP) \qquad \text{(C-9)}$$

$$V_m = k_5(EP)_{max} \qquad \text{(C-10)}$$

The operational definition of the Michaelis constant is the concentration of substrate at which the initial reaction velocity is half of that obtained at a saturating concentration of substrate (equation C-11). This may be converted to equation C-12.

$$v/V_m = (S)/[K_m + (S)] \tag{C-11}$$

$$K_m = (S)[(V_m - v)/v] \tag{C-12}$$

Thus for any model or treatment, evaluation of $(V_m - v)/v$ allows us to write an expression for K_m. Substituting into equation C-12 from equations C-9 and C-10, we obtain equation C-13.

$$K_m = \frac{[(EP)_{max} - (EP)](S)}{(EP)} \tag{C-13}$$

To obtain (EP), a straightforward partition treatment is required. Note that $(EP)_{max}/(E)_T = (EP)/[(ES) + (EP)]$ when (E) approaches zero. Substituting equation C-8 into equation C-6 to eliminate (EP), we obtain equation C-14.

$$\frac{(ES)}{(E)} = (S)\left[\frac{k_1(k_4 + k_5)}{(k_2 + k_3)(k_4 + k_5) - k_3 k_4}\right] \tag{C-14}$$

Similarly eliminating (ES), we obtain equation C-15.

$$\frac{(EP)}{(E)} = (S)\left[\frac{k_1 k_3}{(k_2 + k_3)(k_4 + k_5) - k_3 k_4}\right] \tag{C-15}$$

Then, since $(E)_T = (E) + (ES) + (EP)$, it follows that

$$(E)_T = (E)\left[1 + (S)\left(\frac{k_1(k_3 + k_4 + k_5)}{(k_2 + k_3)(k_4 + k_5) - k_3 k_4}\right)\right] \tag{C-16}$$

and

$$\frac{(EP)}{(E)_T} = \frac{k_1 k_3(S)}{k_1(k_3 + k_4 + k_5)(S) + (k_2 + k_3)(k_4 + k_5) - k_3 k_4} \tag{C-17}$$

When substrate is at a saturating level, the concentration of free enzyme approaches zero and we obtain equation C-18.

$$\frac{(EP)_{max}}{(E)_T} = \frac{(EP)}{(EP) + (ES)} = \frac{1}{1 + [(k_4 + k_5)/k_3]} = \frac{k_3}{k_3 + k_4 + k_5} \tag{C-18}$$

As noted above, regardless of which step is rate limiting, if (P) is close to zero the velocity of the overall reaction is proportional to the concentration of EP (equation C-19). Substituting equations C-17 and C-18 into equation C-19, we obtain a large equation that simplifies to equation C-20.

$$(V_m - v)/v = [(EP)_{max} - (EP)]/(EP) \qquad \text{(C-19)}$$

$$(V_m - v)/v = \frac{k_2(k_4 + k_5) + k_3 k_5}{k_1(k_3 + k_4 + k_5)(S)} \qquad \text{(C-20)}$$

Multiplying this expression by (S) (see equation C-12), we obtain the general expression for the Michaelis constant for any reaction that is adequately described by equation C-1*:

$$K_m = \frac{k_2(k_4 + k_5) + k_3 k_5}{k_1(k_3 + k_4 + k_5)} \qquad \text{(C-21)}$$

When k_3 and k_4 are small relative to k_5, equation C-21 reduces to the Briggs-Haldane expression, equation C-22.

$$K_m = (k_2 + k_3)/k_1 \qquad \text{(C-22)}$$

When in addition k_3 is small relative to k_2, equation C-21 reduces to the Michaelis expression, equation C-23.

$$K_m = k_2/k_1 \qquad \text{(C-23)}$$

The algebraic analysis thus, necessarily, leads to the same conclusions that we reached above: the Briggs-Haldane expression for the Michaelis constant is valid only when k_5 is much larger than k_3 and k_4 (EX‡ is higher than EP‡) and the Michaelis expression is valid when both k_2 and k_5 are much larger than k_3 and k_4 (EX‡ is higher than both ES‡ and EP‡). Because of the interchange of k_5 and k_2 when the reverse reaction is considered, it follows as before that there is no reaction for which the Briggs-Haldane treatment is valid in both directions but for which the Michaelis treatment is not also valid.

It seems likely that the step in which bonds are broken and formed will usually be slower than steps involving dissociation or association, and that thus the Michaelis treatment will apply to most enzymic reactions. Of course the facts that most reactions involve more than one substrate, and that there may be interactions between substrate-binding sites, or between sites that bind substrates and sites that bind positive or negative modifiers, does not

---

* Haldane (55) derived this equation in connection with a discussion of reversibility in enzyme-catalyzed reactions, when he found it necessary to take the EP complex into account. He did not point out, however, and later authors apparently have not recognized, its relevance to the Briggs-Haldane treatment, which had been published five years earlier.

alter the essential Michaelis character of any enzyme for which the free enzyme, free ligands, and enzyme-ligand complexes remain close to equilibrium during the catalytic reaction. But it is not necessary that the Michaelis treatment be applicable to every enzymic reaction; the situation of a relatively high EX‡ barrier seems intrinsically likely on chemical grounds, but evolutionary design may have produced other energy profiles if they were biologically useful in special cases. Any profile, such as profile C of Figure C-1, in which EP‡ is not significantly lower than EX‡ would require the full expression of equation C-21 for the Michaelis constant, and neither the Briggs-Haldane nor the Michaelis expression would be valid in such cases.

For the purposes of this book the important conclusion of this appendix is that there is no case for which the Briggs-Haldane treatment is valid in both directions to which the Michaelis treatment does not also apply. The Briggs-Haldane expression for the Michaelis constant is of severely limited applicability; it applies uniquely only to the situation illustrated by profile B of Figure C-1, and only in the forward direction. It would be trivial to point out that the Briggs-Haldane expression is also valid whenever the Michaelis expression is valid, since in that case the numerator $k_2 + k_3$ approaches k_2, and nothing is to be gained by including a factor that is negligible. Because of its triviality, the Briggs-Haldane expression for K_m should be dropped from textbook treatments of enzyme kinetics. Until that happens, we may well ignore it, and we need not hesitate to infer probable affinities of enzymes for substrates from kinetic Michaelis constants.

Bibliography

1. Adair, G. S. (1925). *J. Biol. Chem.* **63,** 529.
2. Adolf, E. F. (1961). *Physiol. Rev.* **41,** 737.
3. Alberty, R. A. (1969). *J. Biol. Chem.* **244,** 3290.
4. Atkinson, D. E. (1966). *Annu. Rev. Biochem.* **35,** 85.
5. Atkinson, D. E. (1968). *Biochemistry* **7,** 4030.
6. Atkinson, D. E. (1969). *Annu. Rev. Microbiol.* **23,** 47.
7. Atkinson, D. E. (1969). *Curr. Top. Cell. Regul.* **I,** 29.
8. Atkinson, D. E. (1970). *In* "The Enzymes" (P. D. Boyer, ed.), 3rd ed., Vol. I, p. 461. Academic Press, New York.
9. Atkinson, D. E. (1971). *Metab. Pathways, 3rd Ed.* **5,** 1.
10. Atkinson, D. E. (1971). *Adv. Enzyme Regul.* **9,** 207.
11. Atkinson, D. E. (1972). *In* "Horizons of Bioenergetics" (A. San Pietro and H. Gest, eds.), p. 83. Academic Press, New York.
12. Atkinson, D. E. (1975). *In* "Control Mechanisms in Development" (R. H. Meints and E. Davies, eds.), p. 193. Plenum, New York.
12a. Atkinson, D. E., Hathaway, J. A., and Smith, E. C. (1965). *J. Biol. Chem.* **240,** 2682.
13. Atkinson, D. E., Roach, P. J., and Schwedes, J. S. (1975). *Adv. Enzyme Regul.* **13,** 393.
14. Baldwin, R. L. (1968). *J. Dairy Sci.* **51,** 104.
15. Ball, W. J., Jr. (1974). Ph.D. Thesis, University of California, Los Angeles.
16. Ball, W. J., Jr., and Atkinson, D. E. (1975). *J. Bacteriol.* **121,** 975.
17. Banks, B. E. C. (1969). *Chem. Br.* **5,** 515.
18. Banks, B. E. C., and Vernon, C. A. (1970). *Chem. Br.* **6,** 541.
19. Banks, B. E. C., and Vernon, C. A. (1970). *J. Theor. Biol.* **29,** 301.
20. Barnes, L. D., McGuire, J. J., and Atkinson, D. E. (1972). *Biochemistry* **11,** 4322.
21. Bauchop, T., and Elsden, S. R. (1960). *J. Gen. Microbiol.* **23,** 457.
22. Beck, C., Ingraham, J., Maaløe, O., and Neuhard, J. (1973). *J. Mol. Biol.* **78,** 117.
23. Bigler, W. N., and Atkinson, D. E. (1969). *Biochem. Biophys. Res. Commun.* **36,** 381.
24. Blaxter, K. L. (1962). "The Energy Metabolism of Ruminants." Thomas, Springfield, Illinois.
25. Brody, S. (1972). *J. Biol. Chem.* **247,** 6013.
26. Chagoya de Sánchez, V., Brunner, A., and Piña, E. (1972). *Biochem. Biophys. Res. Commun.* **46,** 1441.

284

27. Chance, B., Greenstein, D. S., and Roughton, F. J. W. (1952). *Arch. Biochem. Biophys.* **37,** 301.
28. Chapman, A. G., and Atkinson, D. E. (1973). *J. Biol. Chem.* **248,** 8309.
29. Chapman, A. G., and Atkinson, D. E. (1977). *Adv. Microbiol. Physiol.* **15** (in press).
30. Chapman, A. G., Fall, L., and Atkinson, D. E. (1971). *J. Bacteriol.* **108,** 1072.
31. Chapman, A. G., Miller, A. L., and Atkinson, D. E. (1976). *Cancer Res.* **36,** 1144.
32. Chen, R. F., and Plaut, G. W. E. (1963). *Biochemistry* **2,** 1023.
33. Chibnall, A. C. (1966). *Annu. Rev. Biochem.* **35,** 1.
34. Chulavatnatol, M., and Atkinson, D. E. (1973). *J. Biol. Chem.* **248,** 2712.
35. Cleland, W. W. (1963). *Biochim. Biophys. Acta* **67,** 104.
36. Cleland, W. W. (1963). *Biochim. Biophys. Acta* **67,** 173.
37. Cleland, W. W. (1963). *Biochim. Biophys. Acta* **67,** 188.
38. Cleland, W. W. (1967). *Annu. Rev. Biochem.* **36,** 77.
39. Coe, E. L. (1966). *Biochim. Biophys. Acta* **118,** 495.
40. Cori, G. T., Colowick, S. P., and Cori, C. F. (1938). *J. Biol. Chem.* **123,** 375.
41. Cori, G. T., Colowick, S. P., and Cori, C. F. (1938). *J. Biol. Chem.* **123,** 381.
42. Cornish-Bowden, A., and Eisenthal, R. (1974). *Biochem. J.* **139,** 721.
43. Danielson, L., and Ernster, L. (1963). *Biochem. Z.* **338,** 188.
44. Davison, J. A., and Fynn, G. H. (1974). *Anal. Biochem.* **58,** 632.
45. Dowd, J. E., and Riggs, D. S. (1965). *J. Biol. Chem.* **240,** 863.
46. Eisenthal, R., and Cornish-Bowden, A. (1974). *Biochem. J.* **139,** 715.
47. Garland, P. B. (1968). *Biochem. Soc. Symp.* **27,** 41.
48. George, P. (1953). *Arch. Biochem. Biophys.* **45,** 21.
49. Gerhart, J. C., and Pardee, A. B. (1962). *J. Biol. Chem.* **237,** 891.
50. Ginsburg, A., and Stadtman, E. R. (1973). *In* "The Enzymes of Glutamine Metabolism" (S. Prusiner and E. R. Stadtman, eds.), p. 9. Academic Press, New York.
51. Ginsburg, A., and Stadtman, E. R. (1975). *In* "Subunit Enzymes" (K. E. Ebner, ed.), p. 43. Dekker, New York.
52. Goldbetter, A. (1974). *FEBS Lett.* **43,** 327.
53. Gunsalus, I. C., and Shuster, C. W. (1961). *In* "The Bacteria" (I. C. Gunsalus and R. Y. Stanier, eds.), Vol. 2, p. 1. Academic Press, New York.
54. Guynn, R., and Veech, R. L. (1973). *J. Biol. Chem.* **248,** 6966.
55. Haldane, J. B. S. (1930). "Enzymes," p. 81. Longmans, Green, London.
56. Hathaway, J. A., and Atkinson, D. E. (1963). *J. Biol. Chem.* **238,** 2875.
57. Hathaway, J. A., and Atkinson, D. E. (1965). *Biochem. Biophys. Res. Commun.* **20,** 661.
58. Hommes, F. A., Drost, Y. M., Geraets, W. X. M., and Reijenga, M. A. A. (1975). *Pediatr. Res.* **9,** 51.
59. Hopfield, J. J. (1974). *Proc. Natl. Acad. Sci. U.S.A.* **71,** 4135.
60. Huisman, W. H. (1975). Ph.D. Dissertation, University of California, Los Angeles.
61. Klungsøyr, L., Hageman, J. H., Fall, L., and Atkinson, D. E. (1968). *Biochemistry* **7,** 4035.
62. Kornberg, A. (1962). *In* "Horizons in Biochemistry" (M. Kasha and B. Pullman, eds.), p. 251. Academic Press, New York.
63. Kornberg, A., and Pricer, W. E. (1951). *J. Biol. Chem.* **189,** 123.
64. Koshland, D. E. (1958). *Proc. Natl. Acad. Sci. U.S.A.* **44,** 98.
65. Koshland, D. E. (1969). *Curr. Top. Cell. Regul.* **1,** 1.
66. Koshland, D. E., Némethy, G., and Filmer, D. (1966). *Biochemistry* **5,** 365.
67. Krebs, H. A. (1954). *Bull. Johns Hopkins Hosp.* **95,** 45.
68. Krebs, H. A. (1964). *Proc. R. Soc. London, Ser. B* **159,** 545.

69. Krebs, H. A. (1966). *In* "Current Aspects of Biochemical Energetics" (N. O. Kaplan and E. P. Kennedy, eds.), p. 83. Academic Press, New York.
70. Krebs, H. A., and Veech, R. L. (1969). *Adv. Enzyme Regul.* **7**, 397.
71. Kuehn, G. D., Barnes, L. D., and Atkinson, D. E. (1971). *Biochemistry* **10**, 3945.
72. Liao, C.-L., and Atkinson, D. E. (1971). *J. Bacteriol.* **106**, 37.
73. Lienhard, G. E. (1973). *Science* **180**, 149.
74. Lipmann, F. (1941). *Adv. Enzymol.* **1**, 99.
75. Lipscomb, W. N. (1974). *Tetrahedron* **30**, 1725.
76. Lomax, C. A., and Henderson, J. F. (1973). *Cancer Res.* **33**, 2825.
77. Low, P. S., and Somero, G. H. (1975). *Proc. Natl. Acad. Sci. U.S.A.* **72**, 3305.
78. Lyon, J. B., and Porter, J. (1963). *J. Biol. Chem.* **238**, 1.
79. Maaløe, O., and Kjeldgaard, N. O. (1966). "Control of Macromolecular Synthesis." Benjamin, New York.
80. Mansour, T. E. (1963). *J. Biol. Chem.* **238**, 2285.
81. Mansour, T. E., and Mansour, J. M. (1962). *J. Biol. Chem.* **237**, 629.
82. McComb, R. B., and Yushok, W. D. (1964). *Cancer Res.* **24**, 198.
83. Miller, A. L., and Atkinson, D. E. (1972). *Arch. Biochem. Biophys.* **152**, 531.
84. Milligan, L. P. (1971). *Fed. Proc., Fed. Am. Soc. Exp. Biol.* **30**, 1454.
85. Mitchell, R. A., and Russo, J. A. (1975). *Biochem. Educ.* **3**, 34.
86. Monod, J., Wyman, J., and Changeux, J.-P. (1965). *J. Mol. Biol.* **12**, 88.
87. Morgan, H. E., and Parmaggiani, A. (1964). *J. Biol. Chem.* **239**, 2440.
88. Overgaard-Hanson, K. (1965). *Biochim. Biophys. Acta* **104**, 330.
89. Passonneau, J. V., and Lowry, O. H. (1962). *Biochem. Biophys. Res. Commun.* **7**, 10.
90. Payne, W. J. (1970). *Annu. Rev. Microbiol.* **24**, 17.
91. Penning de Vries, F. W. T., Brunsting, A. H. M., and van Laar, H. H. (1974). *J. Theor. Biol.* **45**, 339.
92. Pittendrigh, C. S. (1958). *In* "Behavior and Evolution" (A. Roe and G. G. Simpson, eds.), p. 394. Yale Univ. Press, New Haven, Connecticut.
93. Platt, J. R. (1964). *Science* **146**, 347.
94. Preiss, J. (1969). *Curr. Top. Cell. Regul.* **1**, 125.
95. Quiocho, F. A., and Lipscomb, W. N. (1971). *Adv. Protein Chem.* **25**, 1.
96. Raivio, K. O., Kekomäki, M. P., and Mäenpää, P. H. (1969). *Biochem. Pharmacol.* **18**, 2615.
97. Ramaiah, A., Hathaway, J. A., and Atkinson, D. E. (1964). *J. Biol. Chem.* **239**, 3619.
98. Ramsey, J. B. (1957). *J. Electrochem. Soc.* **104**, 691.
99. Roach, P. J., Warren, K. R., and Atkinson, D. E. (1975). *Biochemistry* **14**, 5445.
100. Roberts, R. B., Abelson, P. H., Cowie, D. B., Bolton, E. T., and Britten, R. J. (1955). *Carnegie Inst. Washington Publ.* **607**.
101. Roseman, S. (1972). *Metab. Pathways, 3rd Ed.* **6**, 41.
102. Rossmann, M. G., Moras, D., and Olsen, K. W. (1974). *Nature (London)* **250**, 194.
103. Saroff, H. A., and Minton, A. P. (1972). *Science* **175**, 1253.
104. Schonbaum, G. R., and Chance, B. (1976). *In* "The Enzymes" (P. D. Boyer, ed.), 3rd ed., Vol. 13, p. 363. Academic Press, New York.
105. Schramm, V. L., and Leung, H. (1973). *J. Biol. Chem.* **248**, 8313.
106. Scrutton, M. C., and Utter, M. F. (1968). *Annu. Rev. Biochem.* **37**, 249.
107. Segal, H. L. (1959). *In* "The Enzymes" (P. D. Boyer, H. Lardy, and K. Myrbäck, eds.), 2nd ed., Vol. 1, p. 1. Academic Press, New York.
108. Shen, L. C., and Atkinson, D. E. (1970). *J. Biol. Chem.* **245**, 3996.

109. Shen, L. C., and Atkinson, D. E. (1970). *J. Biol. Chem.* **245,** 5974.
110. Shen, L. C., Fall, L., Walton, G. M., and Atkinson, D. E. (1968). *Biochemistry* **7,** 4041.
111. Simmons, M. W. (1974). Ph.D. Thesis, University of California, Los Angeles.
112. Stent, G. (1971). "The Coming of the Golden Age: A View of the End of Progress." Nat. Hist. Press, Garden City, New York.
113. Straus, O. H., and Goldstein, A. (1943). *J. Gen. Physiol.* **26,** 559.
114. Swedes, J. S., Sedo, R. J., and Atkinson, D. E. (1975). *J. Biol. Chem.* **250,** 6930.
115. Talwalkar, R. T., and Lester, R. L. (1973). *Biochim. Biophys. Acta* **306,** 412.
116. Thompson, F. M., and Atkinson, D. E. (1971). *Biochem. Biophys. Res. Commun.* **45,** 1581.
117. Trevelyan, W. E. (1958). *In* "The Chemistry and Biology of Yeasts" (A. H. Cook, ed.), p. 369. Academic Press, New York.
118. Umbarger, H. E. (1956). *Science* **123,** 848.
119. Walker-Simmons, M., and Atkinson, D. E. (1977). *J. Bacteriol.* **130,** 676.
120. Watari, H., and Isogai, Y. (1976). *Biochem. Biophys. Res. Commun.* **69,** 15.
121. Williams, J. F., and Clark, M. G. (1971). *Search* **2,** 80.
122. Williamson, J. R., Browning, E. T., Thurman, R. G., and Scholz, R. (1969). *J. Biol. Chem.* **244,** 5055.
123. Williamson, J. R., Scholz, R., and Browning, E. T. (1969). *J. Biol. Chem.* **244,** 4617.
124. Williamson, J. R., Scholz, R., Browning, E. T., Thurman, R. G., and Fukami, M. H. (1969). *J. Biol. Chem.* **244,** 5044.
125. Wilson, D. F., Stubbs, M., Veech, R. L., Erecińska, M., and Krebs, H. A. (1974). *Biochem. J.* **140,** 57.
126. Woods, H. F., Eggleston, L. V., and Krebs, H. A. (1970). *Biochem. J.* **119,** 501.
127. Wyman, J. (1964). *Adv. Protein Chem.* **19,** 223.
128. Yates, R. A., and Pardee, A. B. (1956). *J. Biol. Chem.* **221,** 757.

Index